Current

Surgical

Management III

A Book of Alternative Viewpoints on Controversial Surgical Problems

EDITORS

EDWIN H. ELLISON, M.D.
Marquette University School of Medicine

STANLEY R. FRIESEN, M.D.
University of Kansas Medical Center

JOHN H. MULHOLLAND, M.D.
New York University College of Medicine

WITH CONTRIBUTIONS BY 104 AUTHORITIES

W. B. Saunders Company

Philadelphia and London

Reprinted November, 1965

Current Surgical Management III

Contributors

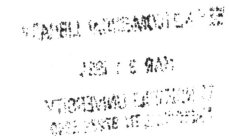

ADAMS, HERBERT D., M.D.
Director, Lahey Clinic Division, Lahey Clinic Foundation, Inc.; Surgeon-in-Chief, New England Baptist Hospital, Boston; Chairman, Medical Administrative Board, and Surgeon, New England Deaconess Hospital; Consultant, United States Naval Hospital, Chelsea, Massachusetts.

APPLEMAN, ROBERT M., M.D.
Resident in Surgery, Mayo Graduate School of Medicine, University of Minnesota; Mayo Clinic and Mayo Foundation, Rochester, Minnesota.

BEAHRS, OLIVER H., M.D.
Associate Professor of Surgery, Mayo Graduate School of Medicine, University of Minnesota; Consultant, Section of Surgery, Mayo Clinic, Rochester, Minnesota.

BELL, JAMES E., M.D.
Instructor in Radiology, Marquette University School of Medicine; Radiologist, Milwaukee County Hospital, Milwaukee, Wisconsin.

BERNARD, HARVEY R., M.D.
Associate Professor, Department of Surgery, Washington University School of Medicine; Surgeon, Barnes and Allied Hospitals, St. Louis City Hospital, Homer G. Phillips Hospital, and John J. Cochran Veterans Administration Hospital, St. Louis, Missouri; Consultant, United States Air Force Hospital, Scott Air Force Base, Belleville, Illinois.

BOWERS, RALPH FIRESTONE, M.D.
Professor of Surgery, University of Tennessee College of Medicine; Chief of Surgical Service, Veterans Administration Hospital, Memphis, Tennessee.

BUTCHER, HARVEY R., JR., M.D.
Professor of Surgery, Washington University School of Medicine; Surgeon, Barnes and Affiliated Hospitals; Consultant, St. Louis City, Cochran Veterans, and Ellis Fischel State Cancer Hospitals, St. Louis, Missouri.

COLE, JACK WESTLEY, M.D.
Professor and Chairman, Department of Surgery, Hahnemann Medical College and Hospital; Chief, Hahnemann Surgery Service, Philadelphia General Hospital; Consultant, Veterans Administration Hospital, Philadelphia, Pennsylvania.

CRILE, GEORGE, JR., M.D.
Head, Department of General Surgery, Cleveland Clinic, Cleveland, Ohio.

DARIN, JOSEPH C., M.D.
Assistant Professor of Surgery, Marquette University School of Medicine; Attending Surgeon, Milwaukee County General Hospital; Consulting Surgeon, Columbia, St. Luke's, St. Joseph's and West Allis Memorial Hospitals, Milwaukee, Wisconsin.

DELANEY, JOHN PATRICK, M.D., PH.D.
Medical Fellow, Department of Surgery, University of Minnesota Hospitals, Minneapolis, Minnesota.

DENNIS, CLARENCE, M.D., PH.D.
Professor and Chairman, Department of Surgery, State University of New York Downstate Medical Center; Surgeon-in-Chief, Kings County Hospital Center, Brooklyn, New York.

DOBERNECK, RAYMOND CLEMENS, M.D.
Medical Fellow, Department of Surgery, University of Minnesota Hospitals, Minneapolis, Minnesota.

DOUBILET, HENRY, M.D.*
Associate Professor of Surgery, New York University College of Medicine; Visiting Surgeon, Bellevue Hospital (Third Division); Attending Surgeon, University and Goldwater Hospitals, New York.
* Deceased.

DUMONT, ALLAN ELIOT, M.D.
Associate Professor of Surgery, New York University School of Medicine; Associate Attending Surgeon, Bellevue Hospital; Associate Visiting Surgeon, University Hospital; Attending Surgeon, Manhattan Veterans Administration Hospital, New York, New York.

DUNPHY, J. ENGLEBERT, M.D.
Professor and Chairman, Department of Surgery, University of California School of Medicine, San Francisco, California.

EFFLER, DONALD BRIAN, M.D.
Chief, Department of Thoracic and Cardiovascular Surgery, Cleveland Clinic, Cleveland, Ohio.

EISENBERG, M. MICHAEL, M.D.
Assistant Professor of Surgery, University of Florida College of Medicine; Attending Surgeon, University Hospital and Clinics, Gainesville, Florida; Attending Surgeon, Veterans Administration Hospital, Lake City, Florida.

ELLIOTT, DAN W., M.D.
Formerly Professor of Surgery, Ohio State University; Presently Professor of Clinical Surgery, University of Pittsburgh; Director of Surgery, Western Pennsylvania Hospital, Pittsburgh, Pennsylvania.

ELLISON, EDWIN H., M.D.
Professor and Chairman, Division of Surgery, Marquette University School of Medicine, Milwaukee, Wisconsin; Director of Surgery, Milwaukee County General Hospital; Senior Consultant in Surgery, Wood Veterans Administration Hospital; Consulting Surgeon, The Milwaukee Children's, Columbia, St. Joseph's, Mt. Sinai, and St. Mary's Hospitals; Honorary Medical Staff, St. Luke's Hospital; Lecturer-Consultant, U. S. Navy, Great Lakes Naval Hospital.

ENGLE, JAMES COLEMAN, M.D.
Medical Fellow, Department of Surgery, University of Minnesota Hospitals, Minneapolis, Minnesota.

FARRIS, JACK MATTHEWS, M.D.
Assistant Clinical Professor of Surgery, Medical School of the University of California at Los Angeles; Staff Surgeon, Hospital of the Good Samaritan, Los Angeles; Consultant, Veterans Administration Hospitals; Senior Consultant in Surgery, Long Beach Veterans Hospital, Long Beach, California.

FAYOS, JUAN V., M.D.
Assistant Professor of Radiology, University of Michigan School of Medicine; Radiologist, University of Michigan Medical Center, Ann Arbor, Michigan.

FERGUSON, DONALD JOHN, M.D., PH.D.
Professor of Surgery, University of Chicago School of Medicine, Chicago, Illinois.

FERRIS, DEWARD OLMSTED, M.D.
Professor of Clinical Surgery, Mayo Graduate School of Medicine, University of Minnesota, Rochester, Minnesota; Head, Section of Surgery, Mayo Clinic; Surgical Staff, St. Mary's Hospital and Methodist Hospital, Rochester, Minnesota.

FORREST, A. P. M., M.D.
Professor of Surgery, Welsh National School of Medicine; United Cardiff Hospitals, Cardiff, Wales.

FRIESEN, STANLEY R., M.D., PH.D.
Professor of Surgery, University of Kansas School of Medicine; Surgeon, University of Kansas Medical Center, Kansas City, Kansas.

GARLAND, L. HENRY, M.D.
Clinical Professor of Radiology, University of California Medical School, San Francisco; Chief Consultant in Radiology, San Francisco General Hospital, Letterman Army Hospital and St. Joseph's Hospital, San Francisco, California.

GILLESBY, WILLIAM JAMES, M.D.
Clinical Associate Professor of Surgery, University of Illinois College of Medicine; Chief, Surgical Service, Veterans

Administration West Side Hospital, Chicago, Illinois.

GLAS, WAYNE W., M.D.
Associate Clinical Professor of Surgery, University of Michigan Medical School; Director of Surgery, Wayne County General Hospital, Eloise, Michigan.

GOODALE, ROBERT LINCOLN, JR., M.D.
Medical Fellow, Department of Surgery, University of Minnesota Hospitals, Minneapolis, Minnesota.

GRANT, GEORGE N., M.D.
Assistant Professor of Surgery, Creighton University Medical School; Creighton Memorial Saint Joseph Hospital, Omaha, Nebraska.

GRIFFEN, WARD O., JR., M.D., PH.D.
Assistant Professor, Department of Surgery, University of Minnesota School of Medical Sciences; Staff Surgeon, University of Minnesota Hospitals, Minneapolis, Minnesota.

HARKINS, HENRY N., M.D., PH.D.
Professor of Surgery, Department of Surgery, University of Washington Medical School; Attending Surgeon, University Hospital; Consultant, Seattle Veterans Administration, King County and Bremerton Naval Hospitals, Seattle, Washington.

HOERR, STANLEY O., M.D.
Instructor in Surgery, Cleveland Clinic Educational Foundation; Staff Surgeon and Chairman, Division of Surgery, Cleveland Clinic Foundation, Cleveland, Ohio.

HOLDER, THOMAS MARTIN, M.D.
Assistant Professor of Surgery and Head of Section of Pediatric Surgery, University of Kansas School of Medicine and Medical Center; Consultant, Munson Army Hospital, Fort Leavenworth, Kansas and Menorah Medical Center and The Children's Mercy Hospital, Kansas City, Missouri.

HORSLEY, GUY W., M.D.
Associate Clinical Professor of Surgery, Medical College of Virginia; Attending Surgeon, St. Elizabeth's Hospital, Richmond, Virginia.

HORSLEY, J. SHELTON, III, M.D.
Clinical Instructor in Surgery, Medical

College of Virginia; Attending Surgeon, St. Elizabeth's Hospital, Richmond, Virginia.

HOWE, COLIN T., B.M., B.CH.
Lecturer in Surgery, University of Birmingham; Surgeon, Queen Elizabeth Hospital, Birmingham, England.

HUNT, THOMAS KNIGHT, M.D.
Assistant Professor of Surgery, University of California School of Medicine, San Francisco, California.

JESSEPH, JOHN E., M.D.
Visiting Associate Scientist, Brookhaven National Laboratory Medical Research Center, Upton, L. I., New York.

JOHNSON, LLOYD P., M.D.
Senior Research Fellow, Department of Surgery, University of Washington School of Medicine, Seattle, Washington.

KARLSON, KARL E., M.D., PH.D.
Professor of Surgery, State University of New York Downstate Medical Center; Visiting Surgeon, Kings County Hospital Center, Brooklyn, New York.

KENNEDY, CHARLES S., M.D.
Emeritus Professor of Surgery, Wayne State University; Consulting Surgeon, The Grace Hospital, Detroit, Michigan.

KITTLE, C. FREDERICK, M.D.
Associate Professor of Surgery, University of Kansas Medical Center, Kansas City, Kansas; Consultant, Veterans Administration Hospital, Kansas City, Missouri.

KLASSEN, KARL P., M.D.
Professor of Surgery, Ohio State University Medical School; Attending Staff, Ohio State University Hospitals, Columbus, Ohio.

KRAMER, PHILIP, M.D.
Assistant Professor, Boston University School of Medicine; Associate Visiting Physician, Massachusetts Memorial Hospitals; Chief, Gastroenterology Clinic, Boston City Hospital, Boston, Massachusetts.

KRIPPAEHNE, WILLIAM W., M.D.
Associate Professor of Surgery, University of Oregon Medical School, Eugene, Oregon.

LAMPE, ISADORE, M.D., PH.D.
Professor of Radiology, University of Michigan School of Medicine; Radiologist, University of Michigan Medical Center, Ann Arbor, Michigan.

LARGIADER, FELIX A., M.D.
Medical Fellow, Department of Surgery, University of Minnesota Hospitals, Minneapolis, Minnesota.

LAUFMAN, HAROLD, M.D., PH.D.
Professor of Surgery, Northwestern University Medical School; Attending Surgeon, Passavant Memorial and Veterans Administration Research Hospitals, Chicago, Illinois.

LAWRENCE, WALTER, JR., M.D.
Associate Clinical Professor of Surgery, Cornell University Medical College; Associate Attending Surgeon, Memorial Sloan-Kettering Cancer Center; Surgical Staff, The New York Hospital, New York.

LEVITAN, RUVEN, M.D.
Assistant Professor of Medicine, Tufts University School of Medicine; Associate in Medicine, Boston University School of Medicine; Director of Gastroenterological Research, New England Center Hospital; Associate Physician, Massachusetts Memorial Hospitals; Assisting Physician, Boston City Hospital, Boston, Massachusetts.

LILLEHEI, RICHARD C., M.D., PH.D.
Associate Professor, Department of Surgery, University of Minnesota School of Medical Sciences; Staff Surgeon, University of Minnesota Hospitals, Minneapolis, Minnesota.

LUI, ALFRED, M.D.
Assistant Clinical Professor of Surgery, University of Michigan Medical School; Assistant Director of Surgery, Wayne County General Hospital, Eloise, Michigan.

MADDEN, JOHN L., M.D.
Clinical Professor of Surgery, New York Medical College Metropolitan Hospital Center; Attending Surgeon and Director of Department of Surgery, St. Clare's Hospital; Attending Surgeon, Flower and Fifth Avenue Hospitals, Metropolitan Hospital Center, New York.

MAHONEY, EARLE B., M.D., D.Sc.(HON.)
Professor of Surgery, University of Rochester School of Medicine and Dentistry; Surgeon, Strong Memorial Hospital, Rochester, New York.

MARKS, CHARLES, M.D.
Associate Professor of Surgery, Marquette University School of Medicine; Attending Surgeon, Milwaukee County Hospital, Wood Veterans Administration Hospital, Columbia, Milwaukee, Mt. Sinai, and Milwaukee Children's Hospitals, Milwaukee, Wisconsin.

MARTIN, LESTER W., M.D.
Associate Professor of Surgery, College of Medicine, University of Cincinnati; Director of Pediatric Surgery, Cincinnati Children's Hospital, Cincinnati, Ohio.

McDONALD, WILLIAM M., M.B., B.S. (MELB.)
Formerly Special Research Fellow in Surgery, Lahey Clinic Foundation, Boston, Massachusetts; Presently Surgeon, Footscray and District Hospital; and Assistant Surgeon, Alfred Hospital, Victoria, Australia.

McVAY, CHESTER BIDWELL, M.D., PH.D.
Associate Professor of Anatomy and Clinical Professor of Surgery, University of South Dakota School of Medicine, Vermillion, South Dakota; Chief of Surgery, Sacred Heart Hospital, Yankton, South Dakota.

MONCRIEF, JOHN ARTHUR, M.D.
Assistant Clinical Professor of Surgery, University of Texas Medical Branch, Galveston, Texas; Commander and Director, U.S. Army Surgical Research Unit, Brooke Army Medical Center, Fort Sam Houston, Texas.

MONK, ROBERT S., M.D.
Assistant Professor of Clinical Surgery, Marquette University School of Medicine; Active Staff, Waukesha Memorial Hospital and West Allis Memorial Hospital; Surgical Staff, Milwaukee County General Hospital; Courtesy Staff at Milwaukee Passavant Hospital, Milwaukee, Wisconsin.

MUELLER, C. BARBER, M.D.
Professor of Surgery and Chairman of Department, State University of New York Upstate Medical Center; Attending Surgeon and Chief of Service, State University Hospital; Attending Sur-

geon, Syracuse Memorial Hospital; Consulting Surgeon, Syracuse Veterans Administration Hospital, Crouse-Irving Hospital, and St. Joseph's Hospital, Syracuse, New York.

MULHOLLAND, JOHN H., M.D.
George David Stewart Professor, Chairman of Department of Surgery, New York University School of Medicine; Director, New York University Surgical Divisions, Bellevue Hospital; Director of Surgery, New York University Hospital, New York.

NARDI, GEORGE L., M.D.
Associate Clinical Professor of Surgery, Harvard Medical School; Associate Visiting Surgeons, Massachusetts General Hospital, Boston, Massachusetts.

NICOLOFF, DEMETRE M., M.D.
Instructor in Surgery, University of Minnesota Medical Center, Minneapolis, Minnesota.

NYHUS, LLOYD M., M.D.
Professor, Department of Surgery, University of Washington School of Medicine, Seattle, Washington; Attending Surgeon, University, King County, and Veterans Administration Hospitals, Seattle; Surgical Consultant, Madigan Army Hospital, Tacoma, and Bremerton Naval Hospital, Bremerton, Washington.

OBERHELMAN, HARRY ALVIN, JR., M.D.
Professor of Surgery, Stanford University School of Medicine; Surgeon, Palo Alto Stanford Hospital, Palo Alto, California.

OGILVIE, HENEAGE, M.D.
Guy's Hospital, London, England.

PALMER, EDDY D., M.D.
Gastroenterology Service, Brooke General Hospital, Fort Sam Houston, Texas.

PATTON, RICHARD, M.D.
Associate Clinical Professor of Surgery, Ohio State University School of Medicine; Attending Staff Surgeon, Ohio State University Hospital and Riverside Methodist Hospital, Columbus, Ohio.

PESSAGNO, DANIEL JAMES, M.D.
Professor of Clinical Surgery, University of Maryland School of Medicine; Chief of Surgery, Mercy Hospital; Surgical Staff of St. Agnes Hospital, Bon

Secours Hospital, and Hospital for Women, Baltimore, Maryland.

PETERS, RICHARD M., M.D.
Professor of Surgery, Department of Thoracic and Cardiac Surgery, University of North Carolina School of Medicine; Attending Physician, North Carolina Memorial Hospital, Gravely Sanatorium, Chapel Hill, North Carolina; Regional Consultant in Thoracic Surgery, Veterans Administration.

POTH, EDGAR J., M.D., PH.D.
Ashbel Smith Professor of Surgery, University of Texas Medical Branch, University of Texas; Chief Surgeon, University of Texas Medical Branch Hospitals, Galveston, Texas.

PUESTOW, CHARLES BERNARD, M.D., PH.D.
Clinical Professor of Surgery, University of Illinois College of Medicine; Chief, Surgical Service of the Veterans Administration Hospital, Hines, Illinois; Senior Surgeon, Henrotin Hospital; Consulting Surgeon, Presbyterian-St. Luke's Hospital; Attending Surgeon, Illinois Research and Educational Hospitals, Chicago, Illinois.

RANDALL, HENRY THOMAS, M.D., Sc.D. (MED.)
Professor of Surgery, Cornell University Medical College; Chairman, Department of Surgery, and Attending Surgeon, Memorial Sloan-Kettering Cancer Center, New York.

RAVITCH, MARK M., M.D.
Associate Professor of Surgery, Johns Hopkins University School of Medicine; Surgeon-in-Chief, Baltimore City Hospital, Baltimore, Maryland.

SALZMAN, EDWIN WILLIAM, M.D.
Instructor in Surgery, Harvard Medical School; Assistant in Surgery, Massachusetts General Hospital, Boston, Massachusetts.

SCHULTE, WILLIAM J., M.D.
Instructor in Surgery, Marquette University School of Medicine; Attending Surgeon, Milwaukee County General Hospital, Milwaukee, Wisconsin.

SHAW, ROBERT STETSON, M.D.
Assistant Clinical Professor of Surgery, Harvard Medical School; Associate Visiting Surgeon, Massachusetts General Hospital, Boston, Massachusetts.

SHERMAN, CHARLES D., JR., M.D.
Clinical Associate Professor of Surgery, University of Rochester School of Medicine and Dentistry; Surgeon, Strong Memorial Hospital and Highland Hospital, Rochester, New York.

SLOOP, RICHARD D., M.D.
Chief Resident, General and Thoracic Surgery, Los Angeles County Harbor General Hospital, Torrance, California.

SMITH, GORDON K., M.D.
Clinical Professor of Surgery, University of Southern California School of Medicine; Surgeon, Hospital of the Good Samaritan, Los Angeles County General Hospital, and Methodist Hospital of Southern California, Los Angeles, California.

SMITH, ROBERT B., III, M.D.
Instructor and Chief Resident, Department of Surgery, Columbia University College of Physicians and Surgeons, New York.

SOERGEL, KONRAD H., M.D.
Assistant Professor of Medicine, Marquette University School of Medicine; Chief, Gastroenterology Service, Milwaukee County General Hospital, Milwaukee, Wisconsin; Attending Gastroenterologist, Veterans Administration Hospital, Wood, Wisconsin.

SPITTELL, JOHN A., JR., M.D., M.S. (MED.)
Assistant Professor of Medicine, Mayo Graduate School of Medicine, University of Minnesota; Consultant and Head of a Section of Medicine, Mayo Clinic, Rochester, Minnesota.

STATE, DAVID, M.D., PH.D.
Professor and Chairman, Department of Surgery, Albert Einstein College of Medicine, Bronx, New York; Director of Surgery and Chief of Cardiovascular and Thoracic Surgery, Bronx Municipal Hospital Center, New York.

STEVENSON, JOHN K., M.D.
Associate Professor of Surgery, University of Washington School of Medicine, Seattle, Washington; Staff Surgeon, University Hospital; Attending Surgeon, Childrens Orthopedic Hospital; Consultant, Swedish Hospital, Seattle, Washington; Consultant, Madigan General Hospital, Tacoma; Consultant, Veterans Administration Hospital; Attending Surgeon, King County Hospital, Seattle, Washington.

STRODE, JOSEPH E., M.D.
Emeritus Chief of Surgery, Straub Clinic and Queens Hospital, Honolulu, Hawaii.

SWENSON, ORVAR, M.D.
Professor of Surgery, Northwestern University School of Medicine; Chief of Surgery, The Children's Memorial Hospital, Chicago, Illinois.

TIDRICK, ROBERT T., M.D.
Professor and Head, Department of Surgery, College of Medicine, University of Iowa, Iowa City, Iowa.

USHER, FRANCIS COWGILL, M.D.
Associate Clinical Professor of Surgery, Baylor University College of Medicine; Attending Surgeon, Methodist, Ben Taub, and Veterans Administration Hospitals, Houston, Texas.

WANGENSTEEN, OWEN H., M.D., PH.D.
Professor and Chairman, Department of Surgery, University of Minnesota School of Medical Sciences; Chief, Surgical Services, University of Minnesota Hospitals, Minneapolis, Minnesota.

WANGENSTEEN, STEPHEN L., M.D.
Formerly Chief Resident and Instructor in Surgery, Columbia University, College of Physicians and Surgeons; Presently Assistant Chief, Surgical Research Branch, Research and Development Command, Office of the Surgeon General, United States Army, Washington, D.C.

WANTZ, GEORGE E., JR., M.D.
Clinical Associate Professor of Surgery, Cornell University Medical College; Attending Surgeon, The New York Hospital, New York, New York.

WARREN, KENNETH W., M.D.
Chairman, Department of Surgery, Lahey Clinic Foundation, Boston, Massachusetts.

WEINBERG, JOSEPH A., M.D.
Clinical Professor of Surgery, University of California, Los Angeles; Chief, Surgical Service, Veterans Administration Hospital, Long Beach, California.

WEISEL, WILSON, M.D.
Clinical Professor of Surgery and Chairman of the Department of Thoracic-Cardiovascular Surgery; Mar-

quette University School of Medicine; Surgical Staff, Milwaukee Children's Hospital, St. Joseph's Hospital, and Columbia Hospital; Chairman of the Department of Surgery, St. Joseph's Hospital; Consultant, Veterans Administration Hospital, Milwaukee County General, St. Luke's, and St. Michael Hospitals, Milwaukee, Wisconsin.

WELCH, C. STUART, M.D., PH.D.
Professor of Surgery, Albany Medical College of Union University; Attending Surgeon, Albany Medical Center Hospital; Consultant, Veterans Administration Hospital; Courtesy Staff, Memorial and St. Peter's Hospitals, Albany, New York.

WILLIAMS, ROGER D., M.D.
Professor of Surgery, Ohio State University College of Medicine; Attending Staff, University Hospital, Courtesy Staff, Columbus Children's Hospital, Columbus, Ohio; Consultant, Veterans Administration Hospital, Dayton, Ohio.

WITTE, MARLYS HEARST, M.D.
Instructor in Medicine, New York University School of Medicine; Assistant Attending Physician, Bellevue Hospital; Assistant Visiting Physician, University Hospital, New York, New York.

WOMACK, NATHAN A., M.D.
Professor and Chairman, Department of Surgery, University of North Carolina School of Medicine; Surgeon-in-Chief, North Carolina Memorial Hospital, Chapel Hill, North Carolina.

WOODWARD, EDWARD R., M.D.
Professor and Head, Department of Surgery, University of Florida College of Medicine; Attending Surgeon, University Hospital and Clinics, Gainesville, Florida; Consultant in Surgery, Veterans Administration Hospital, Lake City, Florida.

WORMAN, LEONARD W., M.D.
Assistant Professor of Thoracic and Cardiovascular Surgery, Marquette University School of Medicine; Assistant Director of Surgery, Milwaukee County General Hospital, Milwaukee, Wisconsin.

ZIFFREN, SIDNEY E., M.D.
Professor of Surgery, University of Iowa College of Medicine; Attending Surgeon, University Hospitals, Iowa City, Iowa.

ZOLLINGER, ROBERT, M., M.D.
Professor and Chairman, Department of Surgery, Ohio State University School of Medicine, Columbus, Ohio.

Preface to the Original Volume

Early textbooks on surgery were authoritative and final because the views and experiences of one individual were recorded. This was possible when the content of surgical knowledge was limited and one surgeon could meet with the whole subject in his activities. Wider knowledge and scope have made such a simple orderly course impractical. New information fragments the literature into segments and at the same time reduces the absolute authority of individual authors. The most searching investigator in a narrow field is likely to be the most uncertain of his ground. The more he learns the more he appreciates what there is still to be learned.

It is a curious paradox that writings on surgery in the period of relative ignorance could be dogmatic, whereas in the present period of great knowledge controversy is accepted. It was possible at the beginning of this century to lay down rules of conduct to meet most situations, so that the practicing surgeon had only to do what the book said should be done. Need for thinking about individual problems was reduced to a minimum. Countless discoveries and accomplishments have brought with them more speculation and more responsibility for thinking rather than less. The mechanical surgeon who might read rules and apply them by formula is farther away than ever before. A surgeon must remain a student and, to paraphrase a statement by Flexner, "employ his senses, aided and unaided, to elicit data that when put together enable him to construct a picture, the outstanding feature of which he tentatively labels. To visualize and solve problems, no two of which are ever alike—that is the concern alike of the practicing surgeons as of the University investigator."

Surgery is an inexact science. If all were known about surgical diseases, there would be little need for surgeons. Search for the truth about obscure diseases will inevitably bring controversy and difference of opinion. When a conviction is arrived at by study and evaluation of experience, it is presented in the literature isolated and on the basis of factual data. There is overpowering and unjustified authority in a viewpoint so stated without rebuttal. This book is an attempt to present, side by side, varying viewpoints on certain surgical topics about which there is controversy.

In some instances, concepts are at variance because of fundamental differences, in others because of less basic disagreements such as the choice of, or timing of, an operation. The subjects chosen seemed to the editors to have legitimate divergence. While the book does not comprehensively cover all surgical problems, the topics selected should add up to those questions which commonly beset a surgeon.

It is impressive to find that what appears on the surface to be marked difference of opinion is not so marked when the ideas are more deeply probed. There are difficulties in communication which create conflict. For instance, even though an entity has a name which would be well understood by all, the controversialists may not be talking about the same thing. The bare term "peritonitis" may mean different things to different people; "radical operation" may mean only what the user intended it to mean. Also, comparison of statistical analyses of results of treatment may not be valid because samples used are not comparable. For example, patients screened from amongst many seeking treatment and who, because of complexity of disease, economic status, or some other factor, are sent to a special clinic or center cannot be collectively compared with the whole group.

A book such as this does not provide answers. It does demonstrate how certain authorities arrived at their own answers. Thus, a reader might be guided in that difficult and unavoidable decision which he must make for each patient he treats. Many factors in the decision cannot be written in a book and are concerned with the sick individual. The training and experience of the surgeon, facilities such as those for anesthesia, ancillary help and many other matters must be weighed in choosing a course.

The notion for the creation of this volume arose out of the inclination of surgeons to argue their differences. The very successful "panel discussions" conducted by the American College of Surgeons are valuable to participants and audience alike because of controversies. All recognize that things are not settled, that knowledge is imperfect, and that there may be different ways to achieve an objective.

Contributors to the volume entered into the spirit and purposes with a zeal that made the editors' task wonderfully instructive. Many contributors seemed to welcome an opportunity to take up a specific argument in writing. It appeared that discussions face to face were more productive of understanding and that factual detached papers in the formal literature were unsatisfactory from the controversy standpoint. The aroused tone of some of the contributors, which makes for exciting reading, came about because the author was not knocking a straw man down, but actually coming to grips. The editors are grateful to all the contributors, not only for the writings, but also for decisive understanding of the purposes of the book.

The editors endeavored in introductions to sections to relate forethoughts regarding the controversies. An attempt has been made in these preambles to avoid arbitration or the taking of sides—sometimes a difficult commission.

The order of presentation of subjects is unusual. In the conventional book on surgery, it is customary to use regional anatomy as the basis for arrangement of chapters. Here, because the emphasis is on problems in general surgery the material is organized in some approximation of the magnitude of the problem in a general surgeon's experience.

In such a cooperative venture, acknowledgments and thanks must be widespread. Of special moment in this respect is our gratefulness to the W. B. Saunders Company for the original idea and for continued interest and help. The contributors in many instances also gave advice and suggestions which are acknowledged gratefully.

JOHN H. MULHOLLAND
EDWIN H. ELLISON
STANLEY R. FRIESEN

Introduction

Current Surgical Management III is the result of appeals from practicing surgeons and residents that further controversial matters be considered, as in Volumes I and II. Such enthusiastic acceptance of the publications confirms the original views of the editors and publishers that while surgeons in practice agree on objectives, they differ in ways of achieving these objectives.

Education of a surgeon at the outset is often a dogmatic process. More or less rigid rules of conduct are set down and enforced; things are done in one way and in no other. Justification for this attitude is frequently offered in the view that one sound method should be mastered for the management of each surgical condition likely to be encountered. But maturity brings the realization that there is no one perfect way, and that there will be none without perfect understanding of background processes of disease. Surgery has progressed to enormous achievements by the development and improvement of methods. But the great steps are taken because of more knowledge. More knowledge in turn requires changes in methods, changes in attitudes and the resiliency to adapt to change.

The editors of Current Surgical Management were aware of the risk that publication of successive volumes and extension of controversial discussions might lead to considerations of fruitless trivialities. But in the few years since 1957, when the first volume was issued, changes in understanding have redirected controversies on subjects discussed in that volume to new planes. For example, the painful decisions regarding management of massively bleeding esophageal varices were discussed in Current Surgical Management I, and are again considered in this volume. But the direction of controversy has shifted noticeably because a realization has come about that hepatic lymph flow is an important factor in the disturbed vascular dynamics of cirrhosis of the liver. Similarly controversy over the matter of surgical treatment of duodenal ulcer and its complications is unremitting. But eight years have changed the perspective of differences. The argument now seems to be more about which effective operation will best preserve functioning gastric mucosa than whether a major segment of the stomach should be removed.

It would be nice to look back and find at least one of the 1957 controversies about which we could say: "This question is settled; there is no more need for troubling indecision; do this in this way every time and it will be right." Passing years seem more to have shaken what relatively solid bases there were than to have firmed our ground. Faint sounds from immunologists now indicate that the appendix, that surgically dispensable organ, has an obscure but important protective function related to that of the thymus. In another few years we may be debating operative methods for preserving a germinal center of lymphoid tissue in an inflamed appendix, certainly a complicating new twist to a simple surgical concept. As a matter of fact, search for a controversial matter which is *probably* settled for good led back to a textbook of surgery published in 1876. Whether or not the use of new-fangled general anesthesia was proper was still being argued. What is apparently a clinching point in the argument is quoted thus: "A review of capital (major) operations, 2586 performed without and 1847 performed with anesthesia, showed that the rate of mortality had not been increased by administration of the anesthetic."

Controversy will go on. The editors are once more indebted to enthusiastic contributors for acknowledging this premise to surgical thought by their gracious participation.

JOHN H. MULHOLLAND

Contents

Treatment of

Early Carcinoma

of the Mid-Esophagus

Introduction

In the recent past a high operative mortality and poor end results characterized the surgical treatment of carcinoma of both the upper and mid-esophagus. Furthermore, conventional x-ray therapy, either alone or as an adjunct to operative intervention, had also proved to be ineffectual. This truly dismal picture is now being challenged by more extensive esophageal resections combined with improved and safer techniques for restoring gastrointestinal continuity. The use of staged procedures in selected patients continues to be of importance. Supervoltage and high energy (CO^{60}) radiotherapy also has been under intensive study and is summarized.

A review of this section gives one an improved insight into the reasonings behind these concepts of therapy and allows a beginning comparison of their relative values.

Both authors advocating operative management have properly emphasized the importance of wide resection, including appropriate removal of lymph nodes draining the esophagus. Adams has advocated immediate esophagogastrostomy and postoperative supervoltage roentgen therapy to the cervical, mediastinal, and subdiaphragmatic areas with an absolute 5-year survival of 9 per cent, but makes no reference to the operative mortality. Mahoney prefers construction of a temporary cervical esophagostomy and gastrostomy following a near-total resection; interposition of the right colon is delayed until nutrition and risk are improved. The reported operative mortality of 15.3 per cent is quite satisfactory, and 3 of the 47 surviving operation are living nearly 5 years.

Lampe reports on 53 patients receiving a complete course of CO^{60}, including 8 patients referred for operation after failure of radiotherapy, with a 5-year survival of 5.7 per cent. The editors agree that comparison of these data with surgical results is difficult, and preferably should include follow-up on all patients resected. Here again radiotherapy is at a disadvantage, since it would be hard to identify those patients who would have had a resectable lesion.

E. H. E.

Experience with High Energy (Cobalt-60) Radiotherapy of Carcinoma of Upper and Middle Thirds of the Thoracic Esophagus

Isadore Lampe *and* Juan V. Fayos

University of Michigan Medical Center, Ann Arbor, Michigan

Program of Treatment

A consistent program of high energy (cobalt-60) radiotherapy of carcinoma of the upper and middle thirds of the thoracic esophagus has been in progress since 1955 at the University of Michigan Medical Center. Because of the high mortality rate and poor results of surgical treatment, this program was initiated when cobalt-60 radiation became available at this institution. Experience with orthovoltage x-ray irradiation prior to 1955 had also been unfavorable. The high energy radiotherapy program was limited to lesions of the upper and middle thirds of the thoracic esophagus, with only occasional attempts at radiotherapy of lesions of the lower third of this organ, attempts which largely have not proved fruitful; most such lesions continue to be treated surgically.

From 1955 through 1958, 75 patients with upper and middle third lesions were seen; these patients had not received prior surgical or radiation treatment. A minimum of 4 years' follow-up observation is available in these patients.

As seen in Table 1, of the 75 patients presenting with this disease at the Alice Crocker Lloyd Radiation Therapy Center, 15 were not treated for the reasons detailed in the table. In 11 of the 15 this was because of disease which, in our judgment, made any attempt at radiotherapy a futile gesture. In 4 patients only metastatic sites were irradiated as a palliative effort and, one may add, with little benefit. Radiotherapy of the primary tumor was started in 56 patients, but completed in only 53; the reasons for discontinuing irradiation are shown in Table 1. In this discussion our chief

TABLE 1.   CARCINOMA OF UPPER AND MIDDLE THIRDS OF THORACIC ESOPHAGUS: PREVIOUSLY UNTREATED PATIENTS (1955 through 1958)

		Number
Patients seen but not treated		15
Patient refused treatment	2	
Patient left for treatment elsewhere	1	
Patient accepted for radiotherapy but surgery (by-pass) done	1	
Not accepted for radiotherapy	1	
Massive supraclavicular metastasis	1	
Extension into lung and pleura	1	
Mediastinal metastasis distant from primary site	1	
Subcutaneous metastasis	1	
Sinus into mediastinum, mediastinitis	1	
Supraclavicular metastasis and mediastinitis	1	
Tracheoesophageal fistula	1	
Bronchoesophageal fistula	1	
Invasion of trachea; fungating tracheal lesion	1	
Esophageal perforation into mediastinum	1	
Age 78, weight 78 lb., condition extremely poor		4
Patients accepted for treatment of metastases only	2	
Bone metastases	2	
Mediastinal metastases remote from primary site		
Patients accepted for radiotherapy of primary lesion:		3
Radiotherapy incomplete		
Death from hemorrhage at tumor dose 2900 r in 21 days	1	
Treatment discontinued at tumor dose 309 r in 5 days because of mediastinitis and abscess	1	
Treatment discontinued at tumor dose 809 r in 7 days because of severe deterioration of general condition	1	
Radiotherapy completed		53
Total		75

concern will be with the 53 patients, 70.6 per cent of all the patients seen, who completed the planned course of radiotherapy.

The treatment was carried out with cobalt-60 radiation. Fifteen patients were treated with fixed field techniques, usually opposed anterior and posterior fields, and 38 with a rotational technique. Except for some of the cases treated early in the period, before a rotational technique had been developed, the rotational technique was used whenever, with the patients in the horizontal position, the esophageal lesion could be placed along the axis of a horizontal cylinder of high radiation dose. The tumor dose usually was about 6000 r in 6 weeks; the calculation of dose disregarded traversed air volumes, so that in the rotationally treated patients the actual dose was somewhat greater.

Results

An additional feature of the program consisted of careful assessment with respect to the possibility of operative intervention when it became apparent that radiotherapy had failed to control the lesion. For the period reported 8 patients were operated on (15.1 per cent). In 6 patients it proved possible to perform esophagectomy. These patients were operated on 2 months to $2\frac{2}{3}$ years after irradiation. Two of these patients died postoperatively. Two other patients died of the neoplasm 8 and 10 months after operation. One patient, on whom operation was performed 3 months after radiotherapy, died of hemorrhage $3\frac{1}{12}$ years after irradiation. It is possible that the hemorrhage was caused by benign ulceration associated with colon transplant. One of the patients on whom resection was done is alive $4\frac{1}{4}$ years after irradiation, the operation having been done 3 months after radiotherapy.

In 2 more patients nonresectability limited operative intervention to by-pass procedures, which were performed 2 and 4 months after irradiation. Both patients died postoperatively. The total operative mortality was 50 per cent; 33 per cent in the esophagectomy cases.

Miscellaneous data that may be of interest are presented in Table 2. Two of the lesions located in the middle third of the esophagus were adenocarcinoma. There was no esophagoscopic or radiographic abnormality of the esophagus from the lower end of each of these lesions to and including the gastric cardia. One of these patients died $1\frac{1}{4}$ years after radiation, 10 months after esophagectomy; the other 4 months after radiotherapy. (A third patient with adenocarcinoma of the middle third of the esophagus was irradiated in 1962. The patient was 79 years old, and was asymptomatic with restoration of the esophageal lumen for over 1 year, but with recurring dysphagia at $1\frac{1}{2}$ years.)

TABLE 2. CARCINOMA OF UPPER AND MIDDLE THIRDS OF THORACIC
ESOPHAGUS: MISCELLANEOUS DATA
(1955 through 1958)

		Number of Patients
Age:	40–49	3
	50–69	29
	70–82	21
Sex:	Male	45
	Female	8
Race:	White	48
	Negro	5
Location:	Upper third	14
	Middle third	39
Histopathology:		
Adenocarcinoma		2
Squamous cell carcinoma		48
Carcinoma, unspecified		2
Cytologic examination positive		1*

* One patient without a histologic diagnosis, but with positive cytologic findings, died 4 months after irradiation.

The results are presented under 2 aspects: (1) assessment of palliative benefit and (2) survival.

Palliation

Table 3 presents data on palliative accomplishment by radiotherapy. For this tabulation the 2 patients alive 5 and 6½ years after irradiation are excluded. The patients on whom postirradiation surgery was performed are rated on the basis of such palliation as may have been obtained by the radiotherapy, not by the surgical procedure. Thus 51 patients are evaluated, all dead except 1 post-surgical case alive at 4¼ years.

TABLE 3.   CARCINOMA OF UPPER AND MIDDLE THIRDS OF THORACIC ESOPHAGUS: PALLIATION OF SWALLOWING OBTAINED BY RADIOTHERAPY* (1955 through 1958)

Duration of Palliation	Number of Patients	Per Cent
0	31	60.8
3 to 6 months	4	7.8
6 to 12 months	3	5.9
1 to 2 years	6	11.8
2 to 3 years	4	7.8
3 to 4 years	3	5.9
Total	51	100.0
Palliation 3 months to 4 years	39.2 per cent	
Palliation 1 to 4 years	25.5 per cent	

* Excluding 2 patients alive 5 and 6½ years later.

Palliation is defined as improved swallowing function to a degree permitting adequate nourishment by mouth for at least 3 months. Adequate nourishment implies at least the ability to take liquids, soft foods, and ground meat without difficulty. One-fourth of the patients achieved palliation for 1 to almost 4 years, and 39 per cent for 3 months to almost 4 years.

Survival

Survival is computed from the time of initiation of radiotherapy. The survival experience is presented in Table 4. The overall 4-year survival rate is 5.7 per cent: 2 patients alive at 5 and 6½ years after radiotherapy only; 1 patient alive at 4¼ years after irradiation, esophagectomy having been performed 3 months after irradiation (residual carcinoma was present at the primary site). For radiotherapy alone, the 4-year survival rate is 3.8 per cent (2 patients), but these are living and well at 5 and 6½ years after treatment; therefore, the 5-year survival rate is the same, 3.8 per cent.

Irradiation or Surgery or Both

The use of high energy radiotherapy in the treatment of carcinoma of the esophagus has not resulted in survival rates that can be considered satis-

TABLE 4.   CARCINOMA OF UPPER AND MIDDLE THIRDS OF THORACIC
ESOPHAGUS: SURVIVAL EXPERIENCE
(1955 through 1958)

	Per Cent Survival				
	1 yr.	2 yrs.	3 yrs.	4 yrs.	(5 yrs.)
Radiotherapy and surgery	32.0	22.6	13.2	5.7*	
Radiotherapy†	28.3	18.8	9.4	3.8‡	(3.8)

* 1 patient alive at 4¼ years, esophagectomy at 3 months after irradiation; 1 alive at 5 years and 1 at 6½ years after radiotherapy only.

† For this computation 2 surgical patients, 1 dead at 3¹⁄₁₂ years and 1 alive at 4¼ years, were counted as dead at the time the post-irradiation recurrence became evident, 3 months in each case.

‡ 1 patient alive at 5 years and 1 at 6½ years after radiotherapy only.

factory; the disease is still a dread one. Nevertheless, apparent cures can be produced in an occasional patient, and a significant record of palliation can be demonstrated. In our experience, this exceeds what we were able to accomplish with orthovoltage x-ray radiation in 80 patients treated prior to 1955. In this group, the 1-year survival rate was 12.8 per cent, the 2- and 3-year rates were 1.3 per cent, and the 4-year rate was 0 per cent. To this extent high energy radiotherapy represents an advance, although a modest one, in what we have been able to achieve in the radiation treatment of this disease. As stated before, we have not undertaken a consistent program of radiotherapy of carcinoma of the lower third of the thoracic esophagus, believing that surgery has more to offer for this lesion.

Comparison of our results with surgical accomplishment as reported in the literature in the treatment of carcinoma of the upper and middle thirds of the thoracic esophagus is in order. Difficulties stand in the way of making a comparison which is meaningful. In only a few papers are the data so presented as to make it possible to determine precisely the number of patients with upper and middle third lesions. In still fewer publications are follow-up data extending over a period of 4 or 5 years available.

In 1954, Sweet[3] presented such data in the form of per cent survival for 1 to 5 years, based on the number of patients surviving resection. The upper third and middle third lesions are dealt with separately, but can be combined. The computation of survival for each of the 5 years is made on the basis of the number eligible: 117 resected cases eligible for calculation of 1-year survival, 112 for 2 years, 101 for 3 years, 93 for 4 years, and 76 for 5 years.

It is our belief that comparison of radiotherapy and surgery is best based on the number of patients completing the planned course of irradiation versus the number of patients on whom esophagectomy was performed. To compare those irradiated with only those surviving esophagectomy is erroneous; failure to survive the operation is a failure of the treatment method. Even this method of comparison is very likely creating a bias against radiotherapy, since it is virtually certain that all the patients irradiated could not have had the disease in a resectable stage. Therefore, Sweet's survival data have been recomputed to arrive at the percentage of esophagectomy patients surviving 1, 2, 3, 4, and 5 years. This is readily done, since the required data are clearly presented. Only one uncertainty exists. Six upper third lesions were resected and it is stated, "There have been no long survivals. One patient lived 2 years and 2 months. The operative mortality is high; 3 of the 6 patients on whom a resection was performed died." For the recomputation it is assumed that only 1 patient survived 1 and 2 years; it is known that none survived 3 years. The operative mortality for upper and middle third lesions was 26.2 per cent. The result of the recalculation appears in Table 5.

TABLE 5.   CARCINOMA OF UPPER AND MIDDLE THIRDS OF THORACIC ESOPHAGUS: SURVIVAL AND OPERATIVE MORTALITY RATES

| | Per Cent Survival | | | | | Operative Mortality (Per cent) |
	1 yr.	2 yrs.	3 yrs.	4 yrs.	5yrs.	
Sweet, 1954	51.3	19.6	11.9	4.3	2.6	26.2
Mustard and Ibberson, 1956	29.6	11.1	3.7	3.7	3.7	66.7
University of Michigan:						
Radiotherapy and surgery	32.0	22.6	13.2	5.7	—	33.3
Radiotherapy only	28.3	18.8	9.4	3.8	(3.8)*	

* The radiotherapy survivors are living at 5 and 6½ years, therefore the 5-year rate is the same as the 4-year one, whereas the surgical survivor is alive at 4¼ years and cannot enter a 5-year calculation.

Pertinent data were presented in 1956 by Mustard and Ibberson.[1] Twenty-seven esophagectomies for upper and middle third thoracic lesions are reported with 18 postoperative deaths (66.7 per cent), and the yearly survival rates are shown in Table 5. Study of Table 5 reveals that high energy radiotherapy has produced results entirely comparable to those reported by surgeons of skill and experience in this field. Indeed the radiation results actually may be superior; it is most unlikely that all of the irradiated cases presented the type of neoplasm that would have permitted resection.

One might indeed argue that the patients treated by irradiation, if one includes those in whom treatment could not be completed, are more comparable to the group of patients subjected to surgical exploration than to the group on whom resection could be performed. If the 5-year survival rate for the patients irradiated is computed on this basis, it is 3.6 per cent, whereas for the surgical series, the rate is 2.2 per cent for that of Mustard and Ibberson, and 1.7 per cent for that of Sweet. This suggests superiority of the radiotherapeutic attack, but this line of argument does not merit being pushed too far, since the results are poor by either approach.

It is evident from our experience that the use of surgery when radiation failure occurs has added something to the salvage rate (Table 4). The price of this gain was high: a 50 per cent operative mortality rate. But these patients were doomed to die of the disease if nothing more was done. It is encouraging to note that in 6 of the 8 patients subjected to surgery, esophagectomy could be accomplished, and that the operative result obtained was significant in 2 patients. One patient survived $3\frac{1}{12}$ years after irradiation, having been operated on 3 months after radiotherapy. The cause of death in this case was hemorrhage, possibly from benign ulceration at the junction of the colon transplant and stomach. The second patient is alive and apparently well $4\frac{1}{4}$ years after initial treatment. This policy seems to be worthwhile.

In view of the low survival experience with radiotherapy alone the question immediately arises: Why not operate on every case after irradiation? It is not possible to predict the result of such a program, but a few comments are in order. Were every case operated on after radiotherapy the possibility exists that the patients who would have survived with radiotherapy alone might succumb to the high operative mortality rate. It would be naive to believe that it would be possible to carry out resection in every patient after irradiation. Review of our cases, excluding the 8 that were in fact operated on, indicates in our judgment that half of these patients could not have been operated on or would have been exceedingly poor candidates for operation because of the following existing conditions: (1) in several, preirradiation thoracotomy had already demonstrated the situation to be inoperable; (2) a number were of advanced age and in poor general condition; (3) in a number of patients evidence of spread of the disease, as shown by vocal cord paralysis, Horner's syndrome, and supraclavicular metastasis, indicated inoperability; (4) in still others abnormality of the tracheal bronchial tree pointed to mediastinal invasion and extension, which would have prevented resection; and (5) a number of patients died within 1 to 2 months after completion of irradiation, and these certainly could not have been subjected to surgery.

What the fate of the other half of the group would have been if subjected to immediate postirradiation operation is conjectural. Our limited experience does not warrant optimism in the direction of expecting greatly improved survival rates. At present we hold the opinion that an attempt at routine postirradiation operation should await the time when reasonable operative mortality rates can be achieved and not before. At the moment it seems to us that the best that can be achieved is to operate when radiation failure is evident.

One exception to the uniform world-wide situation of high operative mortality exists in the work and reports of K. Nakayama. Using a multi-stage resection procedure, Nakayama[2] reported in 1960 an operative mortality of 8.5 per cent in 271 patients with upper and middle thoracic esophageal lesions. Also exceptional is the reported 16.4 per cent 5-year survival in 71 patients so treated. Included in the treatment program is irradiation of the esophageal primary lesion, just prior to resection, with a radiation dose of 2000 to 3000 r administered in about 2 weeks.

Precise comparison of this 5-year survival rate with those cited above cannot be made because the base used for the computation is not clearly stated. We are unable to determine whether the rate is based on the number explored, the number resected, or the number surviving resection. But in any event, this rate certainly appears to exceed that obtained by any other worker in the field, and is a tribute to unusual surgical skill, perhaps aided by the physical characteristics of the patients so treated.

On the basis of other experience in radiotherapy, we believe that the kind of radiotherapy used in this work is considerably less important for the end result than the surgical skill exhibited, and that a more efficient use of radiotherapy might be to employ it to full dose preoperatively. Should this low operative mortality rate become a universal phenomenon in the surgical attack on this disease, there is little question that postirradiation resection should be employed frequently.

Summary

1. Of 75 patients with carcinoma of the upper and middle thirds of the thoracic esophagus seen at the Alice Crocker Lloyd Radiation Therapy Center from 1955 through 1958, 53 completed a planned course of high energy (cobalt-60) radiotherapy to the primary tumor.

2. Eight patients were operated on for recurrence subsequent to irradiation: in 6, esophagectomies were performed; in 2, by-pass procedures.

3. Palliation enduring 3 months to almost 4 years was obtained in 39.2 per cent; 1 to almost 4 years in 25.5 per cent, excluding 2 patients surviving after radiotherapy for 5 and 6½ years.

4. With radiotherapy only, 28.3 per cent were alive at 1 year, 18.8 per cent at 2 years, 9.4 per cent at 3 years, 3.8 per cent at 4 and 5 years. With radiotherapy and surgery 32.0 per cent were alive at 1 year, 22.6 per cent at 2 years, 13.2 per cent at 3 years and 5.7 per cent at 4 years.

5. Comparison of the radiotherapeutic results with 2 surgical series demonstrates that these results are at least as good as those achieved by operative procedures performed by surgeons skilled and experienced in this field.

6. The policy of attempting operation when radiotherapy failed produced a slight but worthwhile improvement in salvage rate. In the face of the current high mortality rates of esophagectomy, it does not seem advisable to embark on a program of routine postirradiation surgery. This opinion is subject to revision should the low operative mortality rate obtained by Nakayama become standard.

References

1. Mustard, R. A., and Ibberson, O.: Carcinoma of the esophagus. A review of 381 cases admitted to Toronto General Hospital 1937–1953 inclusive. Ann. Surg., *144*:927, 1956.
2. Nakayama, K.: Erfahrungen bei etwas 3000 Fallen von Oesophagus und Kardiacarcinom. Langenbecks Arch. klin. Chir., *295*:81, 1960.
3. Sweet, R. H.: Late results of surgical treatment of carcinoma of the esophagus. J.A.M.A., *155*:422, 1954.

Resection and Esophagogastrostomy
in the Treatment of Early
Carcinoma of the Mid-Esophagus

Herbert D. Adams

Lahey Clinic Foundation, Boston

Prognosis

Past experience with the surgical management of carcinoma of the esophagus antedating the antibiotic era, when infection was a prohibitive factor to resection and definitive surgery as we know it today, has left a lasting impression and influence on the present modern management of this disease. At that particular time, when a multistaged presternal reconstruction was done following a transthoracic resection, results were particularly discouraging. Even if resection was successful and the patient survived without serious intrathoracic complications, re-establishment of a good functioning upper gastrointestinal tract was rarely possible. In addition, even if a reasonably satisfactory function had finally been obtained with these multistaged presternal skin tubes, the patient soon succumbed from his carcinoma. I mention these facts to stress these major points that still are of primary concern in our present management of carcinoma of the esophagus, namely, how may we consistently attain good function after resection of the esophagus, and how can we improve the overall prognosis in this discouraging disease?

When we consider the criteria for early or favorable carcinoma at the level of the mid-esophagus, we are concerned with factors that are involved in an early diagnosis and a lesion that is favorable for a curative resection. In a recent review of our results in the surgical management of carcinoma of the esophagus, the outstanding facts remain: there has been no appreciable improvement in patients seen at an earlier clinical stage or in patients reaching definitive treatment at a more favorable pathologic stage.

Measures for Early Diagnosis

Despite all efforts to educate the public concerning the signs and symptoms of carcinoma in general, the serious significance of dysphagia as a symptom of esophageal obstruction, and the possibility that carcinoma is its cause, most of these patients reach us, even today, after months of progressive and marked dysphagia. By the time they come to us for specific treatment, the majority have reached such an advanced stage of difficulty in swallowing that they can take liquids only. Certainly it is well accepted that, in the very early stages of this disease in the esophagus, and particularly at the cardia, x-ray studies may not demonstrate any significant diagnostic change, and therefore such studies tend to discount the seriousness of the situation, and treatment is delayed.

Other concurrent lesions, such as a hiatus hernia, diverticulum, or other potentially obstructing lesions, further confuse the issue and prolong the delay in making the diagnosis and instituting definitive treatment. Therefore, esophagoscopy remains the most specific and valuable diagnostic measure in this serious disease, and in the presence of progressive dysphagia, it should be used far more frequently and earlier than it is at present. Usually, however, this diagnostic measure also is delayed, and we continue to see patients with large, advanced, extensive lesions that are most unfavorable from the standpoint of management as well as prognosis.

We cannot define an early lesion satisfactorily because a grossly small lesion may, histologically, be highly undifferentiated, and minimal clinical symptoms may be associated with it. In contrast, a well differentiated epidermoid carcinoma may be a large bulky tumor before it causes appreciable symptoms of obstruction. In addition, because of the intimate anatomic relationships of the esophagus to other vital structures in the mediastinum, almost any extension beyond the esophageal wall will profoundly influence resectability and curability. In other words, there are no satisfactory criteria of an "early" lesion, that is, a favorable pathologic lesion in this region, and therefore the prognosis at best is usually unfavorable. It is for this reason also that there has been so much discouragement in general with the treatment, particularly of the high lesions (mid- and upper esophagus), to a point that the question has frequently been raised whether the surgical management of carcinomas at these levels is ever curative and is always only palliative.

Argument for Resection and Esophagogastrostomy

Since the advent of antibiotics has made possible refined and definitive surgery, and since these lesions are frequently unfavorable pathologically at a very early stage or because of prolonged delay in diagnosis, I have carried out resection in a great proportion of these cases. I meticulously re-establish the continuity of the upper gastrointestinal tract using the stomach, and

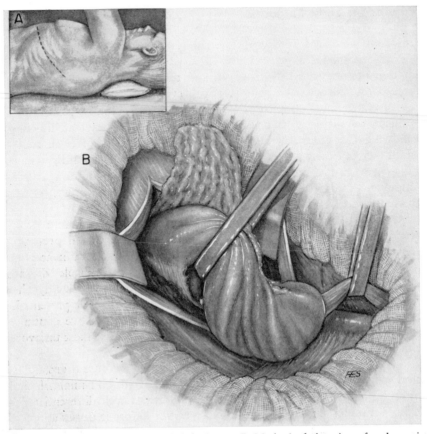

Fig. 1. *A,* Incision used through left thorax. *B,* Method of elevation of and traction on stomach through the diaphragm and esophagus from the mediastinum to avoid trauma to these structures.

supplement this with supervoltage x-ray therapy to the entire regional lymphatics in the mediastinum, and to subdiaphragmatic and low cervical lymphatic systems. Using this procedure, we have almost doubled our resectability, increasing it to 65 per cent, and the only present contraindications to resection are direct invasion of adjacent major vascular structures or a major bronchus and widespread distant metastasis.

Technique

With the proper technique, i.e., utilizing the stomach to bridge the resected defect in the esophagus, the function will be consistently excellent. In my opinion, the key to obtaining excellent function of the reconstructed upper gastrointestinal tract is placing the maximum emphasis on the technique that will consistently preserve good function in the stomach, which has been displaced into the chest, and will also prevent the common complications, either early or late, related to the anastomosis. Results related to the re-establishment of satisfactory function are so variable when the stomach is utilized without regard for function that other structures are sometimes substituted in bridging the defect.

Excellent function can be obtained only if the details of the technique are worked out with extreme care in order to preserve the maximal blood supply and to avoid even minimal trauma to the stomach as it is being mobilized and anastomosed in its new position. It is for these reasons that I prefer to carry out this resection through the left side of the thorax and through the left diaphragm, in order to tailor the mobilization of the stomach to the exact requirements for bridging the defect of the resection without tension.

Only the necessary amount of stomach is mobilized, the maximum amount of blood supply is retained, and direct traction to the stomach wall with gauze or instruments is completely avoided during this procedure. The stomach and esophagus are elevated by means of Penrose tubing, as shown in Figure 1. In addition, a meticulous anastomosis must be carried out with two layers of fine, interrupted, nonabsorbable sutures which, with adequate antibiotic coverage, will prevent immediate complications at the anastomosis, such as leakage and infection, and late complications, such as strictures.

Evaluation of Results

It is my opinion that, by using the stomach in this manner, the best possible function can be obtained. Unless, however, the stomach has been meticulously handled, the maximum amount of blood supply has been preserved, and trauma to the stomach wall has been completely avoided, good function will not be obtained, and results may not be as satisfactory as when some other form of replacement has been utilized. Through this approach, also, extremely adequate resections can be accomplished, with wide resection of the esophagus under direct vision, together with the major portion of the regional lymphatics. By supplementing the resection with supervoltage x-ray therapy delivered to the mediastinum, the subdiaphragmatic periaortic and celiac axis group, and low cervical lymph nodes, our absolute 5-year survival rate has been doubled, being raised from approximately 4 per cent to 9 per cent. Likewise, our resectability rate has increased from approximately 40 per cent 10 years ago to 65 per cent at the present time. Unfortunately, these tumors, as we see them today, are still extensive and advanced, and formerly many would have been considered inoperable. The combination, therefore, of a wide resection of the majority of these lesions and the re-establishment of the continuity of the upper gastrointestinal tract using the stomach, with careful attention to the technical details that preserve function, gives the best results in my hands with respect to return of good function and a more favorable prognosis relating to the cancer itself.

Treatment of Early Carcinoma
of Mid-Esophagus by Resection
with Interposition Reconstruction

Earle B. Mahoney *and* Charles D. Sherman

*University of Rochester School of Medicine and Dentistry,
Rochester, New York*

The first successful resection of carcinoma of the mid-esophagus was performed by Thorek in 1913.[1] This patient was managed by near-total esophagectomy and survived eleven years. In the United States the initial successful resection of the thoracic esophagus with immediate anastomosis of the stomach and esophagus was performed by Adams and Phemister in 1938.[2] This same procedure had been performed first by Oshawa in Japan about 1925,[3] and was usually performed for carcinoma of the cardia. Since 1938, resection of the esophagus for carcinoma occurring at any level, with immediate or delayed reconstruction, has become a commonly performed procedure, but the overall results are disappointing. The operative mortality rate for resectable lesions is fairly high; the long-term survival rates are extremely poor; and frequently the palliative effects of surgery leave much to be desired.

Early carcinoma of the mid-esophagus presents a most challenging problem, since this is the most common site of primary esophageal cancer and is readily amenable to surgical attack. This is the lesion which we feel should be managed by near-total esophagectomy with interposition reconstruction.

The definition of "early carcinoma" is directly related to early diagnosis, the common problem of all malignancies, and implies a small lesion with no metastases and with only very limited immediate extension. This sharply limits the number of patients who will fall in this category because the pathological characteristics of the tumor make early diagnosis difficult. Dysphagia is the primary symptom and, during the early stage of development, depends upon the extent of luminal encroachment by the tumor. The bulky polypoid lesion produces early obstruction, but the more scirrhous type may have very limited mucosal involvement or ulceration and spread longitudinally in the submucosa. Thus this latter type gives minimal symptoms, while it silently becomes an extensive and often inoperable lesion.

Diagnostic Criteria of Early Carcinoma of the Esophagus

The manifestations of this tumor vary so widely that clinical evaluation may be misleading. Under the following conditions, however, one hopes to find a favorable lesion. The gross appearance of the lesion by x-ray and by esophagoscopy should suggest limited involvement of the esophagus. The esophagus should be mobile in the region of the lesion with no esophagoscopic evidence of fixation, and bronchoscopy must show no evidence of involvement of the trachea, carina, or major branches. There should be no x-ray evidence of mediastinal node involvement and no evidence of involvement of the recurrent laryngeal nerve. A scalene node biopsy must be negative for tumor, and there should be nothing to suggest distant metastases. Weight loss is not always evidence that the lesion is far advanced, for as has been pointed out, a polypoid lesion may cause high grade obstruction and yet involve a relatively small amount of esophageal wall. Weight loss with the scirrhous, slowly constricting lesion usually indicates an extensive tumor.

Operative Management

A near-total resection of the esophagus should be performed for all resectable lesions of the middle third. The primary objective is resection of the lesion, that is, removal of the carcinoma at the initial operation, with reconstruction immediately or delayed as a second operation, depending on the patient's general condition. The esophagectomy is performed through a right posterolateral thoracotomy, usually at the sixth interspace, with division of the ribs posteriorly as required for adequate exposure. The lower esophagus is removed with a cuff of the stomach and the cardia is closed. The mobilized esophagus is brought out through a cervical incision and divided just below the junction with the pharynx, essentially a total esophagectomy. If the reconstruction is planned for the initial stage, the right colon is mobilized through an abdominal incision and transplanted in a *substernal tunnel* as previously described. The proximal end of the transplant is anastomosed to the cervical esophagus and the distal end to the stomach.

The operation may be readily modified, depending on the condition of the patient and the lesion encountered. Many of these patients have lost weight; they are anemic and have hypoproteinemia with electrolyte imbalance, the result of their esophageal obstruction. A staged procedure is preferred for these patients, with the resection of the esophagus as the initial procedure; a gastrostomy and cervical esophagostomy complete this stage. The reconstruction is performed later when the patient is in better condition. This can be accomplished with only an abdominal incision, blind tunneling beneath the sternum, and a cervical esophagocolostomy. Another modification is the use of an upper midline abdominal incision, which is extended into the right chest through the costal arch and seventh interspace. This exposure gives the added advantage of the opportunity of resecting the lymph node area about the celiac axis in lower esophageal lesions.

We have preferred the right colon transplant,[4] but the left colon is preferred by others.[5] Recent experience has resulted in the use of the terminal ileum and ascending colon, with an anastomosis of the ileum to the cervical esophagus rather than with the cecum as originally described. It is important to bring the middle colic vascular pedicle behind the stomach to prevent obstruction of the pylorus due to pressure. The cologastrostomy usually lies in better position if the anastomosis is located at the midportion of the stomach on either the anterior or posterior wall. A pyloroplasty is performed for adequate gastric emptying. Frequently the proximal end of the colon or ileum will appear dusky and edematous when pulled through the substernal tunnel, but since this will subside in a few days, a delayed anastomosis is used. The technique of the entire procedure demands the utmost care and delicacy in the handling of tissue: fine silk is used for the anastomosis and tension on suture lines must be avoided. It should be emphasized that the venous circulation of the transplant must be as carefully preserved as the arterial.

Advantages of Resection with Interposition Reconstruction

The right thoracic approach has definite advantages over the left approach for middle third lesions. The entire esophagus is easily exposed and operability can be quickly determined. The excellent exposure allows careful removal of adjacent nodes and soft tissue, with minimal danger of damaging the great vessels or trachea. This approach also provides the ideal method for a multiple stage procedure. The carcinoma is removed at the initial procedure, and many patients gain rapidly, especially when gastrostomy feedings are begun immediately. The reconstruction can be performed as soon as the patient's condition has improved, as indicated by gain in weight and metabolic stabilization. There is good reason to believe that extensive removal of the esophagus is of the utmost importance in the surgical treatment of carcinoma.[6] These lesions have a propensity to spread in the submucosa, and the malignant cells often extend far beyond the gross limits of the tumor. The margin of resection beyond the tumor may be compromised if the surgeon is concerned over his ability to perform the reconstruction, and the high incidence of recurrence in the anastomotic suture line testifies to this inherent danger. Near-total esophagectomy decreases this danger, and we have not encountered any patient where reconstruction could not be accomplished by colon interposition.

The rehabilitation of these patients is usually rapid, and many can live comfortable and useful lives even though recurrence may later develop. Their appetites return rapidly with minimal digestive complaints, and esophagitis has not been a problem.

Evaluation of Resection with Interposition Reconstruction

It is difficult to make a strong case in favor of any one method of therapy for carcinoma of the esophagus because the overall end results are poor under any circumstances. The five-year survivals reported for surgical therapy average less than 10 per cent.[7, 8, 9, 10] We do not have a large enough series followed for sufficient time to give accurate survival rates, but at least three patients are now alive, with no recurrence, about five years after resection. We are hopeful, but as yet do not have evidence to prove, that routine near-total esophagectomy will result in improved survival statistics.

The mortality rate of this procedure compares favorably with that of other methods, especially when performed in two stages: resection followed by colonic interposition reconstruction. Fifty-eight patients had the first-stage resection with two deaths, a mortality rate of 3.4 per cent. Fifty-four patients had the second-stage reconstruction, and seven died as a result of the procedure, a mortality rate of 13 per cent. The initial mortality rate of the one stage procedure was about 25 per cent, and this has largely been replaced by the two-stage operation. Gregory and Otherson[11] reported a small series of esophageal resections with colon replacement in one stage in which the mortality rate was 14.3 per cent, but these were not all performed for malignant disease. The mortality rate for other techniques varies but generally ranges above 30 per cent for carcinoma in the middle third. Nakayama[12] has reported excellent mortality rates, 9.3 per cent, for antethoracic esophagogastric anastomoses, but 33.3 per cent for the intrathoracic anastomoses.

We feel justified in continuing to use near-total esophageal resection with colon interposition because: (1) the two stage procedure carries a low mortality rate in poor risk patients; (2) the rehabilitation is relatively rapid, and patients may take a normal diet without discomfort; (3) postoperative esophagitis has not been a problem; and (4) near-total esophagectomy more nearly fulfills the requirements of a cancer operation than procedures employing a more limited segmental resection. The surgeon attacking carcinoma of the esophagus must be motivated by optimism and anxious to embrace new methods or combinations of therapeutic procedures as they may develop.

References

1. Thorek, F.: First successful case of resection of the thoracic esophagus. Surg., Gynec. and Obst., *16:*614, 1913.

2. Adams, W. E., and Phemister, D. B.: Carcinoma of the lower thoracic esophagus. Report of a successful resection and esophagogastrostomy. J. Thoracic Surg., 7:621, 1938.
3. Oshawa, T.: The surgery of the esophagus. Arch. jap. Chir., 10:605, 1933.
4. Mahoney, E. B., and Sherman, C. D.: Total esophagoplasty using intrathoracic right colon. Surgery, 35:937, 1954.
5. McBurney, R. P.: Total esophagoplasty by utilizing the colon. South. M. J., 531:513, 1960.
6. Scanlon, E. F., Morton, D. R., Walker, J. M., and Watson, W. L.: The case against segmental resection for esophageal carcinoma. Surg., Gynec. and Obst., 101:290, 1955.
7. Kay, S.: A ten year appraisal of the treatment of squamous cell carcinoma of the esophagus. Surg., Gynec. and Obst., 117:167, 1963.
8. Saegesser, F., and Hofstetter, J.: Surgical treatment of cancer of the esophagus. Helvet. chir. Acta, 29:542, 1962.
9. Sweet, R. H.: Late results of surgical treatment of carcinoma of the esophagus. J.A.M.A., 155:422, 1954.
10. Nakayama, K.: Statistical review of five year survivals after surgery for carcinoma of the esophagus and cardiac portion of the stomach. Surgery, 45:883, 1959.
11. Gregory, H. B., Jr., and Otherson, H. B., Jr.: Total esophagectomy and esophago-coloplasty. Surg., Gynec. and Obst., 115:153, 1962.
12. Nakayama, K.: Results of Treatment of Carcinoma of the Oesophagus at the Department of Surgery, Chiba University School of Medicine, Chiba, Japan. In Tanner, N. C., and Smithers, D. W. (Eds.): Tumours of the Oesophagus. Vol. 4, p. 305, Edinburgh & London, E. & S. Livingstone, Ltd., 1961.

Palliation of Advanced
Carcinoma of the Esophagus

Introduction

The reader should make reference to the preceding section when evaluating the contributions to the section on palliation of carcinoma of the esophagus, since the treatment employed even in early lesions may prolong life and control unpleasant symptomatology even while failing to control the ultimate growth of the tumor. Furthermore, the data presented by Lampe, in the section on treatment of early mid-esophageal lesions, includes a very excellent discussion of palliation resulting from high energy (Co^{60}) radiotherapy for carcinoma of the upper and mid-esophagus, at an institution where all patients with carcinoma of the esophagus were referred for x-ray therapy. In this instance, a defined palliation was noted in 39 per cent of the patients for periods ranging from 3 months to almost 4 years. It is somewhat difficult to compare these data with those reported by Garland, whose patients had been classified as being inoperable because of extent of tumor or condition of the patient. Palliation in this instance had occurred in 26 of 45 patients, or 59 per cent, with tumors of the upper and mid-esophagus for periods of 1 to 16 months and averaging 4.7 months. The use of cobalt-60 resulted in palliation for as long as 2 years in 18.8 per cent of those treated. This parallels but does not exceed the results reported by surgeons with a particular interest in this problem.

Two of the contributors have supported mechanical means for palliation, including oral intubation or gastrostomy. Weisel stresses the high frequency of recurrence of inoperable lesions due to local extension, distant metastasis, or complicating illness, including malnutrition, and reports on the use of peroral intubation as a method for preventing the collection of secretions proximal to the tumor and for oral feeding. An average survival of 8 months in 388 patients suggests that aspiration and malnutrition are the major factors influencing palliation, and raises the question whether this procedure might not be useful as a preliminary approach in many patients, regardless of the eventual choice of definitive therapy. Its value in the temporary control of esophagorespiratory fistulas deserves special mention.

Patton supports a valvular gastrostomy over jejunostomy as a means of maintaining nutrition, either during radiation therapy or in preparation for additional operative intervention. The technique employed overcomes several of the objections of other contributors to this discussion; and as a result of personal experience in the use of the Patton gastrostomy, one of the editors questions its value in staged operations for carcinoma of the esophagus.

E. H. E.

Palliation of Advanced Carcinoma of the Esophagus by Intubation

Wilson Weisel

Marquette University School of Medicine

Incidence of Disease

A review of the surgical and pathologic literature emphasizes that carcinoma of the esophagus is a relatively frequent and fatal lesion. Various figures of incidence have been quoted, and it has been said that carcinoma of the esophagus accounts for 2 per cent of all malignancies occurring in the body.[1-3] Approximately 4 per cent of carcinomas involving the alimentary tract are primary in the esophagus and squamous cell in type. About 17 per cent of gastric carcinomas extend into the terminal esophagus, and these are adenocarcinomas. The sex incidence of carcinoma of the esophagus shows that it is predominantly a disease occurring in males, with a ratio of 10 males to one female. It can occur at any age in life, but is most common in the sixth decade, with the greatest number of cases reported between the ages of 50 and 70.

In dealing with an individual patient with carcinoma of the esophagus, however, the statistical incidence has little influence on the problem involved, and treatment affects the outcome only slightly.[4] The occurrence of esophageal carcinoma on our Surgical Services seems to fluctuate considerably, but at one time in the past year, we had on one of our teaching services a high census of 16 patients with carcinoma of the esophagus. It was interesting that among these 16 patients, 14 were clearly inoperable at the time they were admitted to the Surgical Ward. Their inoperability was determined on the basis of distant metastasis, extensive mediastinal extension, or the presence of complicating serious medical problems, including extensive emphysema, severe cardiac disease, and terminal cirrhosis. Two of the 16 patients were considered to have lesions amenable for surgical extirpation, and both of these patients had esophagectomy with continuity of the alimentary tract restored by esophagogastrostomy. Of the

Page 23

14 patients considered inoperable, two showed only minimal obstructive symptoms and signs, and were treated by irradiation therapy. Of the remaining 12 patients, three were obviously in terminal phases, and these were treated symptomatically and with intermittent dilatation. Of the nine patients remaining, two had tracheoesophageal fistulas and the other seven showed progressive obstructive signs. These nine patients were considered for utilization of peroral palliative intubation.

Development of Method

One of the most distressing features of carcinoma of the esophagus is the obstruction to the normal progress of saliva and the various secretions accumulating in the upper pharynx and esophagus. The irritation caused by constant regurgitation and aspiration of this material is one of concern and worry to the patient. Krishaber, in 1881,[5] and Symonds, in 1887[6] described methods of esophageal cannulation for the relief of these patients. There was a resurgence of popularity for this method of therapy occasioned by a paper by Souttar in 1922.[7] Since that time, there have been sporadic periods of interest in this type of therapy for the patient with this progressive debilitating disease, but they have been abandoned largely because of complications of the treatment.

A review of our experience indicates that about 75 of every 100 patients with this lesion will require some type of palliative procedure for obstruction.[8, 9] We have utilized a number of operative techniques in handling these patients, but it is our opinion that gastrostomy falls short, in most cases, of providing comfort to the patient because of persistence of obstructive symptoms. The various bypass procedures have not been uniformly efficient, and all of the operative approaches carry mortality rates and morbidity that we consider excessive for palliative procedures.[10] It was in search of a simple, safe technique that we turned to a method for palliative peroral intubation.

Technique of Intubation

The procedure we have used most frequently is the utilization of a semirigid plastic tube fashioned for the particular patient we intend to treat. The tube is usually made of polyethylene and has a wall approximately 1 to 2 mm. in thickness (Fig. 1). It is thermolabile and has an inside diameter averaging 13 mm. The patient is prepared by preliminary bougienage, usually up to the size where a No. 38 French bougie may be passed through the lesion.

Then under local or general anesthesia, depending on the patient's physical and psychologic status, a bougie, such as the Jackson filiform or a silk-woven Plummer, is passed through the lesion. Over the bougie, the plastic tube is inserted down into the upper esophagus. Then, with the esophagoscope, usually a Roberts esophageal speculum, being used as obturator, the plastic tube is seated into the lesion. Under direct vision, the proximal flange is left about 1 to 2 cm. above the upper portion of the exophytic tumor (Fig. 2). The esophagoscope is then disengaged from the proximal end of the plastic tube and the bougie withdrawn. The tube is carefully inspected with the esophagoscope, and if the prosthetic position is satisfactory, the scope is withdrawn.

The average length of the tubes that we have employed has been

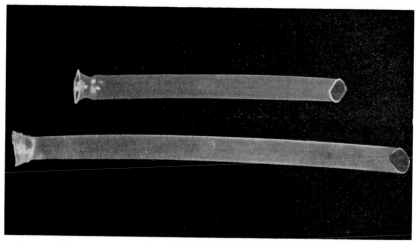

Fig. 1. Polyethylene tubes prepared with proximal flange by heat and pressure and fashioned oblique distal end.

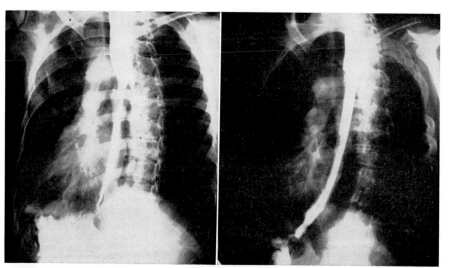

Fig. 2. Esophagograms showing obstructive carcinoma of mid-esophagus (left) and after peroral palliative intubation (right) demonstrating extension of tube above and below lesion.

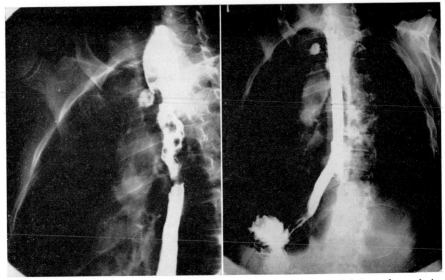

Fig. 3. Preoperative (left) and postoperative esophagogram (right) performed the day following palliation peroral intubation for inoperable carcinoma of the upper esophagus.

between 8 and 12 cm., although some have been as long as 25 cm. The tube is fashioned in such a manner that it will extend above and usually at least 2 cm. below the distal portion of the tumor. On the day following its insertion, the tube is checked by radiographic methods (Fig. 3) for position and patency, and if no other contraindications are present, oral feedings of liquid are begun on the first or second day.

Evaluation of Results of Treatment

In our experience this method has carried a relatively low morbidity and mortality, and has provided satisfactory palliation. Most of these patients have been able to continue normal oral feedings up to the time of the terminal phase of their disease. The type of diet has varied from a perfectly normal diet to liquids or foods that did not require chewing. This method of palliation was utilized on 388 patients up to January, 1963. It was found that the average survival time following intubation was approximately eight months and the longest survival in this group was 30 months. Patients on whom this method has been utilized have varied in age from 40 to 87 years. The obstructing lesion has been in the upper third of the esophagus in 48 patients, in the middle third in 169, and in the distal third in 171. One of the advantages of this method is that it may be utilized at the time of thoracotomy or abdominal exploration, when inoperable lesions are found, and this combined method of peroral intubation was used in 42 patients. It has also been used in conjunction with radiation and chemotherapy and may be effective in controlling esophago-respiratory fistulas, as others have also described (Fig. 4).[11]

The ease with which this method can be applied has another advantage in that the hospitalization period for many of these patients is relatively short. It is not unusual for the patients to go home after five or six days of hospital residency.

The primary complication following peroral intubation has been a probable mediastinitis, resulting from fracture of the esophageal lesion. This has been interpreted from the fact that temperature elevations after intubation have been noted in 32 patients, although in none of these has there been a necessity for mediastinal drainage or other thoracic surgery. We have encountered 14 patients in whom intubation could not be performed for one reason or another, usually because of technical difficulties.

In nine patients the prostheses have become dislodged, and this has required repositioning of the tube. Six patients have had postintubation obstruction of the tube, and in five of these, this was due to the swallowing of a food bolus larger than the diameter of the tube; in the sixth patient obstruction was due to upward growth of the carcinoma and required removal and reinsertion of the prosthesis for relief. The esophagus has actually been perforated in four patients; in three of these, this occurred during insertion of the tube at thoracotomy, and in one during intubation of a distal third carcinoma involving the upper cardia of the stomach. In two of these patients complications developed that led to their demise, although all perforations were closed surgically. There were two patients with lesions in the upper esophagus who developed tracheal obstruction following intubation with acrylic tubes, but this difficulty was resolved

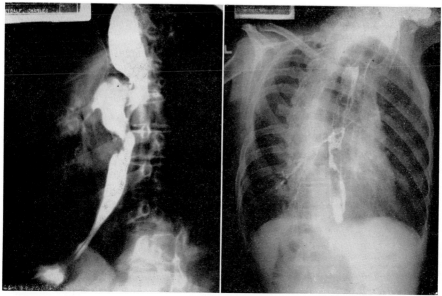

Fig. 4. Mid-esophageal carcinoma with left esophagobronchial fistula (left), treated by peroral intubation (right), showing continued slight spill into fistula later corrected by repositioning of tube.

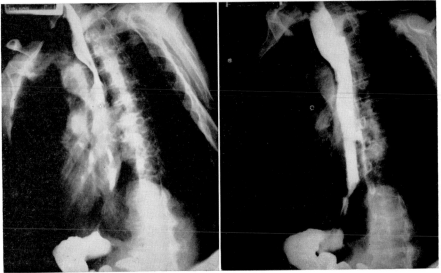

Fig. 5. Upper esophageal carcinoma (left) in patient who could not tolerate acrylic tube because of tracheal compression, but was relieved with replacement by polyethylene prosthesis (right).

by replacing the acrylic prosthesis with a less rigid polyethylene tube (Fig. 5).

In general, it has been our experience that this unfortunate group of patients has shown a most gratifying response to this method of treatment. The primary objections raised to this method have been the danger of esophageal perforations, the small rigid lumen for alimentation, and various problems concerned in treating a progressively fatal disease. It has been our experience, however, that by using a polyethylene thin-walled tube, following careful dilatation, the procedure is safe, and patients have expressed gratitude for relief of their obstruction. Those patients who have been plagued by the harassing cough resulting from regurgitation or respiratory-esophageal fistula have been particularly aided by this method.

We further believe that surgeons trained in endoscopic procedures can utilize this method frequently with topical anesthesia, and will achieve excellent palliative results and a very low mortality and morbidity. It must be reiterated that good results are dependent on an experienced endoscopic operator, a careful planning of the procedure, preparation of the prosthesis, and preliminary dilatation and preparation of the patient.

References

1. Terracol, J., and Sweet, R. H.: Diseases of the Esophagus. Philadelphia, W. B. Saunders Co., 1958.
2. Stout, A. P., and Lattes, R.: Tumors of the Esophagus. Sect. V, Fasc. 20, AFIP, 1957, pp. 44–105.

3. Logan, A.: The surgical treatment of carcinoma of the esophagus and cardia. J. Thoracic Surg., 46:150, 1963.

4. Sweet, R. H.: Late results of treatment of carcinoma of the esophagus. J.A.M.A.. 155:422, 1954.

5. Krishaber, M.: De la sonde oesphagienne a demeurre. Internat. Med. Cong. Trans., 2:393, 1881.

6. Symonds, C. J.: The treatment of malignant stricture of the esophagus by tubage or oral catheterism. Brit. M. J., 1:870, 1887.

7. Souttar, H. S.: Treatment of carcinoma of the esophagus based on one hundred personal cases and eighteen post mortem reports. Brit. J. Surg. 15:76, 1927.

8. Weisel, W., Raine, F., Watson, R. R., and Frederick, J. J.: Palliative treatment of esophageal carcinoma. Ann. Surg, 149:207, 1959.

9. O'Connor, T., Watson, R., Lepley, D., and Weisel, W.: Esophageal prosthesis for palliative intubation. A.M.A. Arch. Surg., 87:275, 1963.

10. Postlethwait, R. L., and Sealy, W. C.: Surgery of the Esophagus. Springfield, Ill., Charles C Thomas, 1961.

11. Kovarik, J. L.: Palliative treatment of a bronchoesophageal fistula. J. Thoracic Surg., 46:252, 1963.

Radiotherapy of
Advanced Cancer of the Esophagus*

L. Henry Garland

University of California Medical School, San Francisco

Most cancer of the esophagus is anatomically advanced at the time of diagnosis. The first symptom noticed by the patient is usually dysphagia —itself a sign of extensive or late disease. The macroscopic findings (by radiology or endoscopy) may suggest a relatively short or localized tumor, but subsequent microscopic studies all too often show submucous infiltration well beyond the apparent margins of the lesion and, frequently, metastatic nodes several centimeters distant thereto. Further, the esophagus has no serosal coat, so that extension of tumor into the surrounding tissues is common, with resultant direct invasion of adjacent structures, such as trachea, bronchus, large blood vessels, or pericardium. Most of the tumors are squamous cell carcinomas; a few (especially at either end of the tube) are adenocarcinomas. Sarcomas, metastatic tumors, and extrinsic tumors invading the esophagus are not rare.

It is worth while to attempt to delineate the gross extent of the primary tumor as accurately as possible. With lesions of marked obstructive nature, this cannot be achieved without exploration or retrograde study at the time of gastrostomy; crude estimate must often suffice.

There is some advantage in classifying tumors according to anatomic site, i.e., tumors of the upper, the middle, and the lower third of the esophagus. Some tumors obviously overlap two adjacent sites, and should be either so classified or arbitrarily assigned to the site of apparent major involvement. Such overlap is especially problematic in lesions of the esophagogastric junction. Some of these are true esophageal squamous cell cancers, some are gastric adenocarcinomas with upward extension, and an occasional case is mixed squamous and adenocarcinoma. Lymphatic drainage of upper third tumors tends to be to the supraclavicular and anterior jugular nodes;

* The author is grateful to the many residents and colleagues who aided with the care of patients described in this report. The follow-up was aided by grants from the California Division of the American Cancer Society and the William Hume–Albert Barrows Cancer Research Fund.

middle third tumors to the retrotracheal, posterior mediastinal, and abdominal nodes; and lower third tumors to the lower mediastinal and abdominal nodes. These facts may be important in planning the size of the irradiation beam. Subdivision of upper third lesions into "cervical" and "intrathoracic" may also be useful, especially in long-necked persons, with apparently small or localized tumors.

Clinical staging of esophageal cancer is of mainly academic value: Stage I, tumor limited to the esophagus; II, tumor with evidence of peri-esophageal spread; and III, tumor with distant metastasis.

Indications for Radiotherapy

The primary indication for radiotherapy is dysphagia due to obstructing tumor. An apparently localized nonobstructing tumor in a patient unsuitable for attempted extirpation also should be treated. Contraindications include terminal status, heavy prior irradiation to the tumor site, and, occasionally, complicating incurable neoplasm of adjacent structures (e.g., larynx, lung, or stomach).

The results of radiotherapy are modest, but it is the only nonsurgical method of treatment currently available that promises some degree of palliation in many cases and long-term arrest in a few.

Methods of Irradiation

The best method of radiotherapy of esophageal lesions is external beam therapy. Interstitial and intracavitary techniques with radioactive sources have been extensively utilized, and almost routinely discarded. The limiting factor in application of external irradiation is not the skin: it is the tolerance of the tumor-adjacent soft parts and the intervening spinal cord. Although it is simpler for the radiotherapist to deliver a desired dose with megavoltage beams, orthovoltage (200 to 300 kv.) beams can deliver all that the normal deep tissues can tolerate. Indeed, the best published results in radiotherapy of cancer of the esophagus have been obtained with careful multiple beam or monitored rotation techniques; orthovoltage being used in each instance.[3]

Depending on the size and thickness of the patient, and on the location of the tumor, two, three, four, or six fields may be used. It is important that the centration of oblique and rotating beams be regularly checked, and that all beams be adequate in length to encompass the entire extent of the lesion. In-site dosimetry is desirable.

For palliation, it is desirable that a tumor dose of about 3000 orthovoltage rads (or 4000 megavoltage rads) be delivered over a period of three to four weeks. For radical treatment, the dose should be between 5000 and 6000 orthovoltage rads, given over a period of five to six weeks (with adequately increased dose when megavoltage beams are used, to allow for the decreased biological efficiency of the latter type of beam).

In elderly and feeble patients there is some advantage to so-called split-dose programs: these are essentially for palliation and consist in delivering about one-half of the planned dose during a period of two to three weeks, then giving the patient two weeks rest, after which the course is resumed for a final two or three week period.

It is desirable to avoid gastrostomy if possible. This may sometimes be achieved by utilizing an indwelling esophageal tube during treatment. Gastrostomy is sometimes recommended with the idea that it is then possible to deliver a larger dose of radiotherapy to the esophagus; this is seldom true, and the fact that the patient is still unable to swallow his saliva renders his status unsatisfactory. In the long run, it is probably a kindness to the patient not to use palliative gastrostomy.

A fistula to the trachea or bronchus, developing during therapy, presents a difficult therapeutic problem. Continued treatment may help the inflammatory component, but seldom controls the undesirable symptoms related to the fistula.

Preoperative radiotherapy, aimed at making an "inoperable" tumor removable, has been extensively tried and usually abandoned.[4] It is not recommended.

Complications

Side effects of radiotherapy include esophagitis, pneumonitis, and pericarditis. They may be minimized by suitable modification of the program. Complications include perforation, mediastinitis, hemorrhage, pericardial tamponage, and stricture. They may be minimized by keeping the tumor dose at a tolerable level (e.g., not over 6000 r orthovoltage in 40 days). We regard the limit of tolerance of thoracic tissues, using 200 r daily tumor dose, to be about 7000 r in 40 days (orthovoltage).

We have previously shown that the relative biological efficiency of megavoltage and telecobalt beams as compared to 200 to 300 kv. x-ray beams is about 80 per cent.[2] That is, one must increase the physical dose of megavolt linear accelerator beams or telecobalt beams about one-fourth to achieve a numerical dose in roentgens equal to that obtained with orthovoltage. In other words, 7500 r telecobalt is biologically equal to about 6000 r of 200 kv. radiation.

Easson,[1] working with Paterson and colleagues at the Christie Hospital in Manchester, England, has shown that under carefully controlled clinical trials, there is *no* improvement in cancer cure rates with megavoltage. The specific tumor sites studied were "deep-seated" lesions—cervix and bladder. He writes: "It is clear that (with 4 mev. x-rays from a linear accelerator) there is no improvement in survival of the cancer patients treated." This conclusion is based on several hundred patients treated with one or other modality and all followed up. At the same time it should be noted that he personally favors megavoltage from the point of view of technical ease of treatment and initial cutaneous status.

Late radiation fibrosis of lung and adjacent tissues is sometimes seen with megavoltage, as with orthovoltage, if the patients survive long enough. However, it is seldom extensive enough to be disabling in patients with esophageal cancer.

Results in Our Studies

The following summarizes our results in 91 patients treated by irradiation for cancer of the esophagus in recent decades. There were 66 patients treated at the San Francisco General Hospital; 11 patients seen in consultation and treated at Letterman Army Hospital; and 14 patients treated in private practice. In all cases the diagnosis was microscopically verified. The majority had squamous cell carcinomas. There were 3 adenocarcinomas. During the same period of time a number of terminal patients was seen in consultation and regarded as unsuitable for radiation treatment.

Most of the treated cases were regarded as inoperable because of either the extent of the tumor or the condition of the patient. None of the described cases had combined surgery and radiotherapy. Three had, or developed in the first week of treatment, tracheo- or bronchoesophageal fistulas. One had concurrent independent cancer of the larynx.

For purposes of clarity, the San Francisco Hospital material will be considered first. There were 66 cases divided as follows:

Upper third tumors   19
Middle third tumors   35
Lower third tumors   12

A majority of the patients were treated by orthovoltage roentgen therapy, in which multiple fixed beams were used. A minority were treated by telecobalt, with either fixed beams or rotation, depending on the individual problem.

Table 1 summarizes our results:

TABLE 1. RESULTS OF RADIATION TREATMENT OF ESOPHAGEAL CANCER AT THE SAN FRANCISCO HOSPITAL

Treatment	Number of Cases	Clinically Improved Cases	Average Survival Following Treatment (Months)	Survival Time (Calculated from Start of Treatment)
Incomplete*	11	1	1.0	2 to 16 weeks
Palliative†	30	11 (37%)	4.2	1 to 12 months
Radical‡	25	20 (80%)	5.0	1 to 16 months
Total	66	32 (48%)	4.0	2 wks. to 16 months

* Less than 1000 r/tumor.
† 1500 r to 3500 r/tumor in 14 to 30 days.
‡ 3500 r to 6000 r/tumor in 21 to 42 days.

In the tables, "clinically improved" means improved ability to swallow, and decrease in pain if present.

Results according to the *location of the tumor* and the *type of treatment* given are shown in Table 2. This reveals the customary relatively better results with upper third tumors as compared to tumors in the other two sites.

TABLE 2.   RESULTS OF RADIATION TREATMENT OF ESOPHAGEAL CANCER BY ANATOMIC SITE OF DISEASE (EXCLUDING INCOMPLETE COURSES)

Treatment	Site	Number of Cases	Clinically Improved Cases	Average Survival (Months)
Palliative	Upper third	8	4	3.6
	Middle third	15	4	4.3
	Lower third	7	3	4.3
Radical	Upper third	9	8	6.0
	Middle third	13	10	4.3
	Lower third	3	2	4.3

Results According to the Modality Used

Orthovoltage roentgen therapy was used in 52 cases; the average survival was 3.8 months. Telecobalt therapy was used in 14 cases; the average survival was 3.2 months. There is of course no significant difference in these results.

If we consider the patients treated by radical radiotherapy, we find the following: in the 19 cases treated by orthovoltage roentgen therapy, the average survival was 5.4 months; in the 6 treated by cobalt teletherapy, the average survival 3.7 months. There is certainly no evidence of improvement in survival rate with cobalt teletherapy in our institution.

Results of radiotherapy in eleven cases of cancer of the esophagus treated at Letterman Army Hospital by irradiation during the last decade, and our experience in private practice during the last two decades are summarized in Table 3.

The range in survival in the 8 "palliatively" treated patients was 3 to 8 months; in the 6 radically treated it was 4 to 22 months. If we limit survival data to data pertaining to *improved cases* (as several authors have done), our figures would range from the 7 to 12 months commonly seen in the literature.

The patients seen in private practice had in general less advanced disease and were in a slightly better state of nutrition than some of those seen at the County Hospital. In our opinion they substantiate the old truism: it is

TABLE 3.   RESULTS OF RADIATION TREATMENT OF ESOPHAGEAL CANCER IN 78 PATIENTS RECEIVING PALLIATIVE OR RADICAL RADIOTHERAPY

Treatment	Location of Patients*	Number of Cases	Average Survival (Months)
Palliative	S.F.H.	30	4.1
	L.A.H.	5	6.0
	Private	8	4.6
Radical	S.F.H.	25	5.0
	L.A.H.	4	4.5
	Private	6	9.3
Incomplete	L.A.H.	2	3 weeks

* S.F.H. is San Francisco General Hospital; L.A.H. is Letterman Army Hospital; Private is author's private office.

the tumor you treat rather than the treatment you give that decides the outcome in many cancer patients.

Table 3 discloses an average survival time of 4.3 months in 43 patients receiving palliative therapy, and of 5.7 months in 35 patients receiving radical radiation therapy. The difference is not impressive, especially when it is noted that survival is calculated from the *start* of radiotherapy, and many programs required 4 to 6 weeks to complete.

Results Reported in the Literature

Watson and Goodner[8] report their experience and that of colleagues with 1484 patients with cancer of the esophagus seen at the Memorial Hospital, New York, between 1926 and 1957. The following summarizes their findings:

        Indeterminate cases: 264
                No biopsy   160
                Lost to follow-up while living   104
        Determinate cases: 1220
                No treatment given   245
                Surgical treatment only   132
                Radiation therapy at
                        Memorial Hospital   727
                Radiation therapy elsewhere   61
                Combined radiation and
                        surgical therapy   55

The average survival of the 727 patients treated by radiotherapy was 6.4 months (*presumably* measured from the date of inception of treatment). The survival varied with tumor location as follows:

> Upper third (190 patients)   7.7 months
> Middle third (363 patients)   5.5 months
> Lower third (171 patients)   6.8 months

Their survival data according to the therapeutic modality employed was as follows:

> Orthovoltage (approximately 200 kv.)
> x-ray therapy   average 7 months
> Orthovoltage x-ray with rotation   4.5 months
> Megavoltage x-ray therapy   6.5 months
> Telecobalt therapy   5.5 months

Two patients received betatron treatment without noteworthy improvement.

Smithers, in a comprehensive article dealing with 314 patients in London, reports the following experience:[5]

> Not treated   65
> Treated by radiation   249

He does not give the average survival in months, but the following data are pertinent:

> Upper third lesions (52 patients) 6, or 11 per cent, survived 5 years
> Middle third lesions (159 patients) 2, or 1 per cent, survived 5 years
> Lower third lesions (102 patients) 2, or 2 per cent, survived 5 years

These results were obtained with radiation, or surgery, or combined treatment. Of 20 patients treated by surgery alone, there was one five-year survival (5 per cent). Of 229 patients treated by radiation, there were seven five-year survivals (3 per cent).

Like other authors, he noted that radiological results tended to be best in upper third lesions, and surgical results best in lower third lesions. He tabulates some remarkable data from 14 centers, covering 6348 patients. These showed an overall five-year survival rate of 1.4 per cent. In the various centers, from 13 to 78 per cent of the patients were untreated; from 0 to 43 per cent were resected; and from 0 to 87 per cent radiated.

Zuppinger reports an experience with an unspecified number of patients treated for cancer of the esophagus by the use of high speed electrons occasionally supplemented by megavoltage x-ray therapy. He employed 30 mev electrons and sometimes a 30-mev x-ray beam. He notes that "improvement did not occur in several patients so treated."

Watson[8] reports observations on 37 patients with cancer of the esophagus (of whom two lacked biopsy validation). Radiation therapy was used in 19 patients; the remainder either had no treatment or had other forms of treatment.

Seventeen patients had a complete course of radiotherapy, followed in a few by postradiation surgery. Four of the 17 patients survived five years, but it is not clear whether (a) one or more of these did not have biopsies or (b) some of these four had supplementary surgery. The average survival time in two patients who had incomplete radiotherapy was 0.8 month, and in the 17 patients who had radiotherapy with or without some surgery, 29 months. The author stresses the need for careful dosimetry and adds, "It should not be assumed that there is any inherent great advantage of super-voltage therapy over orthovoltage in the treatment of cancer of the esophagus. Five-year survivors have been reported with the use of medium voltage machines. . . ." (He refers to a group of 89 patients treated mostly by ortho-voltage radiotherapy and reported as five-year survivors, collected by Tanner and Smithers.)[6]

Summary

Advanced cancer of the esophagus is sometimes benefited by radio-therapy. The average survival time is increased only by a matter of months, but the comfort of the patient (ability to swallow saliva and semisolid food) is often enhanced for at least half the survival period.

Radical radiotherapy should be employed if the apparent extent of the tumor and the condition of the patient warrant it.

Palliative radiotherapy should be used in other patients, assuming that their status is not terminal.

Effective (and relatively inexpensive) radiotherapy can be given by the use of conventional (200 to 300 kv.) orthovoltage roentgen beams. Cobalt units, linear accelerators, and betatrons yield no significant improvement in average survival times, cost the patient much more than orthovoltage therapy, and are sometimes fraught with greater hazard to normal deep structures adjacent to the tumor or in the path of the ionizing beam, because of the absence of tolerance-warning erythema.

One of the most compelling reasons for radiotherapy in this disease is the simple fact that modern medical care of most patients (and their families) requires that something definitive be done—modest though the chances be of significant benefit. When that "something" does not cause undue physical or economic stress, it may be recommended.

References

1. Easson, E. C.: Clinical trials in radiotherapy. Medica Mundi. Philips Eindhoven, 8:64, 1962.
2. Garland, L. H.: The relative biological effectiveness of supervoltage radiation. Am. J. Roentgenol., 86:621, 1961.
3. Garland, L. H.: Radiation therapy of cancer: current results with megavoltage and orthovoltage. Am. J. Roentgenol., 86:621, 1961.
4. Loutat-Jacob, J. L., et al.: Quelles sont les possibilites actuelles du traitment du cancer de l'esophage? Presse Méd., 70:823, 1962.

5. Smithers, D. W.: Treatment of cancer of the esophagus. Ann. Roy. Coll. Surg. Eng., *20*:36, 1957.
6. Tanner, N. C., and Smithers, D. W.: Tumors of the Esophagus. Edinburgh, E. & S. Livingstone, 1961, p. 280.
7. Watson, T. A.: Radiation therapy of cancer of the esophagus. Surg., Gynec. and Obst., *117*:346, 1963.
8. Watson, W. L., and Goodner, J. T.: In Pack, G. T., and Ariel, I. M. (Eds.): Treatment of Cancer and Allied Diseases. New York, Hoeber, 1960.

Permanent Gastrostomy or Jejunostomy for Maintenance of Nutrition in Palliation of Advanced Carcinoma of the Esophagus

Richard Patton

Ohio State University School of Medicine

Indications for Tube Feeding

The reasons for tube feeding in patients with carcinoma of the esophagus are largely negative. When adequate nutrition cannot be taken orally and when esophageal intubation is unwise or unsuccessful, tube feeding is indicated.

Occasionally during the course of irradiation therapy or in the preparation of a debilitated patient for other types of surgery, tube feeding is advantageous.

Gastrostomy vs. Jejunostomy

Rarely is jejunostomy the indicated procedure. Gastrostomy feedings are uniformly better tolerated by the patient. A larger volume of tube feeding as well as a higher caloric intake can be supplied by gastrostomy. The procedure of jejunostomy has no advantages over gastrostomy and should be chosen only when the stomach is not available for gastrostomy.

The Objections to Gastrostomy

"One of those wet messy things that smells and has a tube hanging out of it," is a common reaction to gastrostomy.

The classic serous-lined gastrostomy, as represented by the Stamm, Senn, and Witzel operations, does require a permanent tube. It is satisfactory as a temporary procedure of a few weeks' duration. For a longer period, the permanent tube meets with serious objection.

The classic valvular gastrostomy (Janeway), with a gastric flap and a tract lined with gastric mucosa, is indeed subject to continual seepage. The mucosa lining the tract leading from stomach to skin secretes an irritating mucous discharge that keeps the opening moist and excoriates the skin. It can well be viewed as a "messy thing."

Advantages of the Modified Valvular Gastrostomy

Gastrostomy as a feeding method need have neither of the above disadvantages. With two modifications the valvular gastrostomy can be formed so that it does not leak, and the tract does not seep and excoriate the skin.[1] First, the valve, which functions to prevent reflux from the stomach, is thin. It is formed of two layers of mucosa rather than two full-thickness layers of gastric wall. Since the valvular action is that of a flutter valve, the thinner the valve wall the more effective the valve in preventing leakage after feeding. Second, the tract leading from skin to stomach is formed of the seromuscular layer of the gastric wall and is not full thickness. There is no mucosa to cause seepage from the tract and excoriate the skin. The gastrostomy stoma stays dry.

The procedure is done under local anesthesia, and although somewhat more complicated than the classic gastrostomy, it is by no means difficult, nor does it carry unusual risk.

These advantages have led to less hesitation in recommending a tube feeding procedure. If the anticipated survival time is more than a few weeks, the modified valvular gastrostomy is the procedure of choice. It is not unusual for esophageal obstruction to occur in carcinoma, and for function to be restored after a few days of tube feedings. Obstruction will often recur at a later time. This gastrostomy is well adapted to this problem, since one daily dilatation with the feeding tube is all that is required to keep the tract patent and functioning. Thus the patient may take oral feedings when tolerated, and resume the use of the gastrostomy feedings after weeks or months of disuse.

Technique

Local infiltration anesthesia and an upper left rectus incision are used. The stomach is mobilized, and a square area, 4 cm. by 4 cm., is marked on the anterior gastric wall in the lower part of the middle third of the stomach, midway between the curvatures. An incision through the serosal and muscular layers is made along three sides of this square, leaving the fourth side along the greater curvature to serve as the base of the flap. A dissection plane is developed between the mucosa and the muscle layer, and the flap, consisting of serosal and muscular layers, is raised from the mucosa and left attached

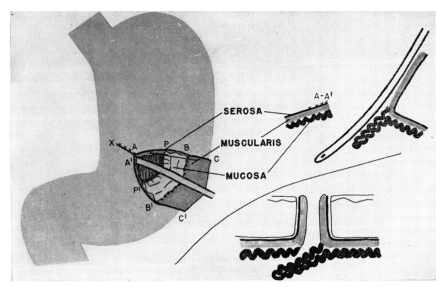

Fig. 1. Technique of permanent gastrostomy for maintenance of nutrition in palliation of advanced carcinoma of the esophagus.

along the greater curvature. Bleeding is controlled by individual ligation of
the vessels. The dissection plane is above the submucous plexus of vessels,
so that the major part of the blood supply is left on the mucosal side. The
4 cm. by 4 cm. area of single thickness mucosa, denuded on the outer surface by raising the flap is used to form the valve (Fig. 1, inset). The interior
of the stomach is entered through an incision in the mucosa along the side of
the square parallel to the lesser curvature. This incision through the mucosa
is then carried along the superior and inferior sides of the square to the
half-way point. This forms a flap 4 cm. wide by 2 cm. deep, which is folded
outward and comes to rest on the other half of the original 4 cm. by 4 cm.
square of mucosa (Fig. 1). It is sutured in place with 0000 nonabsorbable
(silk) sutures. This forms a fold of two thicknesses of gastric mucosa 4 cm.
wide and 2 cm. deep, which serves as the valve. The opening of the gastric
wall is closed transversely over a catheter. Interrupted sutures are taken
through the full thickness of the gastric wall in order to approximate the
superior and inferior sides of the square. A single suture line transverse to
the long axis of the stomach is produced. A second layer of inverting seromuscular sutures is taken to support the suture line. These suture lines complete the valve and form the seromuscular tract around the catheter, which
is brought out through a stab wound just to the left of the incision. The
anterior gastric wall is sutured to peritoneum around the stab wound and
the incision is closed.

Postoperative Care

Continuous suction is applied to the gastrostomy tube for 12 hours, at the end of which time small amounts of water are started through the tube. If the water is well tolerated, the usual feeding formula is administered after 24 to 36 hours. After seven days the tube is removed and inserted four to five times daily for tube feedings. Leakage has not been a problem, and after the feeding has been accomplished, the tube is removed and a small dressing applied.

Tube feedings must be performed at least daily. If tube feedings become unnecessary, the catheter should be inserted daily to prevent closure of the tract.

Summary

All procedures that add to the comfort and well-being of the patient with esophageal carcinoma should be intelligently applied to his management. His nutrition should not suffer, and parenteral alimentation is only adequate for a few days. The modified valvular gastrostomy will function satisfactorily for the life span of the patient with minimal daily care. It should not be delayed when oral feeding fails.

Reference

1. Patton, R.: A modified valvular gastrostomy. A.M.A. Arch. Surg., 70:859, 1955.

Carcinoma
of the Breast

Introduction

Perhaps there is no other field of surgical endeavor where objective evaluation of the results of surgical treatment has been more difficult than in cancer of the breast. In the first volume of Current Surgical Management (1957), controversial aspects of late or metastatic mammary cancer were presented; in the second volume (1960), Haagensen carefully presented an account of comparisons of radical versus simple mastectomy with post-operative irradiation. The additional modalities of treatment, such as chemotherapy and oophorectomy, have complicated comparative studies, but the greatest difficulties probably have come from failure of universal application of classifications of the stage of disease and delay in initiating studies, prospectively, of objective randomization. A good example of a randomized study of simple mastectomy with postoperative irradiation versus extended radical mastectomy was a report from Copenhagen,* in which the absolute 5-year survival rates are practically identical.

Lewison has recently pointed out† that absolute survival rates reported from many areas for different surgical approaches to mammary cancer are strikingly similar, particularly when comparing radical mastectomy with simple mastectomy plus irradiation. Because of the similarity of absolute survival rates it has been suggested that it is safe to carry out prospective randomized clinical studies comparing these two modes of treatment.

An interesting facet of the many investigations being carried out are two observations concerning the premenopausal woman with carcinoma of the breast with proved axillary metastases: (1) Devitt‡ reported a "statistically significant advantage" of conservative operations over radical operations in this group of women; (2) reports from the Surgical Adjuvant Chemotherapy Breast Group indicate that adjunctive chemotherapy has diminished the incidence of early recurrence and metastasis in premeno-

* Kaae et al.: Am. J. Roentgenol., 87:82, 1962.
† Lewison: J.A.M.A., 186:975, 1963.
‡ Devitt: Canad. M.A.J., 87:906, 1962.

pausal women with involved axillary nodes. Because insufficient time has elapsed to permit final conclusions to be drawn from such cooperative integrated studies involving chemotherapeutic agents, no presentation of this controversial aspect is included in this chapter; only surgical operative approaches, with and without irradiation, to the breast, its regional lymphatics, and the ovaries are presented in the following six sections.

S. R. F.

Radical Mastectomy as Therapy for Mammary Cancer

Harvey R. Butcher, Jr.

Washington University School of Medicine

Case for Radical Mastectomy

The thoughtful therapists have questioned the efficacy of radical mastectomy in treating women with mammary cancer principally for two reasons: (1) mortality from mammary cancer per unit population has remained remarkably constant for the past several decades despite the earlier diagnosis of the disease and the more frequent use of radical mastectomy as therapy; (2) the survival rates from mammary cancer after treatment by simple mastectomy and postoperative irradiation,[1] and indeed after simple mastectomy alone[2] or "modified" radical mastectomy,[3] appear to be similar to the survival rates of many series of mammary cancer treated by radical mastectomy.

Actually, it is not possible to accurately measure the relative effectiveness of the variously recommended therapies for mammary cancer from the data at present extant. Until well controlled prospective studies of properly selected population samples are completed, radical mastectomy should be continued as the treatment of choice for carcinoma of the breast. Indeed the efficacy of other therapeutic methods must be compared carefully with the effectiveness of radical mastectomy, since the morbidity and mortality rates from radical mastectomy performed by well trained surgeons are very low. The morbidity associated with simple mastectomy combined with postoperative irradiation surely is no less. Simple mastectomy alone probably is the only currently recommended therapy for mammary cancer that may be associated with morbidity rates that are lower than those for well executed radical mastectomy.

The case for radical mastectomy in the treatment of mammary cancer then rests first upon a demonstration that it is a measurably effective method of therapy; second, upon the ability to show from the facts available that radical mastectomy alone is probably superior to simple mastectomy alone as therapy for mammary cancer; and third, upon the probability that radical mastectomy is at least as effective as simple mastectomy combined with irradiation, radical mastectomy combined with postoperative irradiation, and radical mastectomy to which is added internal mammary or supraclavicular nodal dissections.

Classification and Diagnosis of Mammary Cancer

In order to investigate these ideas we must take into account the biological behavior of mammary cancers. The following biological classification is based upon the cellular growth patterns of the neoplasms using the criteria of Tornberg.[4]

Type I. Nonmetastasizing (Not Invasive)

This type consists of papillary intraductal or comedo carcinoma without stromal invasion. With this type it is often possible to manually express necrotic tumor from enlarged or thickened mammary ducts after incising the biopsy. When this type of neoplasm affects the epithelium of the nipple the signs of Paget's disease of the breast may exist.

Type II. Rarely Metastasizing (Always Invasive)

1. Pure extracellular mucinous or colloid cancer.
2. Medullary cancer with lymphocytic infiltration.
3. Well differentiated adenocarcinoma (Grade I of Tornberg).

The pure mucinous carcinoma of Type II is recognized easily. When the tumor is cut it is seen to be circumscribed and is homogeneously gelatinous. It is soft and has a gray to reddish brown color. The mucin is always extracellular. The medullary cancer of Type II has sharply delimited margins, is uniformly soft, has a light gray color, and may contain small focal necroses. Lymphocytic infiltration is prominent. Medullary cancer may be mistaken grossly for fibroadenoma. Well differentiated Grade I adenocarcinoma microscopically has discretely circumscribed borders and is highly and uniformly cellularly differentiated.

Papillary carcinoma with stromal invasion also is classed as Type II. It is considered Type I when no stromal invasion is demonstrated.

Type III. Moderately Metastasizing (Always Invasive)

1. Adenocarcinoma (Grade II of Tornberg).
2. Intraductal carcinoma with stromal invasion.

Type III tumors comprise those intraductal carcinomas invading the stroma as well as the ordinary infiltrative adenocarcinomas. Actually, all cancers not definitely classified as Types I, II, or IV constitute Type III.

Type IV.   Highly Metastasizing (Always Invasive)

1. Undifferentiated carcinoma (Grade III of Tornberg).

Type IV cancers include the undifferentiated carcinomas having cells without ductal or tubular arrangement and without cellular inflammatory response about them and all types of tumors indisputably invading blood vessels.

The differentiation of mammary cancer into these types can be made *solely* from properly prepared and selected "permanent" tissue sections of the primary tumor. A study of 739 women with unilateral mammary cancer showed that the primary mammary neoplasms of these biological types have different frequencies of axillary nodal metastases, and are associated with widely different mortality rates after radical mastectomy.[5]

Mortality Rates

Women treated by radical mastectomy for Types I and II mammary cancers died at rates which hardly exceeded those expected among women of similar ages without mammary cancer (Fig. 1).

Mortality rates for Types III and IV are much higher. That the lethal potential of Type IV tumors is greater than that of Type III tumors is supported by the observation that the time requisite for a 50 per cent mortality to occur after radical mastectomy for Types III and IV cancers were

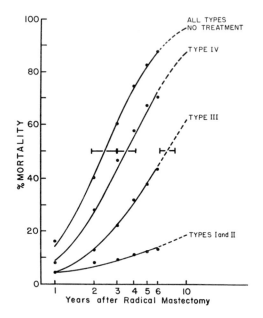

Mortality Expectancy from Mammary Cancer

Fig. 1. This graph compares the mortality expectancy of the different types of mammary cancer treated by radical mastectomy with the untreated series of Greenwood. The lines are calculated from the corresponding fitted probit transformation. The dots about the lines are data points. The confidence limits (95 per cent) for the time of median lethality are represented by the bars to the left and right of the point of 50 per cent mortality. (From Butcher, H. R., Jr.: Ann. Surg., *154*:383, 1961.)

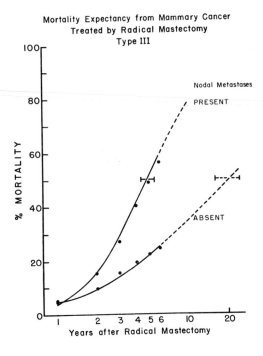

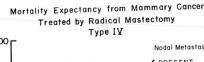

Fig. 2. The mortality expectancy calculated from the respective probit transformations are shown for Type III mammary cancer with and without axillary nodal metastases. (From Butcher, H. R., Jr.: Ann. Surg., *154:*383, 1961.)

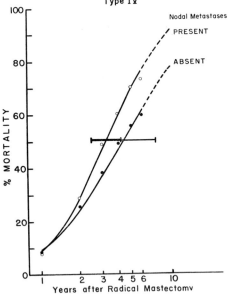

Fig. 3. The mortality expectancy calculated from the respective probit transformations are shown for Type IV mammary cancer with and without axillary nodal metastases. (From Butcher, H. R., Jr.: Ann. Surg., *154:*383, 1961.)

7.1 and 3.5 years respectively. For the most part, the difference in mortality from Types III and IV cancers is ascribable to the different rates with which women with Type III cancer *without* nodal metastases and those with Type III cancer *with* nodal metastases died (Figs. 2 and 3).

Is radical mastectomy a measurably effective way to treat mammary cancer? Radical mastectomy for undifferentiated mammary cancers (Type IV), even when axillary nodal metastases exist, is followed by survival rates significantly better than the survival rates reported by Greenwood in a series of untreated mammary cancers that included all types.

Actually, were it possible to separate the undifferentiated cancers from the other types in Greenwood's series, the mortality rates undoubtedly would be higher than for his total series. Nevertheless, this does not prevent the use of the Greenwood data as a comparison base for ascertaining whether radical mastectomy has appreciable value for the treatment of undifferentiated cancers of the breasts. The use of the Greenwood data in such a comparison serves only to minimize the effectiveness of radical mastectomy. Even so, the time lapse necessary for 50 per cent of the patients with undifferentiated cancers treated by radical mastectomy to die was significantly longer than the time lapse necessary for 50 per cent of Greenwood's

TABLE 1. MORTALITY FROM MAMMARY CANCER*

Treatment	Source	Number	Biological Type	Time of 50% Mortality (years)	95% Confidence Limits (years)	
					From	To
None	Greenwood	651	All	2.4	2.2	2.6
Radical mastectomy	Barnes Hospital	179	IV(N+)†	3.3	2.8	3.7

* Adapted from tables in Butcher, H. R., Jr.: Ann. Surg., *154*:383, 1961.
† Axillary nodal metastases present in all.

untreated series to die (Table 1). Consequently, radical mastectomy, even when used only in cases of undifferentiated tumors with nodal metastases, is a measurably effective way to treat cancer of the breast.

Radical Mastectomy vs. Simple Mastectomy Combined with Irradiation

Although from the available data we cannot really assess the relative effectiveness of radical mastectomy alone and simple mastectomy when combined with irradiation, let us examine the question at least theoretically, using the data just mentioned.

Types III and IV mammary cancers were present in 638 of 739 women. In this group, there were 219 who had no axillary metastases. These are certainly as effectively treated by simple mastectomy and irradiation as by radical mastectomy, and in these the irradiation as well as the axillary dissections were unnecessary. Of the remaining 419 with axillary metastases, 242 died within five years. The question is, would more or less have died if these persons had been treated with simple mastectomy followed by irradiation? It is clear that until we will randomly apply radical mastectomy for one individual and simple mastectomy and irradiation for another, all of whom have been demonstrated to have axillary metastases by biopsy before treatment, the relative merits of these two forms of treatment cannot be assessed certainly. However, from these data an assessment of the relative merits of simple and radical mastectomy can be made. First, simple mastectomy can be reckoned the therapeutic equal of radical mastectomy for the following categories of cases: those persons in whom axillary metastases were absent whether they subsequently died of cancer or not, and those with axillary metastases who died before the point of truncation of the probit line* for their particular tumor. Radical mastectomy must be reckoned superior to simple mastectomy for those cases having axillary metastases who lived beyond their truncation limits. When one considers the problem in this way, it is found that the proportion of women with mammary cancer in a consecutive series who might survive as well after simple mastectomy as after radical mastectomy is approximately 75 per cent. However, simple mastectomy alone is unquestionably biologically inferior to radical mastectomy for the treatment of Types III and IV tumors with axillary metastases; it must leave tumor behind. Consequently, it can be fairly assumed that any individual with axillary metastases treated by simple mastectomy would be likely to die of this residual cancer within the pre-truncation period appropriate to the primary tumor. After radical mastectomy 154 women of 419 who had either Type III or IV tumors with axillary metastases were alive at the truncation point of 6 years—a 6-year cure rate for these two types with axillary metastases of 36 per cent. Undoubtedly, this could not have been achieved by simple mastectomy alone.

Whether irradiation of the axillary supraclavicular and parasternal zones after simple mastectomy would effect as good control of Types III and IV cancers with axillary metastases as radical dissection of the axilla with removal of the breast cannot be answered by the analysis of any extant data. There is no way of knowing how many of the cases treated by simple mastectomy and irradiation had axillary metastases. However, the means of solving this question are now clear.

Actually, the inclusion of individuals having Types I and II mammary cancers in any sample of breast cancer to be used for the assessment of the relative merits of radical mastectomy or any other manner of treatment would be illogical. Only 12 of 101 women who had these types of cancers died within five years after radical mastectomy, and only two of these died of cancer of the breast. Actually, even when the Type III cancers without nodal metastases are included in the sample with the Type I and II, the

* The point of biological truncation is the time when the rate of dying among a group of persons treated for cancer more nearly approximates the death rates of the general population of similar age than the expected rates derived from the mortalities of the afflicted group before this time. It is the point at which the data no longer fit the probit line derived from the antecedent mortality rates of the group.

results of radical mastectomy are so good (92 per cent 5-year, age-corrected survival among 273 cases) that to include this group, which constitutes 37 per cent of the total, in the series treated by such methods as radical mastectomy plus ovariectomy, or radical mastectomy plus cancer chemotherapeutic drugs would be difficult to defend. To include them would merely render the statistics uncertain because one cannot assume that any unclassified sample of mammary cancers would have the same proportions of these cases. In other words, the inclusion of only Type III with lymph node metastases and Type IV with and without metastases would best serve to test the effectiveness of radical mastectomy alone as compared to any other method used.

Irradiation following Radical Mastectomy

The use of postoperative irradiation after radical mastectomy or extension of radical mastectomy to include supraclavicular and internal mammary nodes cannot be justified from the data published. Paterson's well controlled clinical study demonstrated the ineffectiveness of postoperative irradiation as part of the primary therapy for mammary cancer.[6] Similar data from the Barnes Hospital are summarized in Figure 4.[7] Obviously, postoperative irradiation should be reserved for patients who develop proven recurrences or metastases.

Mortality rates following operations that include supraclavicular and intermammary nodes do not seem to differ significantly from those following radical mastectomy (Table 2). Operations more extensive than radical mastectomy should not be considered superior to radical mastectomy for the treatment of mammary cancer until carefully controlled prospective studies

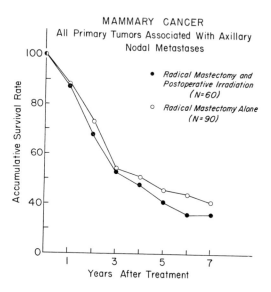

Fig. 4. Accumulative survival rate of all primary tumors with axillary nodal metastases.

TABLE 2.   RESULTS OF TREATMENT IN MAMMARY CARCINOMA; 5-YEAR
SURVIVAL COLUMBIA CLINICAL CLASSIFICATION*

Columbia Clinical Classification	Kennedy & Miller Simple Mast.		Butcher Rad. Mast.		Haagensen & Cooley Rad. Mast.		Dahl-Iversen & Tobiassen Super-Radical	
	No.	Per Cent Surv.	No.	Per Cent Surv.	No.	Per Cent Surv.	No.	Per Cent Surv.
A	115	62	216	76	344	84	277	77
B	34	41	135	48	138	59	61	48
C	18	22	48	48	63	43	20	50
D	45	13	26	11	11	18	8	37
Totals	212	45	425	60	556	72	366	70

* Adapted from data in Haagensen, C. D., et al.: Ann. Surg., *157*:157, 1963.

of properly selected population samples prove that survival rates from mammary cancer are higher after extended operations than they are after radical mastectomy alone.

References

1. McWhirter, R.: The value of simple mastectomy and radiotherapy in the treatment of cancer of the breast. Brit. J. Radiol., *21*:599, 1948.
2. Miller, E. B., and Kennedy, C. S.: Some factors in the choice of treatment of carcinoma of the breast. Ann. Surg., *150*:993, 1959.
3. Crile, G., Jr.: Simplified treatment of cancer of the breast. Ann. Surg., *153*:745, 1961.
4. Hultborn, K. A., and Tornberg, B.: Mammary carcinoma. The biologic character of mammary carcinoma studied in 517 cases by a new form of malignancy grading. Acta radiol. (Stockh.) Suppl. *196*:1, 1960.
5. Butcher, H. R., Jr.: Effectiveness of radical mastectomy for mammary cancer. Ann. Surg., *154*:383, 1961.
6. Paterson, R., and Russell, M. H.: Clinical trials in malignant disease. Part III—Breast cancer: evaluation of postoperative radiotherapy. J. Fac. Radiol., *10*:175, 1959.
7. Butcher, H. R., Jr., Seaman, W. B., Eckert, C., and Saltzstein, S.: An assessment of radical mastectomy and postoperative radiation therapy in the treatment of mammary cancer. Accepted for publication in Cancer.
8. Haagensen, C. D., Cooley, E., et al.: Treatment of early mammary carcinoma, a co-operative international study. Ann. Surg., *157*:157, 1963.
9. Greenwood, M.: The Natural Duration of Cancer. Reports on the Public Health and Medical Subjects. No. 33, His Majesty's Stationery Office, 1926.

Radical Mastectomy with Internal Mammary Node Resection

Donald J. Ferguson

University of Chicago School of Medicine

Progress in Breast Cancer Surgery

Despite efforts of a few unconventional surgeons, the majority of breast cancer patients in this country have been treated for many years by an operation advocated by Halsted and little changed since his day. There are reasons to believe that the surgery of breast cancer has made some progress in the last 60 years, and that Halsted himself would not now be satisfied with "his" operation.

If we are to base our selection of operative procedure today on facts about breast cancer, I think we must include the following among the most relevant:

1. Initial metastases of breast cancer usually develop in the primary lymph nodes: the axillary and internal mammary groups.

2. At operation, about one half of patients have tumor in axillary nodes and one third in internal mammary nodes.

3. Internal mammary nodes, like axillary nodes, may be the only site of metastasis.

4. Although internal mammary nodes are more often invaded from lesions in the medial or central parts of the breast, they can be involved by lesions in any quarter, particularly when the axillary nodes are blocked by metastases.

5. It has not been demonstrated that metastatic cancer can be safely eliminated from internal mammary nodes in any other way than by surgical excision.

6. Surgical mortality and morbidity are not necessarily increased by en bloc resection of internal mammary nodes in addition to radical mastectomy (the Urban operation).

7. Preliminary follow-up results indicate survival without apparent recurrence for 5 to 10 years of about one third of patients who have had en bloc resection of positive internal mammary nodes.

8. Local recurrent cancer after ordinary radical mastectomy may arise in the internal mammary nodes, and the incidence of local recurrence is reduced by the Urban operation.

The conclusion to which these facts lead is fairly obvious, but before stating it let me further discuss some of the points.

The Difference in Surgical Significance between Internal Mammary and Supraclavicular Nodes

The principle of the Halsted radical mastectomy is complete removal of the cancerous breast with surrounding potentially involved skin and muscle, and inclusion of the primary lymph node drainage. The latter is commonly taken to be all the axillary nodes, although it is now clear that internal mammary nodes are also primarily involved from breast cancer. Halsted himself explored the possibilities of anterior mediastinal and supraclavicular node dissection in addition to his standard operation. He abandoned the attack on supraclavicular nodes after about 100 cases, and only a few internal mammary dissections were done on his service. The experience of practically all surgeons with supraclavicular node dissection indicates that it is worthless, because involvement of these nodes with tumor coincides with more distant metastases. Halsted came to the same conclusion earlier. The internal mammary nodes, on the other hand, may be the only site of metastases, and they correspond in surgical importance to the axillary nodes rather than to the supraclavicular.

Mortality and Morbidity of the Urban Operation

Because it is necessary to open the chest and pleural cavity to remove the internal mammary nodes completely, and in continuity with the breast, this approach would have been hazardous in Halsted's day. Results obtained by Urban and by others indicate that radical mastectomy plus anterior mediastinal resection en bloc can be done today without mortality or significant morbidity attributable to the additional dissection. My own experience with extended radical mastectomy began 14 years ago under the direction of Owen H. Wangensteen, who was doing a two-stage operation with removal of both mediastinal and supraclavicular nodes. Results with this procedure were not altogether satisfactory. Subsequently, for the reasons listed previously, I adopted the Urban operation, which I have used since 1957 on every operable breast cancer patient except a few with specific contraindications. There has been no mortality or serious complication, and the only disadvantage I can discover is that up to one hour of additional operating time is required compared to the Halsted operation. Patients only occasionally notice the chest-wall defect, and it does not cause them any difficulty.

It is true that if the procedure were improperly or carelessly done, there would be danger from hemothorax, pneumothorax, or empyema, a risk which is not present with ordinary radical mastectomy. These complications are avoidable, however, and do not occur when the operation is correctly performed. Of course, one would not choose to do the thoracotomy in the presence of extreme age, debility, emphysema, or other intrathoracic disease. The surgeon should have some training in thoracic surgery, and good anesthesia and competent postoperative care are necessary. The Urban operation therefore cannot be recommended for use by all surgeons in all hospitals. Nevertheless, there are increasing numbers of adequately trained surgeons and adequately equipped hospitals where the procedure can be done.

Comparative Results of the Urban and Other Operations

It is regrettable that an operation so well designed as the Urban procedure has not been compared scientifically with ordinary radical mastectomy. If the extended operation has merit, it can be demonstrated unequivocally by controlled study, and probably in no other way. Studies of other extensions of radical mastectomy in which the dissection is not en bloc are not relevant in evaluating the Urban operation. Urban has shown that about one third of patients with positive internal mammary nodes are apparently free of disease 5 years after his operation. One of the unanswered questions, which would be answered in a controlled study, is: how would these particular patients fare after the Halsted operation?

It can hardly be argued that cancer in the internal mammary nodes is innocuous. These nodes are often the first site of local recurrent tumor after radical mastectomy, and they may be the source of distant metastases. It can not be argued that radiation is as good as resection of mediastinal nodes unless it can be shown to eliminate cancer as completely as surgery does and without morbidity. The fact that Urban and others have removed cancerous mediastinal nodes from patients who are well 5 years or more later seems significant in the present state of our knowledge. Considering my own patients with positive mediastinal nodes, I think that even a few long-term cures justify the extra surgical work, since there has been no other penalty attached.

Summary

Breast cancer surgery has remained for many years at the level reached by Halsted. Newer knowledge of surgical, anesthetic, and postoperative techniques allow an extended radical mastectomy to be done without increased mortality or morbidity. At the same time, better knowledge of pathology indicates that internal mammary nodes are primarily involved by metastasis in about one third of breast cancer patients, and are a source of local recurrence after ordinary radical mastectomy. On the basis of these facts, Urban has devised a well conceived operation which has achieved excellent preliminary results, and which appears to be the most satisfactory surgical attack on breast cancer available today.

Reference

1. Urban, J. A.: Surgical excision of internal mammary nodes for breast cancer. Brit. J. Surg., 51:209, 1964.

Modified Radical Mastectomy

A. P. M. Forrest

Welsh National School of Medicine, Cardiff

Since 1890 the standard treatment for primary breast cancer has been radical mastectomy, in which the surgeon removes the whole breast, varying amounts of overlying skin, the axillary fat and lymph nodes, and the pectoral muscles.

In centers in which this operation, with or without adjuvant radiotherapy, forms the basic policy of treatment, the 5-year survival rates of patients with breast cancer approximate 40 per cent.[8] Thus, in the majority of patients with breast cancer, the "radical" operation is but a futile attempt to alter the natural course of the disease (Table 1).

Argument for Modification of Radical Mastectomy

There is no conclusive evidence that extension of the local attack to other nodal areas materially affects these results. Thus, in a randomized study, Paterson and his colleagues in Manchester found that postoperative irradiation of internal mammary and supraclavicular nodes (following radical mastectomy) did not improve survival rates.[3, 18, 19] Surgical removal of these nodes also fails significantly to improve the outlook, for despite encouraging reports by Urban,[24, 25] others have abandoned the so-called extended or super-radical operation in which resection of the internal mammary nodes is added to the standard radical mastectomy.[6, 11]

Conversely, there is growing realization that simplification of local treatment, e.g., to simple mastectomy with or without radiotherapy, or even to local excision, does not reduce survival rates.[7, 14, 17, 21] Unfortunately, attempts to compare the results of McWhirter's regime in Edinburgh with those of radical mastectomy in other centers are impracticable in the absence of information about the histological state of the axillary nodes in patients treated by simple mastectomy. Yet a comparison of the overall results of treating of primary breast cancer in the southeast region of Scotland, where simple mastectomy and radiotherapy is the main treatment policy, with those of other centers in England, where radical mastectomy is practiced, show no difference in 5-year survival rates (Table 2).

TABLE 1. OVERALL 5-YEAR SURVIVAL RATES IN PATIENTS WITH BREAST CANCER SEEN IN CLINICS IN WHICH RADICAL MASTECTOMY, WITH OR WITHOUT RADIOTHERAPY, IS THE MAIN POLICY OF TREATMENT*

England 15,450	Birmingham London Manchester Oxford Bristol	38%
North America 15,556	California Chicago Connecticut Minnesota New York Saskatchewan Toronto	43%
Scandinavia 2419	Oslo Stockholm	40%

* Calculated from Table 1 in Forrest, A.P.M.: Treatment of Cancer of the Breast. *In* Irvine, W. T. (ed.): Modern Trends in Surgery. Vol. I. London, Butterworths, 1962, p. 106.

TABLE 2. COMPARISON OF OVERALL 5-YEAR CRUDE SURVIVAL RATES FOR PATIENTS WITH PRIMARY BREAST CANCER TREATED IN SOUTHEASTERN SCOTLAND[17] AND IN OTHER REGIONS IN ENGLAND[8]

Area	Treatment Policy	No. of Cases	Crude 5-year Survival (per cent)
Southeastern Scotland	Simple mastectomy + radiotherapy	1609	42
England	Radical mastectomy + radiotherapy	15,450	38

A controlled comparison of these two extremes of treatment—extended radical mastectomy and simple mastectomy and radiotherapy—has been reported from Copenhagen where 668 patients with primary breast cancer have been selected randomly for treatment by one or the other operation. Preliminary results suggest that, up to 5 years, recurrence-free survival rates are identical (Table 3 and Fig. 1).[6, 14, 15]

From these facts it seems reasonable to conclude that by the time a large proportion of patients with breast cancer come for treatment, the disease has already spread beyond the limits of local surgery. Even if local surgery is restricted to patients in whom a careful search for metastatic or regional lymphatic spread (including supraclavicular or high axillary and internal mammary node biopsy) proves negative, the results, in terms of cure of cancer, are still unsatisfactory. It would therefore appear that, in the majority of patients with primary breast cancer, the main function of local treatment is to remove the offending lump, protecting against ulcera-

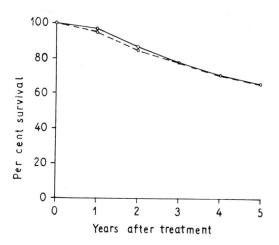

Fig. 1. Crude 5-year survival rates of controlled series of patients treated by simple mastectomy and radiotherapy (———) and extended radical mastectomy (– – – –). (From Kaae, S., and Johansen, H.: Amer. J. Roentgenol., *87*:82, 1962. Charles C Thomas, Publisher.)

TABLE 3.   RANDOMIZED STUDY OF 5-YEAR SURVIVAL IN SIMPLE VS. EXTENDED RADICAL MASTECTOMY[14, 15]

	Operable Cases		All Cases	
	Number	Per Cent 5-year Survival	Number	Per Cent 5-year Survival
Simple mastectomy + radiotherapy	187	67	182	54
Extended radical mastectomy	166	69	182	55

tion, and to prevent local recurrence. As this almost invariably occurs in skin and axilla, adequate removal of skin and clearance of the axillary nodes are of prime importance. The high incidence of local recurrence following radical mastectomy (40 per cent of 507 patients in whom radical mastectomy failed to cure had local recurrence at death[4]) suggests that even this aim is not achieved.

Radical mastectomy eradicates the primary tumor, the overlying skin, the main lymphatic pathways, and the axillary nodes, but not without morbidity from delayed healing, interference with function, lymphedema, and considerable deformity. These disadvantages can be reduced by an operation which, although still "radical" in its removal of diseased or potentially diseased tissue, preserves those normal functional structures in which recurrence of disease is virtually unknown.

Preservation of the Pectoralis Major Muscle

Standard radical mastectomy involves sacrifice of the pectoral muscles, of which the most important is the pectoralis major, which covers the anterior surface of the chest wall. Its functions are dichotomous, in that its clavicular part (which usually is preserved in a radical mastectomy) acts with the anterior portion of the deltoid to raise the arm forward and control its descent. The larger costal part, normally removed in a radical mastectomy, acts in concert with latissimus dorsi and teres major to pull the arm down against resistance or, if the arm is fixed as in climbing, raise the trunk.[16]

To the average woman, removal of this muscle may cause little disability, and although 33.1 per cent of 507 patients complained of functional impairment following radical mastectomy, this was severe in only 1.9 per cent.[26] Of greater consequence to a woman is the loss of the muscle pad below the clavicle which leads to an unsightly hollow, preventing the wearing of low-necked clothes and usually making a surgical prosthetic-containing "bra" necessary. Preservation of the muscle leaves a patient whose appearance is normal when wearing an ordinary "bra" with a simple false breast—even in a "bikini."[12]

Reasons Given for Removal

Two reasons are usually given for removing the pectoralis major as part of radical mastectomy: eradication of deep lymphatic pathways and achievement of adequate access to the axilla. Neither of these is valid.

REMOVAL OF INVOLVED LYMPHATICS. The classic belief that an important lymphatic plexus runs in close relationship to the fascia covering the pectoral muscle has not been supported by recent studies in which Thorotrast[9] and the intravital injections of dyes and radiogold[23] have been used to map out the lymphatic drainage of the breast.

The main lymphatics draining the breast run within its substance toward the axilla and perforate the deep fascia with the axillary tail. Only a few fine channels run deep to the breast in the pectoral fascia, and these probably drain the fascia itself. Lymphatics from the breast do perforate the deep fascia other than in the axilla but only at certain focal points, where they accompany the anterior perforating branches of the internal mammary vessels and the lateral perforating branches of the intercostal vessels. These lymphatics pierce the pectoral and intercostal muscles to gain entry to the thoracic cavity and end in the internal mammary nodes. In the upper part of the chest they pass through the pectoral muscles with the acromiothoracic and other vessels, and may drain into the interpectoral nodes of Rotter.

It is worthy of note that these penetrating channels drain lymph from all parts of the breast to the internal mammary nodes.

These findings suggest that, apart from the removal of the small and probably insignificant interpectoral nodes, removal of the pectoralis major muscle will not give added protection unless it is also intended to remove the underlying chest wall and the intrathoracic lymph nodes.

ACCESS TO INVOLVED LYMPHATICS. Removal of the pectoralis major muscle is not an essential step in gaining full access to the axilla.[11, 20, 22] If the arm is lifted so that the forearm lies in front of and parallel to the chest, and the upper arm at right angles to the chest, the pectoralis major is relaxed and can be retracted to expose the pectoralis minor. Following the division of the pectoralis minor, the upper reaches of the axilla are in full view.[20]

Quite apart from the adequacy of access, it is now doubtful whether high axillary clearance is of great value. From a detailed study of the number and distribution of involved axillary nodes in 107 patients with breast cancer treated by radical mastectomy, Auchingloss concluded that only patients in whom three or less nodes were involved, and these in the lower axillary groups, stand a chance of surviving 5 years. On the basis of this evidence Auchingloss limits the highest point of the axillary dissection to the lower border of the pectoralis minor muscle.

The Modified Operation

Preservation of the pectoralis major muscle in performing a radical mastectomy is not new and, according to Holman, was practiced regularly by J. B. Murphy, who followed the technique of Bryant of Guy's Hospital, London. Detailed descriptions of techniques are to be found in the recent literature.[1, 11, 20] In essence it can be performed by any of the standard techniques used for radical mastectomy and the dissection started either by stripping the breast off the pectoral muscle (from medial to lateral side) or by approaching the axilla first, stripping the nodes and fat downward from the highest point.

It is probably most convenient first to raise the skin flaps and strip the breast and pectoral fascia off the pectoralis major from medial to lateral side. The breast can then be wrapped in a towel or placed in a plastic bag and the axillary tail mobilized upward to the axilla.

The lower border of the pectoralis major is then defined and retracted, the pectoralis minor divided, the fascia over the neurovascular bundle divided, and the nodes and axillary fat stripped from above downward. Alternatively, although perhaps more likely to lead to freeing of cells up into the lymphatics, I have found it convenient to define latissimus dorsi up to its attachment, divide the axillary fascia close to coracobrachialis, and strip the axillary tail and its contiguous lymphatics from below upward, retracting pectoralis major and dividing pectoralis minor to reach the highest point of the dissection. In this way the axillary lymphatics and surrounding tissues can be cored out to the level of the clavicle and first rib.

Whichever method is used, the arm should be separately draped, so that it can be brought forward in the manner described above to relax the muscles and allow access to the upper axilla. It should be noted that, during this maneuver, the neurovascular bundle assumes a vertical, rather than its usual horizontal, course. The postoperative course of patients following modified radical mastectomy is smooth—suction drainage leads to rapid healing of the wound and arm movements can be resumed within a few days. The rarity of delay in healing may account for the lower incidence of lymphedema of the arm noted with the operation.[5]

RESULTS. Several authors have suggested that the results of modified radical operation are comparable to those of radical mastectomy,[2, 5, 11, 13, 20, 22, 27] but no controlled trial of the operation versus radical mastectomy has yet been reported. Modified radical mastectomy was one of the methods surveyed in the cooperative study recently reported by Haagensen et al.,[10] in which the results of treating patients by a variety of methods in different centers were compared. In Table 4 the 5-year survival rates have been calculated for all "operable" cases (Columbia stages A and B) and, where available, the incidence of axillary node involvement, based on *histological* findings, are included.

Although it is not possible to draw definite conclusions from this type of survey, in general the results of modified radical mastectomy are similar to those of standard radical, extended radical, and simple mastectomy with radiotherapy. The high survival rates in Haagensen's own series of cases treated by radical mastectomy cannot be taken as showing superiority of this method of treatment as (a) they do not conform with those of Butcher, (b) stricter criteria of operability (including triple biopsy) have been applied, and (c) the very detailed examination of axillary nodes (including

TABLE 4. RESULTS OF DIFFERENT METHODS OF TREATMENT OF OPERABLE BREAST CANCER*

Treatment	Number	Operable (Columbia A + B) Cases	
		5-yr. Survival (Per Cent)	Axillary Nodes Involvde (Per Cent)
Radical mastectomy			
Butcher (St. Louis)	351	65	49
Haagensen and Cooley (New York)	482	77	45
Simple mastectomy + radiotherapy			
Kennedy and Miller—1000r (Detroit)	149	57	—
Kaae and Johansen—3000r (Copenhagen)	187	67	—
Modified radical			
Handley and Thackray (London)	135	67	59
Williams and Curwen (London)	125	66	—
Extended radical			
Dahl-Iversen and Johansen (Copenhagen)	386	69	37

* Calculated from data of Haagensen, C. D., et al.: Ann. Surg., *157*:157, 1963.

serial section) normally practiced at the Presbyterian Hospital may give a falsely high incidence of axillary node involvement compared to that of other centers in which such complete examination is not normally practiced and small axillary deposits missed.

Conclusions

There is no concrete evidence that removal of the pectoralis major muscle improves the results of standard radical mastectomy in primary breast cancer. Preservation of the muscle reduces morbidity. Since, in the majority of patients, the local attack fails to cure the disease, maintenance of normal appearance and function would appear to be an essential part of rational local therapy.

References

1. Auchingloss, H.: Significance of location and number of axillary metastases in carcinoma of the breast. A justification for a more conservative operation. Ann. Surg., 158:37, 1963.
2. Berg, J. W., and Robbins, S. F.: Modified mastectomy for older poor risk patients. Surg., Gynec. and Obst., 113:631, 1961.
3. Cole, M. P.: The place of radiotherapy in the management of early breast cancer. A report of two clinical trials. Brit. J. Surg., 51:216, 1963.
4. Collins, V. P.: Breast cancer: influence of treatment that fails to cure. Cancer, 9:1177, 1956.
5. Crile, G.: Simplified treatment of cancer of the breast. Early results of a clinical study. Ann. Surg., 153:745, 1961.
6. Dahl-Iversen, E.: An extended radical operation for carcinoma of the breast. J. Roy. Coll. Surg. Edinb., 8:81, 1963.
7. Devitt, J. E.: The local control of carcinoma of the breast. Canad. J. Surg., 6:316, 1963.
8. Forrest, A. P. M.: Treatment of Cancer of the Breast. In Irvine, W. T. (ed.): Modern Trends in Surgery. Vol. 1. London, Butterworths, 1962, p. 106.
9. Gray, J. H.: The relation of lymphatic vessels to the spread of cancer. Brit. J. Surg., 26:462, 1959.
10. Haagensen, C. D. et al.: Treatment of early mammary carcinoma. A co-operative international study. Ann. Surg., 157:157, 1963.
11. Handley, R. S.: An extended radical operation for carcinoma of the breast. Reflections and results. J. Roy. Coll. Surg. Edinb., 8:81, 1960.
12. Handley, R. S.: The early spread of breast carcinoma and its bearing on operative treatment. Brit. J. Surg., 51:206, 1964.
13. Holman, C. C.: Cancer of the breast. The principles of surgical treatment. Lancet, 1:174, 1954.
14. Kaae, S., and Johansen, H.: Breast cancer; 5-year results: two random series of simple mastectomy with postoperative irradiation versus extended radical mastectomy. Am. J. Roentgenol., 87:82, 1962.
15. Kaae, S., and Johansen, H. See Haagensen et al.
16. Lockhart, R. D., Hamilton, G. F., and Fyfe, F. W.: Anatomy of the Human Body. London, Faber and Faber Ltd., 1959.
17. McWhirter, R.: Simple mastectomy and radiotherapy in the treatment of breast cancer. Brit. J. Radiol., 28:128, 1955.

18. Paterson, R.: Breast cancer. A report of two clinical trials. J. Roy. Coll. Surg. Edinb.,
    7:243, 1962.
19. Paterson, R., and Russell, M. H.: Clinical trials in malignant disease. Part III. Breast
    cancer: Evaluation of post-operative radiotherapy. J. Fac. Radiol., *10:175*, 1959.
20. Patey, D. H., and Dyson, W. H.: Prognosis of carcinoma of the breast in relation to
    the type of operation performed. Brit. J. Cancer, *2:7*, 1948.
21. Porritt, A.: Early carcinoma of the breast. Brit. J. Surg., *51:214*, 1963.
22. Ross, J. P. An investigation into the effects of radium upon carcinoma of the breast.
    Brit. J. Surg., 27:211, 1939.
23. Turner-Warwick, R. T.: The lymphatics of the breast. Brit. J. Surg., *46:574*, 1959.
24. Urban, J. A.: Extended radical mastectomy for breast cancer. Am. J. Surg., *106:399*,
    1963.
25. Urban, J. A.: Surgical excision of internal mammary nodes for breast cancer. Brit. J.
    Surg., *51:209*, 1963.
26. Watson, T. A., Bond, A. F., and Phillips, A. J.: Swelling and dysfunction of the
    upper limb following radical mastectomy. Surg., Gynec. and Obst., *116:99*, 1963.
27. Williams, I. G., Murley, R. S., and Curwen, M. P.: Carcinoma of the female breast:
    conservative and radical surgery. Brit. M. J., *2:787*, 1953.

The Place of Simple Mastectomy in the Treatment of Carcinoma of the Breast

Charles S. Kennedy

Wayne State University College of Medicine

In 1918 my observations of radical mastectomies done in Detroit, Chicago, New York, Philadelphia, and at the Mayo Clinic convinced me that these operations could not offer any more hope of 5-year survival from carcinoma of the breast than simple mastectomy. Perhaps it is significant in my conclusion that I did not see William Halsted work. Regardless, my own personal experience and observations in the ensuing 45 years have offered little to change this overall point of view.

The radical mastectomies that I have seen were done with skin flaps of about one centimeter in thickness, no skin grafts, partial preservation of the pectoralis major muscle, retraction of the breast medially, completion in less than three hours and, in general, following Willy Meyer[1] rather than Halsted.

The Halsted[2] radical mastectomy, to the best of my ability to determine, is characterized by skin flaps of the order of 2 mm. in thickness, skin grafting, complete sacrifice of the pectoral muscles, and no retraction of the cancer laden breast, and requires approximately six hours for completion. It is represented best in the world, in my opinion, by the technique described by Cushman Haagensen.[3]

In 1946 my associate, Elmer B. Miller, joined me in the practice of surgery and at once disagreed with the use of simple mastectomy for the treatment of carcinoma of the breast. He began a careful study which has continued to the present.

The clinical grouping of all the cases of carcinoma of the breast treated at The Grace Hospital in Detroit has been accomplished following the Columbia Clinical Classification developed by Haagensen, Stout,[4] and Cooley.[5] As far as I know, this is the only classification based purely on preoperative findings and hence useful in comparison of results, no matter

TABLE 1.   COLUMBIA CLINICAL CLASSIFICATION

Clinical Group	Clinical Features
A	1. No clinically involved lymph nodes 2. No grave signs
B	1. Clinically involved nodes (trans. diam. less than 2.5 cm.) 2. No grave signs
C	Any one of the following five grave signs: 1. Limited skin edema (involvement less than ⅓ skin over breast) 2. Ulceration of skin 3. Solid fixation primary tumor to chest wall 4. Axillary nodes 2.5 cm. or greater in diameter 5. Fixation of axillary nodes to skin or surrounding tissues
D	Any one of the following ten conditions: 1. Any two or more of above five grave signs 2. Edema involving ⅓ or more of skin over breast 3. Satellite nodules in skin over breast 4. Inflammatory carcinoma 5. Parasternal tumor nodules 6. Edema of the arm 7. Distant metastases 8. Microscopically proved supraclavicular metastases 9. Microscopically proved apical axillary metastases 10. Microscopically proved internal mammary metastases

what form of treatment may be decided upon as wise for the individual case. It is presented in Table 1 as used by us at The Grace Hospital.[6]

Studying my cases and subsequently all cases of carcinoma of the breast at The Grace Hospital in Detroit, Miller found that the x-ray therapy used on these patients was of such strength as to have essentially no effect on the survival of the patients, and that unknowingly a series of cases of carcinoma of the breast, treated by simple mastectomy alone, had been compiled. This statement is based on my understanding that good x-ray therapy requires a tumor dose of at least 3500 roentgen units.[7-11]

In general, the cases at The Grace Hospital during the period of study all received far less than this amount, based on a study of the roentgenologist's own charts.[12-15]

The study, as indicated in Table 2, would seem to vindicate my judgment, and that of McWhirter[16] and Kaae,[17] that simple mastectomy compares favorably with the Mayo type of radical mastectomy. That this statement is justified, is substantiated by the fact that the figures recently reported from the Mayo Clinic by Berkson[18] are essentially the same as those for the less than three-hour radical mastectomies done at The Grace Hospital. This is especially true when one takes cognizance of the fact that the Mayo Clinic reports only those cases they can follow and deletes all operative deaths whereas in the other series all cases are included; those cases lost to follow-up being considered as deaths due to cancer.

TABLE 2. FIVE-YEAR SURVIVAL RATES AT THE GRACE HOSPITAL

Columbia Clinical Group	No. of Cases	Five-Year Survival	Percentages
Simple Mastectomy (Kennedy, 1927–1956; The Grace Hosp., 1951–1957)			
A	151	97	64
B	43	18	42
C	26	7	27
D	49	7	14
Total	269	129	48
Survival (excluding clinically inoperable cases)			56
Less than Three-Hour Radical Mastectomy (Grace, 1951–1957)			
A	162	100	62
B	45	12	27
C	29	11	38
D	13	0	0
Total	249	123	49
Survival (excluding clinically inoperable cases)			52

TABLE 3. COMPARISON OF McWHIRTER'S METHOD (BY KAAE) OF TREATMENT OF CARCINOMA OF BREAST TO MAYO TECHNIQUE (USED AT THE GRACE HOSPITAL)

Columbia Clinical Group	No. of Cases	Five-Year Survival	Percentages
McWhirter Method			
A	159	112	70
B	28	14	50
C	9	2	22
D	3	0	0
Total	199	128	64
Survival (excluding clinically inoperable cases)			65
Mayo Method			
A	151	97	64
B	40	10	25
C	22	8	36
D	12	0	0
Total	225	115	51
Survival (excluding clinically inoperable cases)			54

McWhirter[19] has not classified his cases according to the Columbia Clinical Classification. However, Kaae has,[11, 17] and Table 3 shows a comparison of simple mastectomy followed by adequate x-ray therapy as outlined by McWhirter to radical mastectomy of the Mayo type. It must be perfectly clear that the cases treated by the McWhirter method were treated at the Radium Center in Copenhagen, Denmark, and the cases treated by

TABLE 4.   COMPARISON OF McWHIRTER'S METHOD (BY KAAE) OF TREATMENT OF CARCINOMA OF THE BREAST TO RADICAL MASTECTOMY BY HAAGENSEN

Columbia Clinical Group	No. of Cases	Five-Year Survival	Percentages
McWhirter Method			
A	159	112	70
B	28	14	50
C	9	2	22
D	3	0	0
Total	199	128	64
Survival (excluding clinically inoperable cases)			65
Haagensen's Results			
A	228	188	83
B	122	71	59
C	50	19	38
D	10	2	20
Total	410	280	69
Survival (excluding clinically inoperable cases)			70

the Mayo technique were treated at The Grace Hospital in Detroit, Michigan.

It is my belief based on the facts presented, which I believe to be true, that simple mastectomy followed by good x-ray therapy is the treatment of choice for carcinoma of the breast. In consideration of my associate, E. B. Miller, I present Table 4, which compares McWhirter's method to similar cases treated by the meticulous type of Halsted radical mastectomy done by Haagensen.

It is my conclusion that one should treat carcinoma of the breast either by simple mastectomy with adequate x-ray therapy or by the true Halsted type radical mastectomy, and that there is no defense, in my opinion, for the so-called standard radical mastectomy or Mayo Clinic approach.

References

1. Meyer, W.: An improved method of the radical operation for carcinoma of the breast. Med. Rec., *46*:746, 1894.
2. Halsted, W. S.: The results of operations for the cure of cancer of the breast performed at the Johns Hopkins Hospital from June 1889 to January 1894. Johns Hopkins Hosp. Rep., *4*:297, 1894.
3. Haagensen, C. D.: Diseases of the Breast. Philadelphia, W. B. Saunders Co., 1956.
4. Haagensen, C. D., and Stout, A. P.: Carcinoma of the breast. II. Criteria of operability. Ann. Surg., *118*:1032, 1943.
5. Haagensen, C. D., and Cooley, E.: Treatment of early mammary carcinoma (The Columbia Clinical Classification). Ann. Surg., *157*:160, 1963.
6. Dion, R. M., Welsh, G. J., Kennedy, C. S., Miller, E. B., and McLean, D. C.: Grades of mastectomy. Grace Hosp. Bull., *40*:78, 1962.

7. Lenz, M.: Roentgen therapy of cancer of the breast. Radiology, *38*:686, 1942.
8. Lenz, M.: Tumor dosage and results in roentgen therapy of cancer of the breast. Am. J. Roentgenol., *56*:67, 1946.
9. Baclesse, F.: La roentgenthérapie seule employée dans le traitement des cancers du sein, opérables et inopérables. Mem. e Congr. fr. de Chir., Paris, *51*:125, 1948.
10. McWhirter, R.: Simple mastectomy and radiotherapy in the treatment of breast cancer. Brit. J. Radiol., *28*:128, 1955.
11. Kaae, S., and Johansen, H.: Breast cancer. Am. J. Roentgenol., *87*:82, 1962.
12. Miller, E. B., and Kennedy, C. S.: A study of results of treatment of carcinoma of the breast by simple mastectomy followed by x-ray therapy. Grace Hosp. Bull., *35*:1, 1957.
13. Gulick, A. E.: Personal communication, 1958.
14. Miller, E. B., and Kennedy, C. S.: Some factors in the choice of treatment of carcinoma of the breast. Ann. Surg., *150*:993, 1959.
15. Kennedy, C. S., and Miller, E. B.: Treatment of early mammary carcinoma (simple mastectomy for mammary carcinoma). Ann. Surg., *157*:161, 1963.
16. McWhirter, R.: Breast cancer; comparison of results at Mayo Clinic and in Edinburgh. Lancet, 2:1060, 1958.
17. Kaae, S., and Johansen, H.: Treatment of early mammary carcinoma (simple mastectomy plus postoperative irradiation by the method of McWhirter for mammary carcinoma). Ann. Surg., *157*:175, 1963.
18. Berkson, J., Harrington, S. W., Clagett, O. T., et al.: Mortality and survival in surgically treated cancer of the breast. A statistical summary of some experience of the Mayo Clinic. Proc. Staff Meet. Mayo Clin., *32*:645, 1957.
19. McWhirter, R.: Some factors influencing prognosis in breast cancer. J. Fac. Radiologists, *8*:220, 1957.

Simple Mastectomy with or without Radiation in the Treatment of Cancer of the Breast

George Crile, Jr.

The Cleveland Clinic Foundation

For the last eight years I have been treating clinical stage 1 (Manchester classification) breast cancer by simple mastectomy, usually without postoperative irradiation. Clinical stage 2 cancer has been treated either by simple mastectomy extended to include the low and central groups of axillary nodes, or by simple mastectomy followed by McWhirter style radiation to the axilla, supraclavicular region, and internal mammary chain.

The series consists of 251 patients with previously untreated breast cancer seen at the Cleveland Clinic in the years 1955 through 1958. All these patients have been followed for five to eight years and all have been studied prospectively as a clinical experiment. Three questions are raised by this study.

What Is the Efficacy of Radiation When Given Prophylactically to Nodes That Are Involved but Are Still so Small That the Metastases Cannot Be Diagnosed Clinically (Clinical Stage 1)?

Sixteen patients with clinical stage 1 breast cancer were treated by simple mastectomy and prophylactic radiation of the axilla, supraclavicular region, and internal mammary nodes. All these have been followed for five to eight years and in none has there developed any palpable involvement of axillary nodes. Since approximately one third of all patients thought clinically to have stage 1 cancer actually have microscopic deposits in the axillary nodes, 5 of the 16 clinical stage 1 patients treated by simple mastectomy and radiation might have had reappearance of cancer in the axilla if they had not been irradiated. In a larger series of patients treated in the same way since 1958, but not followed so long, no axillary nodes have become palpable. Since no cancers have appeared, it seems that microfoci of breast cancer in axillary nodes are radiosensitive and can be well controlled for periods at least as long as eight years by radiation therapy. McWhirter's vast experience with treatment of this type[1] and the randomized clinical experiment of Kaae and Johansen[2] establish this point beyond reasonable doubt, and suggest that metastases in nodes of the internal mammary chain can be equally well controlled by radiation.

Does Irradiation Control the Growth of Cancer in Palpably Involved Axillary Nodes (Clinical Stage 2)?

My experience with simple mastectomy and radiation for stage 2 cancers has been limited to the more unfavorable cases in which the apex of the axilla or many axillary nodes were involved. I have treated the more favorable cases, with involvement limited to the low and central nodal groups, by extended simple mastectomy, removing the low and central axillary nodes along with the breast but not disturbing the muscles. Because of this selection the survival rate following simple mastectomy and radiation has been lower than that following extended simple or radical mastectomy, but if allowance is made for the factor of selectivity, there is no difference. I employed simple mastectomy and radiation in 69 per cent of my 27 clinical stage 2 cases and had a 50 per cent five-year survival rate while my colleagues employed radical mastectomy (usually with radiation) in 89 per cent of theirs and had a 48 per cent survival rate. This limited experience confirms the impressions of McWhirter[1] and of Kaae and Johansen[2] that, from the standpoint of the patient's survival, radiation of involved nodes is as effective as excision.

In only two cases in this series of clinical stage 2 cancers has radiation therapy failed to control the tumor in axillary nodes during the life of the patient. One of these tumors was a rare and radioresistant squamous-cell cancer and the other inexplicably grew in spite of radiation and caused enough discomfort to warrant axillary dissection.

From these experiences my conclusions are similar to those of Haagensen and Stout,[3] who believe that extensive axillary involvement is best treated by radiation. Minor involvement can be treated equally effectively by surgery or radiation, but since extension of simple mastectomy to include the low and central nodal groups does not increase morbidity it seems simpler to dissect the nodes when involvement is minimal or moderate.

If Simple Mastectomy Is Done and Nodes Later Become Palpably Involved and Then Are Removed, Does the Delay Result in an Increase in the Number of Nodes Involved by Cancer or in a Decrease in the Rate of Survival?

Forty patients with clinical stage 1 breast cancer were treated by radical mastectomy and 13 of these (32.5 per cent) were found by the pathologist to have axillary metastases. An additional 40 patients were treated by simple mastectomy without radiation; 12 of these (30 per cent) later were found to have axillary metastases and were treated by axillary dissections. The time between mastectomy and axillary dissection ranged from 1 month to 6 years, averaging 22 months. In spite of this delay there were more patients with only one node involved, and fewer with 10 or more nodes involved, in the group with delayed dissections than in the group treated initially by radical mastectomy. The rate of five-year survival and the rate of five- to eight-year survival free of disease were higher in the delayed group. After removal of the primary tumor there seemed to be no tendency for breast cancer to metastasize from node to node or from node to distant organs.

Experiments (pending publication) with sarcoma 1 on the feet of strain A mice and with a melanoma implanted on the hind feet of hamsters indicate that there is little or no tendency for these cancers to spread from node to node or to metastasize to the lungs after the primary tumors have been removed. If breast cancer does not tend to spread from node to node after the primary tumor is removed there would not appear to be any urgency about resecting microfoci of cancer in axillary nodes. Much of the morbidity of surgery for breast cancer could be avoided if uninvolved axillary nodes were not removed. Furthermore there is a possibility that lymphocytes in uninvolved axillary nodes are immunized by antigens from the tumor and in some cases act as a part of the host's defense against the systemic spread of cancer.

Discussion

This article does not attempt to compare the results of surgery with those of radiation, but points out that in breast cancer, involvement of the regional nodes can be treated satisfactorily by either method. Since the combination of axillary dissection and radiation tends to destroy more lymphatics and cause more edema of the arm than either of the treatments alone the combination should be avoided.

If the breast is mobilized from the chest wall through a more or less transverse incision that ends up at the hairline of the axilla, the axilla can be opened and explored much as an abdomen is explored before the surgeon commits himself to a method of treatment. If there is extensive axillary involvement the breast can be removed and the axilla left undisturbed as advocated by McWhirter.[1]

If the axillary involvement is limited to a few nodes of the low and central groups an extended simple mastectomy with axillary dissection can be done and radiation is not required.

If there is no apparent involvement of the nodes it is not clear as to whether extended simple mastectomy should be done or the axilla left alone and observed. Our experience indicates that the survival rate will be approximately the same no matter which course is followed, the advantage, if any, lying with the simple procedure.[4]

Perhaps parasternal nodes should be irradiated prophylactically in patients with medial quadrant or central lesions, for involvement of these nodes is difficult to recognize. Although we have not followed this course, and during the time of this study we were not sterilizing patients prophylactically, the 5-year survival rate of patients operated on at the Cleveland Clinic in 1958 for operable cancer of the breast was 71 per cent. During this year 79 per cent of the operations were simple mastectomies, and only 3 per cent of the patients had radical mastectomies with removal of muscles. Year by year, as we have simplified surgical procedures and eliminated postoperative radiation, the crude survival rate of all patients in all stages of the disease, operable and inoperable, has risen from 48 (44 per cent) of 108 patients in 1955 and 1956 to 80 (55 per cent) of 143 patients in 1957 and 1958. The survival rate of the operable stages 1 and 2 cases has similarly risen from 46 (57 per cent) of 81 to 74 (70 per cent) of 105. During the first period 47 per cent of the operations were simple mastectomies and during the second 72 per cent. In both periods 75 per cent of all patients seen were considered to be operable.

The studies reported here have been planned in advance, and all the patients have been followed. What is now required is a larger, randomized study of the survival of patients with clinical stage 1 cancer following simple and radical mastectomies without radiation therapy.

References

1. McWhirter, R.: Discussion: The treatment of cancer of the breast. Proc. Roy. Soc. Med., *41*:122, 1948.
2. Kaae, S., and Johansen, H.: Breast cancer; a comparison of the results of simple mastectomy with postoperative roentgen irradiation by the McWhirter method with those of extended radical mastectomy. Acta radiol., *188*:155, 1959.
3. Haagensen, C. D., and Stout, A. P.: Carcinoma of breast; results of treatment, 1935–1942. Ann. Surg., *134*:151, 1951.
4. Crile, G., Jr.: Results of simplified treatment of breast cancer. Surg., Gynec. and Obst., *118*:517, 1964.

Prophylactic Bilateral Oophorectomy in the Treatment of Carcinoma of the Breast

J. Shelton Horsley, III, *and* Guy W. Horsley

St. Elizabeth's Hospital, Richmond, Va.

Definition

Prophylactic bilateral oophorectomy refers to surgical removal of both ovaries at the time of radical mastectomy in the initial treatment of operable adenocarcinoma of the breast. This is an adjunct to radical mastectomy, performed during or immediately following the closure of the mastectomy wound.

Arguments for Prophylactic Oophorectomy—The Rationale

In removing the ovaries we have attempted to decrease the circulating estrogen available to stimulate growth of tumor cells. Many cells are liberated into the venous blood draining the site of the neoplasm at the time of surgery. Certainly anything done to make the environment of these cells less favorable for growth will be beneficial to the patient.

Many studies have shown the close relationship of estrogen with the pathogenesis of adenocarcinoma of the female breast. The much higher incidence in women than men bears out this relationship. The disease thrives best in laboratory animals in an estrogen-rich environment. Five times as many women with carcinoma of the breast have a late menopause as compared with women without this neoplasm.

A recent study of the epidemiology of breast carcinoma indicated that castration in the premenopausal age group protected against breast cancer, particularly before age 37 years.

Jessiman and Moore, in their study of metastatic carcinoma of the breast in premenopausal and menopausal women, found no patients who did not give some evidence, however slight, of transient worsening when given estrogen for a stilbestrol test. They stated "that virtually all tumors in the young or menopausal age are 'estrogen-stimulated': they will grow less well, for a time, with less estrogen."

Rather striking remissions of metastatic disease following bilateral oophorectomy are not unusual. Despite the fact that all remissions are temporary, they are, nevertheless, impressive and indicate again the close relationship of estrogen with the pathogenesis of breast carcinoma in the premenopausal and menopausal age groups.

There is an increased incidence of cortical stromal hyperplasia of the ovaries of postmenopausal women who have metastatic breast carcinoma. In 100 such women cortical stromal hyperplasia was found in 86 per cent, whereas a control group of postmenopausal women without breast carcinoma showed this change in only 38 per cent. The cells present are similar to those seen in granulosa cell tumors of the ovaries, which produce large amounts of estrogen. There is good evidence to support the hypothesis that these ovaries secrete increased amounts of estrogen; however, this has not been conclusively established.

These factors—the much greater incidence in women than men, the work with estrogen in laboratory animals, the high incidence of late menopause, the protection from breast carcinoma afforded by castration in the premenopausal age, the response both to estrogen stimulation and deprivation in metastatic disease, and the increased incidence of cortical stromal hyperplasia of the ovaries in postmenopausal women with breast carcinoma —all favor the biologic presence of an estrogen-stimulated tumor.

Arguments against Prophylactic Oophorectomy

There is no statistically significant series of random cases available to support the claims of the beneficial effects of prophylactic bilateral oophorectomy. There are several such studies being conducted at the present time that should give us more definite answers in the near future.

A favorable response to therapeutic castration is the most reliable method currently available for selection of candidates for adrenalectomy or hypophysectomy in women with metastatic carcinoma of the breast. This is demonstrated in the report of the Joint Committee on Endocrine Ablative Procedures in Disseminated Mammary Carcinoma. In the group of patients who showed an objective regression after oophorectomy, 45 per cent had a second regression after adrenalectomy or hypophysectomy; however, among the nonresponders to oophorectomy there was only an 11 per cent favorable response.

The disadvantages of an early menopause are well known. In our experience we have had little difficulty controlling symptoms with mild sedatives and reassurance. It is our impression that the patients are so pleased that everything is being done to afford them a cure for their cancer that few complain of any ill effects of their castration.

There is the occasional case that may flare up after oophorectomy; however, there is only one report in the literature of three cases, and although there are doubtless a few more unreported or unrecognized, this must be a rare occurrence.

There is also a suggestive difference in the incidence of earlier and more extensive development of arteriosclerosis in surgically castrated women. This has not been confirmed, however.

Selection of Patients

We recommend surgical castration as an adjunct to radical mastectomy in all women with operable carcinoma of the breast in the premenopausal and menopausal age groups up to and including five years postmenopausal. We have extended this to five years following cessation of menstruation because of the high level of estrogen that frequently persists to that period of time.

We use the menstrual history as our sole determinant. If this has been stopped artificially and ovarian function is still present, we recommend castration through age 55 years.

Technique

We are particularly careful to discuss this procedure in detail with the patient before operation.

The oophorectomy is carried out with a new operative setup during the completion of the mastectomy while the assistant is closing the wound. This adds approximately 20 minutes to the procedure, obviates a second anesthesia and operation, and gives the patient the early beneficial effect of estrogen deprivation.

We favor surgical removal of the ovaries since x-ray may be unreliable and is delayed in its effect. With ovarian irradiation, the urinary estrogen levels usually fall to a low level in 80 to 130 days but may take over 140 days. Despite the cessation of uterine bleeding, significant amounts of estrogen may still be present. Surgical removal is more definitive, and the urinary excretion of estrogen falls to low, often immeasurable, levels in 48 to 72 hours.

Results

It is important to emphasize again that no statistically significant series of random cases has been published. All series have been small except several recent publications in which ovarian irradiation was used. In consideration of all published cases, in which either x-ray or surgical castration was performed prophylactically as an adjunct to radical mastectomy, the five-year survival rates compared to radical mastectomy alone show an overall improvement of 5 per cent to 20 per cent with a mean of approximately 10 per cent. There is less data at 10 years but apparently this improvement is maintained.

Summary

We have presented the arguments for and against prophylactic bilateral oophorectomy as an adjunct to radical mastectomy in the treatment of all operable cases of adenocarcinoma of the breast in the premenopausal and menopausal age groups, including the first five years postmenopausal.

The advantages of bilateral oophorectomy being carried out at the time of the radical mastectomy have been stressed.

The benefits of surgical castration as opposed to ovarian irradiation have been discussed.

The results have been presented emphasizing the fact that to date no statistically significant series of random cases has been published. This reemphasizes the importance of such a study.

Conclusion

On the basis of our present-day knowledge and experience, we believe prophylactic oophorectomy as an adjunct to radical mastectomy is of definite benefit to the patient.

References

1. Alrich, E. M., and P. Hairston: Carcinoma of the Breast: Prophylactic Oophorectomy. Trans. of South. Surg. Assoc., 74:178, 1963.
2. Block, G. E., A. B. Vial and F. W. Pullen: Estrogen excretion following operative and irradiation castration in cases of mammary cancer. Surgery, 43:415, 1958.
3. Cole, M. P.: The Value of Ovarian Irradiation in the Management of Breast Cancer. Paper presented at the Symposium on the Prognosis of Malignant Tumors of the Breast, Paris, 1962.
4. Hirayama, T., and E. L. Wynder: A study of the epidemiology of cancer of the breast: II. The influence of hysterectomy. Cancer, 15:28, 1962.
5. Horsley, G. W.: Treatment of cancer of the breast in premenopausal patients with radical amputation and bilateral oophorectomy. Ann. Surg., 125:703, 1947.
6. Horsley, J. S.: Bilateral oophorectomy with radical operation for cancer of the breast. Surgery, 15:590, 1944.
7. Horsley, J. S., III, and G. W. Horsley: Twenty years' experience with prophylactic bilateral oophorectomy in the treatment of carcinoma of the breast. Ann. Surg., 155:935, 1962.
8. Jessiman, A. G., and F. D. Moore: Carcinoma of the breast: the study and treatment of the patient. New England J. Med., 254:846, 900, 947, 1956.

9. Lewison, E. F.: Prophylactic versus therapeutic castration in the total treatment of breast cancer. Obs. and Gynec. Survey, *17*:769, 1962.

10. MacDonald, I.: Endocrine ablation in disseminated mammary carcinoma. Surg., Gynec. and Obst., *115*:215, 1962.

11. Marcus, C. C.: Ovarian cortical stromal hyperplasia and carcinoma of the endometrium. Obst. Gynec., *21*:175, 1963.

12. Novak, E. R., and Williams, T. J.: Autopsy comparison of cardiovascular changes in the castrate and normal woman. Am. J. Obst. and Gynec., *80*:863, 1960.

13. Paterson, R., and Russell, M. H.: Clinical trials in malignant disease. Part II. Breast cancer, value of irradiation of the ovaries. J. Fac. Radiol., London, *10*:130, 1959.

14. Rosenberg, M. F., and E. M. Uhlmann: Prophylactic castration in carcinoma of the breast. Arch. Surg., *78*:376, 1959.

15. Sommers, S. C., and H. A. Teloh: Ovarian stromal hyperplasia in breast cancer. Arch. Path., *53*:160, 1952.

16. Treves, N.: An evaluation of prophylactic castration in the treatment of mammary carcinoma. Cancer, *10*:393, 1957.

17. Wilson, R. E., Jessiman, A. G., and Moore, F. D.: Severe exacerbation of cancer of the breast after oophorectomy and adrenalectomy. New England J. Med., *258*:312, 1958.

Conservative vs. Operative Management of Severe Nonpenetrating Injuries of the Chest

Introduction

The management of closed chest injuries has and will continue to challenge the judgment and technical skill of surgeons. For purposes of this discussion, conservative treatment will include all therapy, other than operative thoracotomy, that might be required to improve and then to assure normal respiration and circulation; operative treatment, in turn, refers to formal thoracotomy.

Those favoring operative treatment point out that the initial appearance of a patient with nonpenetrating trauma to the chest does not necessarily indicate the extent of the intrathoracic injury, and that unnecessary morbidity and mortality have occurred and continue to occur because of delayed thorough evaluation or lack of aggressiveness in instituting surgical therapy by the responsible physician. The examples cited are numerous and include: intrathoracic rupture of the trachea, laceration or complete separation of a bronchus, severe laceration of a subsegment, segment, or lobe of the lung, either with or without intrapulmonary hematoma, tear of the diaphragm, and finally, rupture of the thoracic aorta.

Those favoring conservative management find it difficult to justify routine or frequent thoracotomy for the sake of the occasional patient when simpler methods will provide effective therapy for most.

One should realize that there is complete agreement that initial treatment of severe closed chest injuries should include not only adequate replacement of diminished blood volume, but also all those measures required to assure adequate ventilation, including laryngoscopy or bronchoscopy, or both, with aspiration of the tracheobronchial tree and, when necessary, tracheostomy. Both advocate stabilization of a flaccid chest wall and employ needle aspiration or closed intercostal catheter drainage for hemopneumothorax.

The only point of disagreement, therefore, lies in the ultimate management of these patients, and arguments for both sides are well presented by the authors.

E. H. E.

Definitive Treatment
of Severe Closed Chest Injuries

K. P. Klassen

Ohio State University College of Medicine

Nonpenetrating injuries of the chest bring to the emergency room patients whose excellent clinical appearance shortly after the accident frequently does not indicate the severity of the intrathoracic trauma or allow for prognostication without a complete and thorough evaluation of each case. A compressive force or sudden de-acceleration may produce tracheal or bronchial rupture, laceration of the lung and diaphragm, and complete severance of the thoracic aorta without suggestive findings on preliminary physical examination. Patients with nonpenetrating thoracic injuries have succumbed in the emergency room because of delayed thorough evaluation or lack of aggressiveness in instituting surgical therapy by the examining physician.

Much can be learned by a rapid determination of the circumstances of the accident and the forces producing the injury. Sudden de-acceleration, with the patient facing the direction of motion, will exert a tremendous force from the sternum to the spine, producing compressive, shearing, and tearing injuries of some or all intrathoracic organs depending on the physical nature of the object immediately in front of the thorax. Sudden compressive forces, such as explosions, compression between heavy objects, and falls from great heights, will produce similar forces and injuries.

The external appearance of the patient at first glance permits rapid evaluation of the case. State of consciousness, cyanosis, pallor, patency of the airway, and the ventilating function of the thorax are appreciated at a glance, while pulse rate, blood pressure, altered breath sounds, dullness, and mediastinal shift are noted on rapid physical examination. In cases of dyspnea and cyanosis, laryngoscopy and bronchoscopy must be performed to determine the cause of the airway obstruction and to aspirate the tracheal and bronchial fluid. An upright film of the chest is obtained, and blood is drawn for hemoglobin and hematocrit determination and crossmatching. The briefly outlined evaluation of the patient takes only a few minutes, but may establish the diagnosis and set the stage for definitive surgical intervention. In general, efforts must be directed toward restoration of a patent airway, effective ventilation, and adequate blood volume.

Patency of Airway

Obstruction of the airway is immediately apparent. Respiratory stridor and intercostal retraction are usually present. Blood in the nasopharynx may originate from facial injuries. If no source is found, laryngoscopy and bronchoscopy with repeated aspiration will establish the site of bleeding of the tracheobronchial tree. Tracheal and bronchial lacerations can be diagnosed readily by such endoscopic procedures. In the absence of such injury, aspiration of the blood and vomitus from the trachea and bronchi will solve the airway problem.

Hemoptysis is usually present, although blood may be absent in the tracheobronchial tree, with laceration and complete tear of a major bronchus. Subcutaneous emphysema of the anterior mediastinum and chest wall appears early, and sometimes bilateral pneumothorax may be present. Upright films of the chest will demonstrate mediastinal and subcutaneous emphysema. The presence of mediastinal, subcutaneous emphysema and pneumothorax by itself does not indicate tracheobronchial disruption or laceration; this finding, more frequently, is the result of rib fractures with laceration of the lung. Adequate intercostal catheter suction will bring about rapid expansion of the lung when air leakage is due to laceration of the lung, while in bronchial tear and disruption, the lung will remain collapsed. The failure of the lung to expand with adequate intercostal suction and the endoscopic visualization of laceration and disruption of the trachea or bronchus will establish the diagnosis without difficulty.

The treatment of tracheobronchial tears or lacerations must be accomplished in the immediate post-trauma period to prevent prolonged morbidity, subsequent stenosis, and difficult reparative procedures. Neglected bronchial trauma may lead to destruction of the involved lung, eventually requiring resection. Laceration of the cervical trachea is usually incomplete, and immediate repair can be accomplished through a low transverse neck incision with intratracheal intubation. A sternotomy may be necessary for adequate exposure. A tracheostomy is established distal to the repair for postoperative aspiration of the tracheobronchial tree as well as for protection of the repaired trachea from cough pressure. In such injuries, there usually is no loss of tracheal substance, and no difficulties are encountered in primary closure and maintenance of tracheal patency.

Intrathoracic rupture of the trachea may not be associated with pneumothorax. The diagnosis is established by endoscopy, and intubation of the trachea is performed upon recognition of the rupture. A right thoracotomy gives best access to the trachea and is performed through a posterolateral incision through the periosteum of the fifth rib. The necks of the fourth and fifth ribs are sectioned, giving excellent exposure. Repair is performed by direct suture of the defect, using fine silk. Every attempt must be made to utilize the cartilages and fragments of the trachea. Up to three rings can be excised with direct end-to-end anastomosis, while small defects can be bridged with mediastinal pleura and the ligated azygous vein used as a pedicle graft. The mediastinum adjacent to the repair is not closed, and thoracotomy tube drainage is used in the post-operative period. Prompt expansion of the lung will aid in sealing small leaks in the area of anastomosis. The intercostal drainage tubes are removed when the lungs are completely expanded.

Although bronchial laceration of minor degree may escape diagnosis, bronchial rupture, with total separation of the severed ends, can be diagnosed easily by utilizing bronchoscopy and spot film bronchography. Upon diagnosis, intercostal catheter drainage and intratracheal intubation must be established prior to thoracotomy. Suction must be maintained to remove air and blood from the pleural space prior to turning the patient on the contralateral side for the thoracotomy, since flooding of the remaining lung and tension pneumothorax may occur when the anesthetist administers positive pressure.

Upon diagnosis, the repair of the lacerated or completely separated bronchus offers no technical problems. A posterolateral thoracotomy incision is used for adequate exposure. The mediastinum is opened, and bleeding from the bronchial arteries is controlled. Interrupted fine silk sutures are used for repair of the bronchial defect. Reamputation of the bronchial stumps is not necessary, since the tear usually is clean, occasionally leaving the bronchial arteries intact. Mediastinal or parietal pleura is used as sliding or free grafts to reinforce the suture line. The thoracotomy is closed routinely, utilizing an anterior and posterior No. 26 Foley catheter for drainage. These are removed when x-ray films show complete expansion of the lung. A tracheostomy is not mandatory, the intratracheal tube being left in place until the patient is fully conscious with return of his cough reflex. A tracheostomy may contribute toward accidental perforation of the bronchial anastomosis by too vigorous aspiration attempts by untrained personnel in the postoperative period.

Primary repair of lacerated or ruptured bronchi seldom results in stenosis at the site of the anastomosis. In the immediate postoperative period, local edema of the bronchus and bleeding can produce atelectasis of the pulmonary tissue distal to the anastomosis, and may require bronchial aspiration, use of expectorants, and antibiotics.

Adequate Ventilation

Respiratory exchange may become highly ineffective secondary to multiple rib fractures, costosternal separation, and large diaphragmatic tears. The ventilatory mechanism in such closed chest injuries may further be impaired by progressive intrapleural accumulation of blood and air leading to pulmonary compression and mediastinal shift. The respiratory difficulties can readily be ascertained by physical examination and confirmed by an upright film of the chest.

Stabilization of Flaccid Chest

Stabilization of a flaccid chest is usually accomplished by the use of sandbags or the utilization of towel-clip traction of the sternum. Immobilization of the fractured ribs by intercostal suturing with catgut, and by suture of the costal cartilage to the sternum is occasionally utilized when a thoracotomy has been performed for the definitive treatment of intrathoracic injuries.

Prompt Thoracotomy for Hemothorax and Pneumothorax

The initial treatment of hemo- and pneumothorax is essentially the same. Under local anesthesia, a trocar thoracotomy is performed in the sixth interspace, midaxillary line, and a No. 26 French or larger catheter introduced into the pleural space. Suction is established by using a controlled system. Prompt expansion of the lung will occur in most instances, and with approximation of the visceral and parietal pleuras, intercostal, internal mammary, and pulmonary bleeding will stop promptly. In instances of the continuation of bleeding, a thoracotomy is indicated for the definitive treatment of the intrathoracic injury.

Perforated Pleura

Small perforations of the visceral pleura with multiple air leaks, produced by the frequently sharp rib fractures, will seal upon complete expansion of the lung with adequate suction. Severely lacerated subsegments, segments, and lobes are excised, particularly when there is loss of vascular continuity or bronchial laceration. Intrapulmonary hematomas must be evaluated by complete evacuation and removal of severely damaged adjacent parenchyma of the lung. Upon completion of the debridement, increased intratracheal pressure by the anesthesiologist should produce complete aeration of the pulmonary tissue, indicating adequate excision of all severely damaged lung parenchyma. Small air leaks produced during such resection need not be sutured, since they will close with expansion of the lung. Bleeding from an intercostal artery is treated by ligation, while tears in the major pulmonary vessels can be treated by suture repair without loss of vessel continuity.

Chylothorax

Chylothorax following compressive injury of the chest simulates the symptomatology and clinical finding of a hemothorax. The diagnosis is established if chyle is aspirated by thoracentesis. Adequate intercostal suction applied immediately upon recognition has, in our experience, brought about expansion of the lung with sealing of the tear in the thoracic duct. Thoracotomy and ligation of the duct has not been necessary.

Ruptured Diaphragm

Rupture of the diaphragm is usually the result of a compressive force applied to the lower lateral chest wall. Survival in right diaphragmatic tears is infrequent, since it is associated with extensive laceration and rupture of the liver leading to early demise. Left diaphragmatic tear is seen more frequently in the emergency room. It may be associated with severe intra-abdominal bleeding secondary to rupture of the spleen and kidney. The diagnosis of rupture of the diaphragm should be entertained in all cases of splenic rupture. X-ray examination of the chest will indicate a high intrathoracic fluid-gas level, which should be regarded as the intrathoracic stomach or bowel. The differentiation from a traumatic hemopneumothorax is not difficult, since lung markings are present above the fluid level, and air is absent from the upper portion of the thorax. Additional diagnostic procedures that can be performed readily on an emergency basis include contrast studies of the esophagus and stomach. X-ray studies with a radiopaque gastric suction tube in the stomach will also clarify this problem, indicating the intrathoracic position of the stomach. Aspiration of the peritoneum for blood can be followed by the injection of 500 cc. of air, which will clearly demonstrate the continuity of the pleural space with the peritoneal cavity. Repair of the torn diaphragm must be accomplished through a thoracoabdominal incision, which will permit inspection of the abdomen for possible splenic rupture and other injuries.

Rupture of Thoracic Aorta

The most challenging problem in the emergency room is that of rupture of the thoracic aorta. This spectacular injury should be suspected in all automobile drivers involved in rapid de-acceleration accidents. Seat belts do not prevent the compressive force of the steering wheel against the anterior chest wall.

The patient may present himself without symptoms and physical findings. The blood pressure may be normal with some tachycardia. Murmurs usually are absent and the pulsation in the abdominal aorta is quite normal. The injury may be a minimal laceration of the aorta, just distal and anterior to the left subclavian artery, or there may be complete transsection of the aorta at this level. The diagnosis can be established readily.

Progressive widening of the aortic shadow is demonstrated on an upright x-ray film of the chest. The progression of this mediastinal widening may be slow until a break in the mediastinal pleura leads to rapid production of a complete hemothorax and fatal shock. Immediate retrograde aortography, when available, can be utilized to confirm the diagnosis. By this technique, however, the time involved in this procedure and the usual technical inadequacy of such tests, when not done during the routine working hours, contraindicates this procedure in most instances. Obliteration of the aortic arch with progressive widening of the superior mediastinum, in a patient with a steering wheel injury, is sufficient reason for immediate thoracotomy. In our series of eight cases, a correct diagnosis was made in seven patients on the basis of the aforementioned evidence alone; in the eighth patient, the widening of the mediastinum was secondary to fracture of the transverse processes and necks of the second and third ribs on the left, producing a mediastinal hematoma from bleeding intercostal arteries. This condition has been known to progress to massive, fatal hemorrhage while the patient is awaiting an aortogram for confirmation of the diagnosis. The most important factor in the effective treatment of rupture of the aorta is awareness of this condition in steering wheel injuries.

Cardiopulmonary Bypass

Time is of the essence in the surgical treatment of rupture of the aorta. Cardiopulmonary bypass should be made available on diagnosis of rupture of the aorta, and complete cardiovascular instrument sets should be in readiness. Obviously, crossmatching must be performed, and adequate blood must be made available. The thoracotomy should be large and should be performed through the fifth interspace, with section of the third, fourth, and fifth ribs at the neck. This will offer adequate exposure for the superior mediastinum. When the mediastinum is opened, the laceration is found without difficulty. Simple lacerations with a small bleeding point can be controlled with finger pressure until the aortic arch has been immobilized. Umbilical tapes are placed between the left common carotid and subclavian arteries and distal to the tear of the aorta. When the injury is limited to laceration of the aorta up to half its circumference, a partially occluding aortic clamp is placed on the aorta, and the aorta is repaired by direct suturing with fine silk. Dacron felt can be used to reinforce the repair of the aorta. In cases of complete rupture of the aorta, umbilical tapes are secured and clamps placed both proximal and distal to the rupture. Bypass is prepared by utilizing the left atrium and femoral artery. Occasionally, the subclavian artery can be used for a bypass should the cardiac pump bypass setup not be available. We have also occluded the aorta for as long as fifteen minutes without difficulty; this permitted the insertion of an intraluminal tube over which the aorta was repaired.

Summary

The appearance of a patient with nonpenetrating trauma to the chest does not necessarily indicate the extent of the intrathoracic injury or its potentiality. In upper airway obstruction, endoscopy serves to establish the cause of this difficulty and leads to proper treatment. Interference with normal ventilation due to collapse of the lung and shift of the mediastinum by accumulating air or blood can be treated initially by adequate intercostal catheter suction. When this procedure fails to completely expand the lung with control of the air leakage and bleeding, thoracotomy is indicated for definitive repair. In patients with superior mediastinal widening following trauma to the chest, rupture of the aorta should be suspected, and immediate thoracotomy for the repair of the laceration of the aorta is indicated.

Conservative Management
of Severe Closed Chest Injuries

Leonard W. Worman

Marquette University School of Medicine

The conservative management of thoracic trauma encompasses all those measures short of formal thoracotomy that are necessary to restore or maintain ventilation and circulation. These measures can be described by the term, "resuscitation."[4] Any procedure that places an increased burden on the two vital functions of ventilation and circulation must be undertaken cautiously, since they are already necessarily in peril from thoracic trauma. For this reason, and in spite of the enviable record of safety now achieved in the performance of routine thoracotomy, it is difficult to justify routine thoracotomy in the treatment of chest trauma for the sake of the occasional patient when simpler methods will provide effective therapy for most patients. The surgeon's ability to perform an operation is not an indication for surgery. At the Milwaukee County Hospital, a continued emphasis on the nonoperative management of thoracic trauma has not prevented prompt surgical therapy in those instances where the injuries made thoracotomy necessary.[5] Blunt trauma to the thorax produces a variety of injuries, many of which require immediate treatment.

Maintenance of Ventilation

Closed Intercostal Catheter Drainage

Pneumothorax occurs commonly. A large-bore needle thrust into the affected hemithorax will occasionally be a necessary lifesaving maneuver for the relief of tension pneumothorax. More routinely, closed intercostal catheter drainage is used to restore normal intrapleural pressures and empty the pleural space of both blood and air. Under these conditions bleeding from the two most commonly injured structures, the chest wall and the lung, is rarely a continuing problem. Pneumothorax following blunt chest trauma is usually the result of minor damage to the lung. As a rule the air leak is quickly sealed by reparative processes of the pulmonary tissue; the

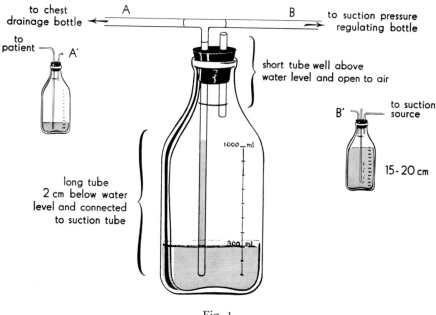

to chest
drainage bottle

A

B

to suction pressure
regulating bottle

to
patient

A'

short tube well above
water level and open to air

B'

to suction
source

1000 _ ml

15-20 cm

long tube
2 cm below water
level and connected
to suction tube

300 ml

Fig. 1

necessity for surgical intervention to close a ruptured bronchus is the
rare exception. With a large air leak the addition of suction will be necessary to keep the lung expanded. The vacuum cleaner type pleural suction
pump has the necessary high instantaneous flow rate and is safe. Other
machines and wall suction form a closed system if mechanical or power
failure occurs. For this reason a safety vent[3] is necessary if they are used
(Fig. 1). The pleural space empty of everything but the properly expanded
lung is not likely to become infected.

Thoracentesis

Where hemothorax is present without pneumothorax, thoracentesis
is indicated and should be repeated if necessary. Usually hemostasis will
have occurred, and sufficient blood can be removed to eliminate the late
problem of lung entrapment. The danger of infection is perhaps less with
thoracentesis than with closed intercostal catheter drainage. Aspiration is
not a very satisfactory way to treat pneumothorax due to trauma because
complete expansion is difficult, the air leak requires more time to seal
itself than is true of clotting in a vascular leak, and one is more likely to
injure the lung with the needle, thus compounding the problem.

Intercostal Nerve Blocks

Local anesthesia to the intercostal nerves effectively relieves chest wall
pain, thereby restoring the mobility necessary for ventilation and effectively
preventing the suppression of the normal cough reflex. Where the latter

reason is the more important, such a pain-free interval once in 24 hours usually seems to be sufficient.

Clear Tracheobronchial Tree

The removal of secretions from the tracheobronchial tree is an absolute necessity. If coughing alone will not suffice, intermittent suction by catheter should be used. If these measures are ineffective, bronchoscopy will be necessary.

Tracheostomy

Tracheostomy may or may not effectively decrease functional dead space and the work of ventilation,[2] but it does diminish the peak intraluminal pressure and will therefore decrease the air leak from an injured bronchus. Tracheostomy is indicated most often in the treatment of blunt thoracic trauma to aid in the removal of secretions and to permit assisted ventilation by means of a mechanical respirator, either volume or pressure controlled. In the latter instance a cuff on the tracheostomy tube is a necessary adjunct. The operation can be efficiently done at the bedside through a small neat transverse incision.

Respirator Assisted Ventilation

This may be mandatory in the treatment of the injured patient with pre-existing pulmonary disease. Standard oxygen therapy is a poor substitute for assisted ventilation in the chest trauma patient. Assisted ventilation is a most useful method of therapy for the patient with a flail chest.

Stabilization of the Flailing Chest Wall

This must be accomplished by traction if respirator-assisted ventilation is not used. Internal fixation requires extensive dissection and is generally ineffective; therefore it is not an indication for thoracotomy.

Maintenance of Circulation

Pericardiocentesis

Pericardial tamponade is a rare complication of blunt chest trauma. A paradoxical pulse is occasionally seen in patients with grunting respirations due to thoracic wall pain, but an elevated venous pressure and a falling arterial blood pressure should make one consider acute pericardial tamponade. Aspiration from the xiphocostal angle is simple and safe—removal of 25 to 50 ml. of blood should give relief. This amount of blood accidentally taken from the ventricle would be of little consequence. If symptoms should recur in a period of hours the procedure can be repeated. However, blood in the pericardium indicates the presence of a significant injury, and resuscitation is best continued in the operating room since early thoracotomy may be necessary.

Replenishing the Blood Volume

This is necessary to restore and maintain circulation. Continued hemorrhage that cannot be simply controlled is the only indication for using uncrossmatched 0-negative blood. The need for 0-negative blood transfusion is rare in blunt thoracic trauma. Frequently, the plasma expanders that are administered while appropriately crossmatched blood is being obtained will restore the blood pressure and pulse to normal. The problem of pulmonary edema's occurring in the course of therapy for shock in these patients is sometimes over-emphasized. Measurement of central venous pressure is a guide that will permit rapid and adequate transfusion with safety.

Since it is the recorded observation of many surgeons that these resuscitative measures frequently suffice to control the result of injury to the chest, they must be considered definitive measures. There would seem to be several other good reasons for emphasizing the nonoperative management of blunt thoracic trauma. Nonoperative measures do not require elaborate equipment. They are easily grasped in principle and simply accomplished in practice, even when taught to physicians outside the field of thoracic surgery. The need to make generally available an efficient therapy for a common problem cannot be ignored. Also, a significant number of patients with thoracic trauma will require operative intervention for the proper therapy of concomitant extrathoracic injuries (Fig. 2). Routine thoracotomy would thus place the patient in double jeopardy.

While initial examination does not often demonstrate the need for early thoracotomy, the possible necessity for early operation should always be considered, and when indicated the approach must be aggressive. Failure of initial resuscitative measures indicates the need for further careful evaluation. Continued bleeding and contamination of the mediastinal and pleural spaces from a damaged esophagus constitute urgent needs for thoracotomy.[5] A continued air leak may indicate the need for thoracotomy, but if the measures already outlined are used, it is difficult to conceive of the need as urgent.

The progress of resuscitation is monitored by recording frequent repeated familiar observations; the blood pressure, pulse, and respiratory rate are the most important. The character of the breath sounds, the skin color, and the temperature are also useful. Hemoglobin and hematocrit changes are not useful indices early in the course of therapy, since they are measures of concentration, and the rate of change depends on the shift of fluid between compartments—not upon the rate of hemorrhage. Parenthetically it is frequently forgotten that infusions of plasma will lower the hemoglobin and hematocrit, and overzealous transfusion has

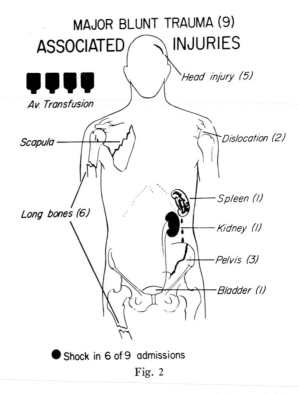

Fig. 2

produced pulmonary edema when the decreased hemoglobin is then mistakenly attributed to mean a volume deficit. Simple manometric measure of central venous pressure is the most useful guide to blood replacement. Blood volume determinations are cumbersome and probably inaccurate in the presence of shock.[1] The rate of bleeding is conveniently measured by noting the rate of drainage accumulating in the chest catheter drainage bottle. The efficiency of drainage is determined by repeated upright portable chest x-rays, which should be employed without shame in this age of modern electronic miracles. The instruments for the measurement of arterial blood pH, pCO_2 and oxygen saturation are rapidly becoming generally available, and the physician should become familiar with them since, at the moment, they represent the most precise index of the adequacy of ventilation and circulation.

Case Report

The following case report is illustrative of the role of conservative therapy in the treatment of serious blunt thoracic trauma.

A 61 year old white male was admitted to the Milwaukee County Hospital on Christmas Eve, 1963, following an automobile accident. There were multiple rib fractures on the right, with extensive subcutaneous emphysema present over the upper half of the body. Chest x-ray showed complete pneumothorax. Closed intercostal catheter drainage was instituted in the emergency room, and a repeat chest film showed the lung expanded. The chest wall was stable, and with intercostal nerve blocks ventilation was adequate. A diagnosis of chronic obstructive emphysema was based on the presence of an increased anterior-posterior diameter of the chest, plus the history of chronic, usually nonproductive cough and moderate dyspnea brought on by mild exertion. Air leak ceased in 12 hours, and the chest tube was removed on the morning of December 26. That evening the patient experienced rather severe respiratory difficulty, and following this a mild flailing of the right chest developed. A chest x-ray showed recurrence of the pneumothorax. Simple traction with one towel clip stabilized the chest wall. The chest tube was reinserted. A diagnosis of ruptured bronchus, originally rejected in view of the known diagnosis of pulmonary emphysema and probable cystic changes, was again entertained; however, the patient did well, and the air leak again stopped in 12 hours. On December 28, a tracheostomy was done to aid in the removal of secretions which had not initially been a problem. On December 30, the patient became nauseated and restless. Examination showed a blood pressure of 60/30, a pulse of 120. Melena was present and blood was obtained by nasogastric tube. Further history compatible with a chronic peptic ulcer was elicited. The blood pressure and pulse returned quickly to normal with the use of whole blood. However, melena continued, and on December 31 suture hemostasis of a chronic duodenal ulcer was necessary, and a vagotomy and pyloroplasty were done. Bronchoscopy was done with this anesthesia, and a 1 cm. laceration of the right upper lobe bronchus, apparently now sealed, was demonstrated. Respirator-assisted ventilation was necessary to maintain arterial blood pH, pO_2, and pCO_2 near normal for the next two weeks. The abdominal wound partly dehisced on the sixth day and evisceration occurred on the seventh postoperative day, making secondary closure necessary. The patient survived and was discharged on the twenty-first hospital day.

Thoracotomy would have enabled us to suture the bronchus, which sealed itself, and to remove a sizable cyst, which previous x-rays, finally obtained, show to have been present for years. In this patient with a chronic duodenal ulcer which bled massively, thoracotomy would not seem to be the necessary operation of choice.

Even while emphasizing the nonoperative management of chest trauma, it is possible to recognize early the indications for thoracotomy necessary to successfully manage esophageal, aortic, and cardiac injuries.[5]

Summary

The choice of the nonoperative versus the operative management of chest trauma is possible only in a restricted sense. Even in civilian practice the physician will encounter some injuries for which only formal thoracotomy will suffice to repair the damage to vital tissues and organs. However, in spite of some arguments to the contrary, a continued emphasis of the nonoperative management of most chest injuries is both logically and experientially sound.

References

1. McLean, L. D.: Blood volume versus central venous pressure in shock. Surg., Gynec. and Obst., *118*:594, 1964.

2. Maloney, J. V., and McDonald, L.: Treatment of blunt trauma to the thorax. Am. J. Surg., *105*:484, 1963.
3. Narodick, B. G.: Personal communication.
4. Shefts, L. M.: The Initial Management of Thoracic and Thoraco-abdominal Trauma. Springfield, Ill., Charles C Thomas, 1956, pp. 3–25.
5. Worman, L. W., Narodick, B. G., and Pemberton, A. H.: Treatment of chest trauma: indications for thoracotomy. J. Trauma, 2:544, 1962.

Cholecystectomy
in Acute Cholecystitis

Introduction

In the first chapter of the first issue of Current Surgical Management (1957), the controversy regarding the "timing" of operation (early versus delayed) in acute cholecystitis is presented. Another controversial aspect of the surgical management of acute cholecystitis is apparent when one considers the method of carrying out a cholecystectomy when the disease is in its acute phase. In addition to the "how to do it" argument there is also the question of "what to do" operatively for these acutely ill patients. Well trained surgeons ought to be facile in doing a cholecystectomy from either of the approaches which are supported in this section, i.e., from fundus to porta, or from porta to fundus. Some surgeons are explicit in their choice and rigidly hold to one of the approaches in acute cholecystitis, others have a definite preference for one over the other but do not exclude the use of the other in some instances, and of course other surgeons do not seem to have a strong preference either way.

It behooves the good surgeon to realize that certain features of operative intervention in acute cholecystitis must be kept in mind—that the appreciation of the pathologic changes in the acute stage of the disease, the awareness that anomalies may be present, and good exposure of the operative field all are mandatory for either approach to cholecystectomy. Secondary only to the primary mission of saving the life of the patient who is acutely ill with substantiated acute cholecystitis is the ever-present obligation of the surgeon consciously to use all his skill in avoiding injury to the main bile ducts with the resultant catastrophe of bile duct stricture.

The personal reasons for preference for each of the surgical approaches to cholecystectomy are presented in this chapter by two surgeons. Both very appropriately emphasize, in addition, that cholecystostomy in certain patients with acute cholecystitis not only is lifesaving, but also is a preventive to traumatic stricture of the bile ducts.

S. R. F.

Cholecystectomy from Porta to Fundus

John L. Madden

St. Clare's Hospital, New York

Before I present my case for the porta-to-fundus cholecystectomy, I should like to discuss certain aspects of cholecystectomy that are generally considered important.

Today, cholecystectomy is one of the most, if not the most, common of all abdominal operations. It is also an operation that may be simple to perform in one patient, but supremely challenging in another.

Anomalies Encountered in Cholecystectomy

Anomalies of the bile ducts and their related vascular structures are so common that the surgeon should consider the anatomy of the region abnormal until proved otherwise. This is also good psychologic preparation for the surgeon in the event that an anomaly is present.

Whenever the performance of a cholecystectomy appears unusually simple, we should pause and take inventory because of the increased likelihood of an anomaly being present. The long, thin, and easily accessible "cystic duct," which is about to be clamped may prove to be the common bile duct. Unfortunately it is almost always the "simplest cholecystectomy that I have ever done" that results postoperatively in a traumatic stricture. It is for this reason that the term "simple cholecystectomy" should not be used at the time of operation. It applies only to the patient whose postoperative course proves completely uneventful.

The high incidence of biliary tract anomalies makes it mandatory to identify absolutely each structure before it is clamped or severed. The cystic duct should not be ligated until the common hepatic duct cephalad and the common bile duct caudad are each clearly seen. Similarly, the right hepatic artery, which is so commonly located anterior instead of posterior to the common hepatic duct, is isolated routinely as an anatomic landmark. When this artery is lateral to the common duct, it is an indication that it has its origin from the superior mesenteric artery rather than the celiac axis. This pattern obtained in approximately 10 per cent of 200 dissected cadaver specimens.[3]

Characteristically the right hepatic artery forms a convex arch from the summit of which one, and occasionally two, cystic arteries arise. In some patients the tortuous right hepatic artery may be in close approximation to the ampullary region of the gallbladder, and if narrow in diameter, it may be mistaken for the cystic artery. Under such circumstances the real cystic artery is usually short and narrow. In fact, it may prove so short as to preclude the double application of clamps. Furthermore, despite the isolation and ligation of a large cystic artery, the possibility of encountering an additional cystic artery during the removal of the gallbladder from its "bed" should always be considered.

Whether the gallbladder is removed from the porta to the fundus or by the reverse technique, the presence of one or more bile ducts between the gallbladder and the liver is always a possibility. When present, these ducts are commonly called aberrant. However, the frequency with which they are found belies the term.

Routine Use of Drain

Finally, a drain is always used. It is surprising how frequently copious bile drainage is observed on the wound dressings in patients in whom the operative field was unusually "dry" preceding the wound closure. Admittedly, in my own experience, the decision not to use a drain is compatible with an uneventful postoperative convalescence. However, the risk to the patient is believed too great to justify this practice. Accordingly, the use of a drain routinely is both recommended and practiced.

The exit of the drain is through the wound, the site varying in the individual patient. This is usually in its mid portion. This practice has proved completely satisfactory, although it is believed that stab-wound drainage lateral to the incision is generally preferred.

Choice of Incision

The incision used will depend upon the preference of the individual surgeon. Regardless of the choice, the basic requirement for any incision is adequacy of exposure.

The Kocher or subcostal incision is universally popular. Many surgeons prefer the transverse incision, particularly in the relatively obese patient with a wide subcostal angle. More recently Holman[1] has repopularized the use of the Kehr incision. However, my own preference is the obliquely longitudinal muscle-splitting incision described by Masson[2] and commonly referred to as the Mayo incision. This incision begins in the right costoxiphoid angle and proceeds obliquely downward to terminate just below and approximately 2 cm. to the right of the umbilicus. For many years the whole of the thickness of the right rectus muscle was retracted laterally, both to lessen the bleeding and to maintain the nerve supply. However, separation of the muscle along the plane of junction of its inner and middle thirds has proved preferable, even though, theoretically, it is less acceptable both anatomically and physiologically.

Choice of Technique

In the performance of a cholecystectomy, the removal of the gallbladder from the porta to the fundus is preferred. However, before further discussion of this preference, the statement must be immediately qualified.

The operation should always be adapted to the immediate and particular requirements of the individual patient and not the patient to a single type of operation. Accordingly, in some patients the findings at operation may preclude the removal of the gallbladder from the porta to the fundus and necessitate its removal from the fundus to the porta. Therefore, the surgeon who undertakes the operation should be able to perform both techniques equally well. In general, however, the findings at operation usually permit the surgeon to perform the technique of election.

There are occasions when a cholecystostomy should be performed rather than a cholecystectomy. This applies regardless of the experience and technical skill of the surgeon. One should never be ashamed to perform a cholecystostomy. Its performance is more often an expression of mature surgical judgment than a lack of surgical skill. The admonition that a living patient may always be operated upon a second time should never be forgotten.

The preference for the porta-to-fundus (retrograde) technique to the fundus-to-porta (antegrade) technique is based on a comparative experience with both methods.

Advantages of Porta-to-Fundus Technique

The advantages of using the porta-to-fundus technique are:

1. The dissection of the cystic duct and related structures is begun in an unobscured and relatively bloodless field.

2. Preliminary ligation and severance of the cystic artery lessens the degree of blood loss during the removal of the gallbladder from its liver "bed."

3. The relatively avascular plane of cleavage between the gallbladder and liver is readily obtained after the cystic duct and cystic artery are ligated and transected.

4. The accidental perforation of the gallbladder during its dissection is less apt to occur.

5. Peritoneal flaps for closure of the liver "bed" are easily formed.

6. The upward traction on the gallbladder as it is being dissected permits a clear exposure of its liver "bed." Accordingly, the so-called aberrant ducts and blood vessels may be readily seen and disposed of as required.

7. When the gallbladder is completely mobilized except for the peritoneal attachment of the fundus to the liver, it may be hung over the wound margin as a traction weight. This facilitates both the inspection of the liver "bed" and the insertion of sutures as needed for hemostasis.

8. There is less danger of dislodging stones from the gallbladder into the common bile duct.

9. When exploration of the common duct is indicated, the isolation and preliminary ligation of the cystic duct is readily performed. This prevents the subsequent passage of gallbladder stones into the common duct after exploration of the common duct is completed. Furthermore, the use of the gallbladder for traction provides a technical expediency and facilitates the common duct exploration.

10. The removal of the gallbladder is surgically clean and not messy as it is based on the primary control of the blood supply and the adequacy of exposure of the gallbladder "bed."

The disadvantage of the porta-to-fundus method is that in some patients there may be extensive inflammatory tissue reaction about the porta which would interdict its use. At times, however, the same interdiction also may apply to the fundus-to-porta technique and permit only the performance of a cholecystostomy.

Fundus-to-Porta Technique

The proclaimed advantage of the fundus-to-porta technique is that it lessens the chance of injury to the common duct or the right hepatic artery. That this is applicable, particularly in the patient with inflammatory induration about the porta, is readily admitted. However, I think it should be emphasized that the common bile duct and the right hepatic artery, either alone or combined, can be and have been injured during the removal of the gallbladder from above-downward. This technique does not provide a magic formula, and its use demands the same precautions as observed in a cholecystectomy from below-upward.

The disadvantages in the fundus-to-porta technique for cholecystectomy are the direct opposites of the advantages for the porta-to-fundus technique previously listed.

Conclusion

This controversy may be concluded by stating that regardless of the technique employed for cholecystectomy, a thorough grounding in surgical anatomy, the acquisition of basic technical skills, mature surgical judgment, and alertness throughout the operation are essential.

References

1. Holman, E.: An incisional approach for cholecystectomy and choledochotomy designed to reduce injury to the common duct. Surg., Gynec. and Obst., 97:344, 1953.
2. Masson, J. C.: Exposure in gallbladder surgery. Ann. Surg., 69:422, 1919.
3. Michels, N. A.: Blood Supply and Anatomy of the Upper Abdominal Organs. Philadelphia, J. B. Lippincott Company, 1955.

Fundus-to-Porta
Technique in Cholecystectomy

Stanley O. Hoerr

The Cleveland Clinic Foundation

Advantages of Fundus-to-Porta Cholecystectomy

The nature of the pathologic process in acute cholecystitis explains my preference for a fundus-downward removal of the gallbladder. In nine out of ten patients the cause of acute cholecystitis is a gallstone, usually impacted in the cystic duct. There follows not only the characteristic tense swelling of the gallbladder itself, with marked edema of the gallbladder wall, and adherence of omentum and intestines (in the later phases) to the gallbladder, but also intense inflammation in the tissues surrounding the cystic duct and its junction with the common bile duct. A relatively prompt result is the obscuring of this vital junction and that of the junction of the cystic artery and the hepatic artery. Since accidental occlusion of the hepatic artery or its right branch may be fatal within a few days, and an unrecognized injury of the common bile duct may produce protracted suffering as well as a delayed fatality, the surgeon is at some pains to avoid these mishaps. Three features of fundus-down cholecystectomy render these accidents less likely to occur:

1. *The gallbladder is eliminated as a source of interference with exposure.* The critical areas of the junction of cystic duct and common bile duct, and the junction of cystic artery and hepatic artery, lie cephalad to the perpendicular projection of gallbladder and right lobe of liver toward the spine. Without retraction, the hands of the surgeon working in this area are beneath the overhang of liver and gallbladder. He is thus hindered by an oblique view of these areas, or must depend on traction inferiorly (toward the feet of the patient) of the proximal gallbladder, and retraction cephalad of fundus of gallbladder and liver, with resulting distortion of normal anatomic relationships.

In a careful fundus-down cholecystectomy, the liver is more easily retracted cephalad, a clamp on the fundus acts as a handle for retraction inferiorly, and as the critical areas are approached exposure gets better and

Page 102

better and direct visibility is accomplished. This dissection is always preceded by trocar decompression of the gallbladder to facilitate the application of clamps.

Bleeding from the gallbladder fossa—cited as the major disadvantage of cholecystectomy prior to control of the principal blood supply—almost invariably is checked by the pressure of a malleable retractor placed over narrow sponges in the fossa. Occasional sutures may be of help. Bleeding from the gallbladder itself may be controlled by hemostats.

Dissection must be carefully done—millimeter by millimeter—and it must stay close to the wall of the gallbladder. In some instances it may be wise to open the gallbladder widely in order to guide this dissection. If cystic artery is cut before it is recognized, it will be at a safe distance from the hepatic artery or its right branch. The same applies to the cystic duct—if it should be very short, cutting into it or the heptaic duct before recognition does not produce irretrievable injury.

2. Junction of ducts and vessels are visualized from the more favorable side. The cystic duct forms a sharp angle with the common bile duct, proximally (cephalad), in contrast to the obtuse angle formed when viewed from the inferior side. It is easier to confuse common bile duct with cystic duct when it is viewed from the distal (inferior) side (right hand side of the surgeon standing on the patient's right side), where they often seem to join in a smooth, confluent fashion. When viewed from the left hand or cephalad side, however, the junction can hardly be missed. *The dissection MUST enter the "crotch" of the junction when carried out in this direction, whether hepatic duct or cystic duct is being dissected, and accidental division of the hepatic duct is thereby avoided.*

3. Cystic artery and cystic duct are identified first and followed to their sources. A sound surgical principle is to proceed from the known to the unknown when anatomy is obscured. In fundus-to-porta cholecystectomy the gallbladder is identified first, then the cystic artery and cystic duct from their junction with the gallbladder, and finally the junction of cystic duct and hepatic duct. (The cystic artery should be ligated as close to gallbladder as possible.) Proceeding in this fashion, *cystic duct may be divided at any convenient point even without positive identification of common bile duct,* and with confidence that common bile duct or hepatic duct has not been encountered.

I was originally taught to remove the gallbladder starting with the isolation, ligation, and division of the cystic vessels and the cystic duct. Having learned that in the so-called difficult gallbladder it was actually easier as well as less nervewracking to start with the fundus and work toward cystic vessels and cystic duct, I have used fundus-down cholecystectomy more and more frequently; I now employ the other method only when deliberately showing a resident a procedure that I feel he should know exists.

Although I use fundus-down cholecystectomy virtually for all cholecystectomies, there are differences in the objectives of surgery for acute cholecystitis which makes this technique especially valuable. In elective operations for gallstones the objective is the removal of the gallbladder. The physical condition of the patient should be at its peak, and the timing of the operation should assure minimum active inflammation in the operative area. Cholecystectomy is thus almost always accomplished with safety irrespective of the method used, and the common bile duct explored if indicated. If technical difficulties arise, the surgeon should have no reluctance in taking extra time to solve them. In operating for acute cholecystitis, on the other hand, the primary objective is saving a life by decompression of the gallbladder. The fact that the gallbladder may be safely removed in most patients does not alter this primary mission.

Indications for Cholecystostomy

In some patients the surgeon will plan deliberately to perform a cholecystostomy, intending to follow this with a cholecystectomy at a later date. In other patients, however, the decision to perform a cholecystostomy may be made during the operation. The reasons for such a decision will be either (1) deterioration of the patient during the operation (from blood loss or prolonged surgery) or (2) unexpected difficulty in identifying the vital structures to be preserved. In attempted cholecystectomy upward from porta hepatis, the train of events leading to cholecystostomy will be initiated by a frustrating and fruitless period spent in attempting to find the common bile duct. The stubbornness and pride of the surgeon help aggravate the situation.

In fundus-down cholecystectomy the operation is easily abandoned at any point for either reason noted above by suturing a catheter (I employ a No. 24 to No. 30 Foley) into the gallbladder and closing the abdomen. On the other hand, if all goes well, it is equally simple to obtain operative cholangiograms and explore for stones in the common bile duct as well as to remove the gallbladder. (In my personal experience there are stones in the common bile duct in only 5 per cent of patients with acute cholecystitis as opposed to 20 per cent in elective cholecystectomy; therefore, omitting exploration in acute cholecystitis will lead to relatively few later operations for retained stones.)

Identification of Structures during Operation

In an occasional patient having elective surgery, not only could I not find the *junction* of cystic duct and hepatic duct, but I could not even find the common bile duct. I cannot agree with those who insist that in every operation for acute cholecystitis the common bile duct must be found, even if this requires disturbing the pancreas. Such an approach in my opinion, would lead to failures, increased morbidity, and an occasional avoidable death from pancreatitis.

In gangrenous cholecystitis, I have occasionally seen the gallbladder become separated from its attachments to hepatic artery and common bile duct after it was surgically detached from the gallbladder fossa, and this without the application of a single clamp, or the use of undue traction. There was no bleeding from cystic vessels which were never seen, and no bile from a cystic duct which was also lost in necrotic tissue. An effort to find these structures as the first step in the operation would have been a nightmare!

The principal argument that can be levelled against fundus-down chole-cystectomy is that it is needlessly bloody. In an experience with over a hundred patients having acute cholecystitis, I have noted really trouble-some bleeding on only one or two occasions. Bleeding from the fossa itself may occur, regardless of whether cystic vessels are first ligated, and must be controlled before the abdomen is closed. Some "ooze" can be accepted while the gallbladder is being removed, provided sponging or suction will keep the exact site of dissection visible.

Not all surgeons enthuse over operating when the gallbladder is in its acute phase. It has been my own practice to operate promptly—within a day or two of hospitalization—once the diagnosis is reasonably certain, and the patient has been properly prepared. I have characterized cholecystec-tomy under these circumstances as "hard on the surgeon but easy on the patient." I feel sure that if I favored preliminary identification of the cystic artery and duct in these patients, I would be much more reluctant to operate promptly, and much more likely to wait for several months and a "quies-cent" phase, performing a deliberate cholecystostomy, if the condition failed to subside with conservative management.

Summary

There are numerous examples in surgery of employment of different techniques for a given operation by surgeons of equal experience and per-formance. It is clear that these differences must stem from personal prefer-ence and are not related to the successful consummation of the surgical mission. If in time one method becomes more commonly employed than others, it will be because it is simpler or quicker or both.

I issue this invitation to surgeons whose objection to fundus-to-porta cholecystectomy is on theoretical grounds: try it in a few elective opera-tions, particularly in obese patients with large livers. If it does not seem to be a better method at the time, you may be surprised nevertheless to find yourself turning to it in a tight spot with acute cholecystitis; at the very least you will acquire background for condemning it!

Congenital
Choledochal Cyst

Introduction

Choledochal cysts are uncommon, but when they are noted at operation the operative management may not be clearly evident to the surgeon. This is due in part to lack of familiarity with the abnormality because of its infrequency, but is due also to inadequate knowledge of its pathogenesis and its subsequent course. Because there is a controversy in the literature regarding the surgical treatment of congenital choledochal cysts, the problem is reviewed and discussed in this section. The question is whether the cyst should be excised or whether it suffices to carry out internal drainage by choledochocyst-duodenostomy or Roux-en-Y choledochocyst-jejunostomy.

S. R. F.

Choledochal Cyst:
Management by
Roux-en-Y Jejunal Drainage

Thomas M. Holder

Kansas University School of Medicine

Incidence and Diagnostic Criteria

The choledochal cyst is not infrequently the cause of biliary tract obstruction in the child. It is seen with less frequency in the infant and in the adult. The symptom complex of intermittent jaundice, abdominal pain, and a right upper quadrant mass is frequently associated with a choledochal cyst. The diagnosis is seldom made when the child is first seen. Most often the diagnosis of hepatitis is entertained, since this is by far the most common cause of jaundice in children. In the neonatal period the infant with a choledochal cyst may present symptoms clinically indistinguishable from biliary atresia, neonatal hepatitis, or the inspissated bile syndrome.

Roentgenographic study of the duodenum with contrast medium will show an extrinsic mass displacing the second portion of the duodenum anteriorly and medially. If an intravenous cholangiogram is done at the same time and the dye adequately concentrated, the mass displacing the duodenum will be visualized.

The operative findings of choledochal cyst should be familiar to all surgeons who operate in the upper abdomen. The common bile duct is markedly dilated; the gallbladder is frequently of normal size. There is no tumor in the region of the lower common duct, and usually there is no direct or indirect evidence of gallstones. A number of published reports indicate that on occasion these operative findings have not been interpreted correctly. An operative cholangiogram is a helpful diagnostic aid.

Rationale of Treatment

The term "idiopathic dilatation of the common bile duct" has been used for this entity and indicates the current status of knowledge of its etiology. The condition is presumably congenital. Why some patients go for years before having symptoms of biliary obstruction is not well understood.

In the treatment of this entity two factors are worthy of note: (1) properly treated this is a benign disease; (2) most of the patients are young and will probably have a number of decades to live if the proper operation is performed. With these thoughts in mind therapy should be planned which is not only safe, but will offer long-term relief of symptoms.

The two forms of treatment which offer some reasonable chance for a good long-term result are: (1) simple internal drainage of the cyst into the duodenum or jejunum or (2) excision of the cyst with drainage of the proximal biliary tract into the intestinal tract. Nonoperative treatment and external drainage have been totally unsatisfactory.

The majority of patients with choledochal cyst have a diffuse dilatation of the common bile duct, extending in some instances back into the intra-hepatic biliary radicles. For this group of patients we prefer Roux-en-Y internal drainage into a defunctionalized jejunal loop. Internal drainage may be carried out to the stomach, duodenum, or small bowel. The stomach has not proved a uniformly satisfactory bile drainage receptacle, and in those instances in which the cyst has been drained into the stomach, there has been a surprisingly high mortality.

Drainage to the Duodenum

Drainage of the cyst into the duodenum has been the most popular form of therapy. It has the advantage of being safe and simple. The close proximity of the dilated common duct as it runs behind the duodenum allows for the easy creation of a stoma of considerable size between the two structures. It also drains the bile into the intestinal tract at its normal level, allow-ing for neutralization of gastric acid just distal to the pylorus.

TABLE 1.   RESULTS OF TREATMENT OF CHOLEDOCHAL CYST*

	No. Patients	Operative Deaths	Operative Mortality	Persistent Symptoms	Failure Requiring Revision of Procedure
Drainage to duodenum	44	1†	2%	9	4
Drainage to jejunum	17	0‡	0	1	1
Excision of cyst	18	3	17%	0	0

* Tabulated from the report of Alonso-Lej, F., Rever, W. B., and Pessagno, D. J.: Int. Abstr. Surg., *108:*1, 1959.

† This patient died 5 days postoperatively of "unrelated causes"; one other patient died one year postoperatively of tuberculosis.

‡ One patient died 4 months postoperatively of appendicitis; another died 18 months postoperatively of carcinoma.

The disadvantage of drainage into the duodenum is a practical and alarming one: ascending cholangitis. The accompanying table is tabulated from the results of the extensive current review of the subject.[1] Since this is a relatively uncommon lesion and the experience of any one individual is insufficient for statistical analysis, I shall refer freely to their findings. Of the 44 patients having choledochoduodenostomy, nine (20 per cent) had persistent symptoms of cholangitis. Four of the 44 had symptoms sufficient to require a revision of the drainage procedure. The operative mortality with this procedure is small. The morbidity is sufficiently great, however, that it is not the preferable form of treatment for the long life most of these patients should expect. Its principal usefulness is for the patient who is seriously ill, since it represents the simplest operative procedure offering adequate drainage.

Drainage to the Jejunum by Roux-en-Y

Drainage of the cyst into the jejunum by a Roux-en-Y technique appears to offer the best chance of complete relief of symptoms with the smallest operative risk. Ascending cholangitis, the main objection to drainage to the duodenum, has not been a problem when the drainage has been to a defunctionalized jejunal limb. The defunctionalized jejunal limb should be 15 cm. in length in the infant and at least 30 cm. in length in the older child or adult. The theoretical objection to drainage into the jejunum is the possibility of increased duodenal ulceration in patients in whom the bile has been diverted past the duodenum. This has not occurred in my own experience or in those patients reviewed by Alonso-Lej et al.

An objection to drainage in general is that the stoma between the cyst and the intestine may close. There is no question that the cyst decreases considerably in size with drainage and there have indeed been instances when the stoma has closed following a drainage procedure. Three of the five revisions indicated in the table were done because of stomal closure; two were to the duodenum and one to the jejunum with a Braun loop. The stoma should be a fairly large one. With a Roux limb a stoma of any desired size can be created easily without fear of reflux of intestinal contents into the biliary tree. Although no incidence of anastomotic closure or stenosis was reported following excision of the cyst, general experience with anastomosis of the biliary tree to the gut would lead one to believe that this particular anastomosis would not be uniquely free of this problem.

In the report of Alonso-Lej et al. the one patient reported to have persistent symptoms after a Roux-en-Y jejunal drainage was a patient with diarrhea. It is somewhat difficult to attribute this to the drainage procedure unless a disproportionate amount of small bowel were excluded from the circuit in creating the defunctionalized limb. The Roux limb drainage to the jejunum has given excellent relief of symptoms. There were no deaths in this group of patients (Table 1).

The Case against Excision of the Cyst

Complete excision of the cyst is an appealing idea since it "removes the pathology." In those few patients who have a diverticulum of the common bile duct with a relatively narrow stalk, as demonstrated by operative findings and operative cholangiography, the best form of treatment is excision of the diverticulum and temporary T-tube drainage of the common duct. This will result in a relatively normal biliary tract with competent sphincter into the duodenum.

If, however, as in the usual case, the entire common duct is involved (and frequently the common hepatic duct), excision of the dilated area of duct increases considerably the magnitude of the operative procedure and appreciably increases the operative mortality. The operative mortality of 17 per cent with partial or total excision of the cyst is excessive compared with the simple drainage of the cyst to the duodenum or jejunum with a 2 per cent mortality (Table 1). After excision of the cyst the question of whether to drain the bile into the duodenum or the jejunum can be argued the same as for the simple drainage procedure. Those patients who have survived excision of the cyst have been relieved of their symptoms.

Summary

It would seem that in most instances the most satisfactory form of therapy for choledochal cyst is simple internal drainage of the cyst into the intestine with a defunctionalized jejunal limb Roux-en-Y procedure. The relief of symptoms is satisfactory and the mortality quite low compared to the reported mortality results when the cyst is excised.

Reference

1. Alonso-Lej, F., Rever, W. B., Jr., and Pessagno, D. J.: Congenital choledochal cyst, with a report of 2, and analysis of 94, cases. Int. Abstr. Surg., *108*:1–30, 1959.

Excision as Treatment of Choice in Congenital Choledochal Cyst

Daniel J. Pessagno

University of Maryland School of Medicine

The multiplicity of surgical procedures in the treatment of congenital cystic dilatation of the common bile duct serves to point out the controversy regarding its treatment.

Four hundred and three authentic cases and 16 doubtful cases of congenital choledochal cyst were collected from the world literature. Ninety-four were newly analyzed and two new cases were presented by us.[1]

The disease is congenital in origin. The etiology consists of a weakness in a specific portion of the common bile duct caused by hyperproliferation and hypervacuolization of that area during embryonic development. Such weakness constitutes a protodilatation status which develops into a clinical entity when the ductal pressure increases because of an obstructive factor.

Choledochal cyst is classified into the following three types. The first type, which is the most common, is classically described by many authors. We agree with Tsardakas and Robnett[2] in proposing that this variety be called congenital cystic dilatation of the common bile duct. Anatomically, the biliary tree presents four features: (1) the intrahepatic tree is normal, (2) the biliary tree above the cystic dilatation is somewhat dilated secondary to the obstructive factor in the distal choledochus, (3) the cystic dilatation begins and ends sharply, and (4) the terminal common bile duct is frequently narrowed.

The second type is the congenital diverticulum of the common bile duct. This is rare. It is characterized morphologically by a diverticulum that arises laterally from the wall of the common bile duct. The biliary tree may be normal or slightly dilated.

The third type offers special peculiarities and the question remains whether it originates from the same etiologic factors. The term, choledochocele, was used for the first time by Wheeler[3] when he commented on

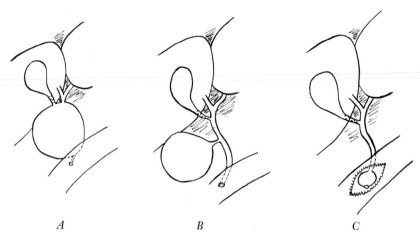

Fig. 1.   A, Congenital cystic dilatation of the common bile duct. *B,* Congenital diverticulum of the common bile duct. *C,* Congenital choledochocele.

a case reported in December 1915 in the Dublin Journal of Medical Sciences, in that the third type of choledochal cyst resembles a congenital ureterocele —anatomically.

The classic diagnostic triad of choleductal cysts are: pain, jaundice, and mass. Intermittence of these symptoms increases the probability of congenital cystic dilatation. Jaundice is absent in the diverticulum type. In a choledochocele, the mass is absent but nausea and vomiting are always present.

We present one of our cases in detail because of some lessons we learned from it:

M.G., an 18 year old, married, white female came to this country from her native country, Italy, on December 20, 1956. She was admitted on February 25, 1957, on the Medical Service of Mercy Hospital with the chief complaint of vague right upper quadrant abdominal pain. Pain had a gradual onset about one week prior to admission. It was non-radiating, unaffected by exercise or food intake, and not relieved by drugs. She complained of mild malaise, anorexia, and vomiting on three occasions during the four days prior to admission. The family noticed jaundice for about three days and there was generalized pruritus. The patient denied chills, fever, intolerance to fatty foods, weight loss, or any previous illnesses. A review of her organic system was completely negative. She had received the routine immunization shots prior to entering the United States. Her family history was noncontributory.

Physical examination revealed the patient to be a well developed, well nourished, white female in no acute distress. Temperature was 97.2° F; pulse 74/minute, and respiration 19/minute. The blood pressure was 120/80. The skin and mucous membranes were markedly icteric. Examination of the head, neck, eyes, ears, nose, and throat revealed normal findings. The lungs were clear to percussion and auscultation. The heart was not enlarged and there was a Grade I systolic murmur at the apex which was not transmitted. Rhythm was normal. The heart sounds were otherwise of good quality. The abdomen was enlarged particularly on the right side. The left side of the abdomen was tympanitic but on the right side the percussion note was dull. No free fluid was noted. The entire right side of the abdomen was slightly tender, but there was no rigidity. The liver was believed to be enlarged but its lower edge could not be delineated in that it seemed to fuse with a large mass which occupied the entire right side of the abdomen, extending well beyond the midline. The mass seemed to be rather fixed except for slight movement with respiration. The mass was firm and smooth. Bowel sounds were active. The rest of the physical examination was within normal limits.

Laboratory data and special studies: Examination of the blood revealed hemoglobin, 12 Gm.; hematocrit, 37 per cent; and white blood cell count, 6350: 62 per cent polymorphonuclears, 37 per cent lymphocytes, and 1 per cent monocytes. The absolute eosinophil count was 33. The bleeding time was 1 minute, and the coagulation time was 8 minutes and 45 seconds. The platelet count was 448,000. The sedimentation rate was 30. The Kahn and Hinton serology test was negative. The serum electrolytes in milliequivalents were: Na^+, 128.5; K^+, 3.75; Cl^-, 102.8; CO_2, 22.1. The serum iron level was 106 micrograms. The urinalysis revealed a clear amber color; specific gravity, 1.020; acid reaction; no sugar or acetone; a trace of albumin; and a negative microscopic examination. Test for the presence of bile was positive. The urobilinogen was 4+ and on the following day was 1+. The bilirubin was 4+. Stool examination revealed that a normal amount of bile was present. The fasting blood sugar was 118 mg.; NPN, 17 mg.; BUN, 8 mg.; serum cholesterol, 360 mg. and the cholesterol esters, 65 mg. The serum albumin was 4.1 Gm., globulin, 3.2 mg. The prothrombin time was 14 seconds with undiluted plasma and 82 seconds with 12.5 per cent diluted plasma. The alkaline phosphatase was 14.7 units and serum amylase 308 units. The van den Berg reaction showed a direct bilirubin of 10.4 mg. per cent in one minute; 12.4 in 30 minutes and a total of 15.8 mg. per cent. The icteric index was 55. The cephalin flocculation was negative and thymol turbidity showed 2+ units. Sigmoidoscopy was negative. EKG was read as a normal variant. Radiologic studies showed chest was negative; flat plate of the abdomen showed a huge rounded mass occupying the upper two-thirds of the right abdomen extending across the midline where it displaced the large bowel to the left. No calcifications were within it. The right kidney shadow could be seen through the mass and appeared to be normal in size. The inferior border appeared to be atypical for the usual type of liver enlargement. There was no evidence of spleen enlargement. The radiologic interpretation was either a large hepatic cyst or tumor.

Preoperative course: During the first 48 hours after admission the jaundice increased, the temperature climbed to 101.4° F and the patient began to vomit bile-stained gastric contents. Surgical consultation was obtained and exploratory laparotomy was advised. Preoperative diagnoses were: (1) pancreatic cyst, (2) hydrops of the gallbladder, or (3) cystic dilatation of the common bile duct.

Operation: On February 28, 1957, the patient was explored. A choledochal cyst was found. Because of the difficulties in dissection and the deterioration of the patient's condition during the operation, a choledocho-cyst-duodenostomy was performed, anastomosing the most dependent part of the cyst to the second portion of the duodenum. The stoma measured 6 cms. A Foley catheter was then placed in the cyst and brought out of the abdomen through a stab wound for further x-ray studies and for drainage purposes.

Postoperative Course: The initial postoperative course was stormy. As jaundice cleared an intravenous cholangiogram was performed, which did not demonstrate the biliary tree. Injection of radiopaque dye through the catheter into the cyst failed to reveal the opening that was demonstrated at the laparotomy, or any dye in the duodenum. The patient was discharged one month after the operation and was followed in the outpatient department. She remained slightly jaundiced. The fistula continued to drain and the patient complained of right upper abdominal pain. A second attempt was made to visualize the biliary tree through the fistula and cyst. This was unsuccessful except to show that the cyst had decreased in size. It was believed that the anastomosis had closed, and the patient was re-admitted for definitive surgery.

Reoperation: On July 2, 1957, the patient was re-explored. The anastomosis was found to have completely closed. The cyst, together with the gallbladder and cystic duct, was excised. The common hepatic duct, which measured 18 mm. in diameter, was anastomosed to the second portion of the duodenum. No internal support was used. The patient's postoperative course was again stormy, but the patient responded to combative measures. She was discharged one month after surgery. She has been followed in

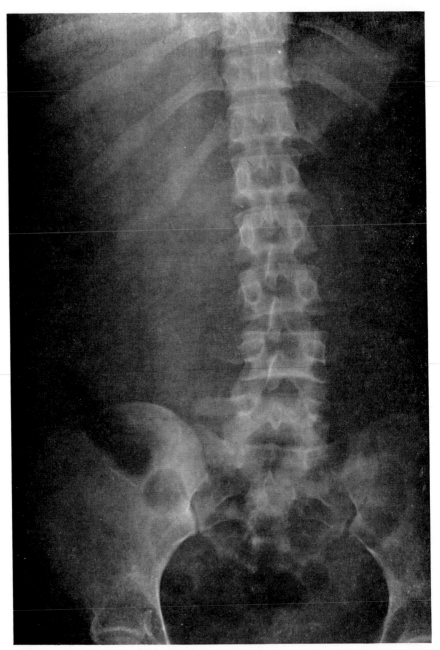

Fig. 2. Flat film of the abdomen shows a huge mass occupying the upper two thirds of the right abdomen and extending across the midline where it displaces the large bowel to the left.

the outpatient department. When seen in March, 1957, she was completely asymptomatic, gained weight, not jaundiced, and, when a gastrointestinal series was performed using Gastrografin, no opaque material could be forced into the biliary tree. In November, 1958, the patient was seen in the obstetrical clinic completely asymptomatic and 5 months pregnant.

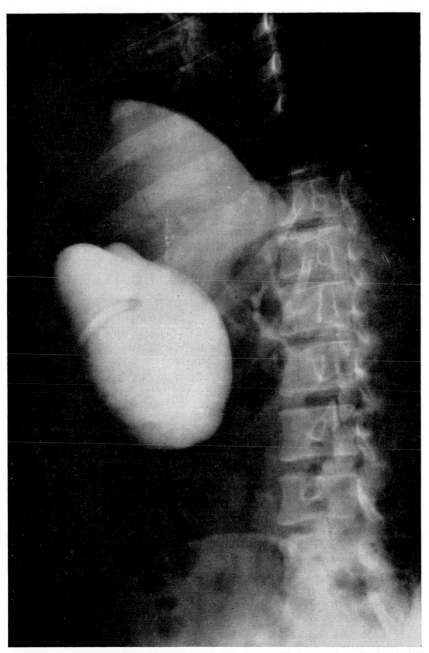

Fig. 3. Injection of radiopaque dye into the choledochal cyst through the draining fistula fails to reveal the opening that was demonstrated at laparotomy or any dye in the duodenum. Film was obtained three weeks following a choledochocyst-duodenostomy.

A choledochocystenterostomy is analogous to a gastroenterostomy with a patent pylorus, in which case the secondary opening, the cyst enterostomy in the former and the gastroenterostomy in the latter, frequently ceases to function. This was described in the foregoing case report; Glove[4] reported a similar occurrence. In the same report Glove pointed out that another reason for the failure of such an anastomosis is the absence of epithelial lining in the cyst. With excision of the cyst the nidus of infection is removed; the culture media, so to speak is obliterated. Choledochocystenterostomy, which is primarily a drainage procedure, never adequately drains the cyst (the location of the anastomosis may make a difference). A fluid level is often seen in the erect film. Infection and ascending cholangitis occur frequently. Hertzler and McGuire[5] reported that the size of the cyst did not change eleven years after a choledochocyst-duodenostomy. McWhorter,[6] in 1935, performed an autopsy on his patient who had been subjected to excision of the cyst in 1922 and could not find any clinical or histological evidence of cholangitis. Lesser morbidity is closely related to the lessened incidence of infection and cholangitis. The cyst, per se, is potentially or actively infected at the time of operation. If this is not removed, as in choledochocystenterostomy, the natural course of the disease progresses, i.e., infection and ascending cholangitis. Secondly, when the anastomosis is made the normal bacterial flora of the small intestine comes in contact with an ideal culture media, and bacteria may grow rapidly in the new environment and account for the increased morbidity. For the second and third type of choledochal cyst, it is quite obvious that excision is the treatment of choice; no argument need be presented.

There is considerable controversy regarding the treatment of congenital cystic degeneration of the common bile duct as is indicated by the multiplicity of surgical procedures advocated.

The sine qua non for adequate treatment is the recognition of the lesion at the operating table.

Alternative Procedures

Among the many surgical procedures reported in the literature the following were analyzed by us:
1. Complete removal of the cyst and anastomosis of the remaining biliary tree to the intestinal tract
2. Anastomosis of a portion of the intestinal tract to the cyst
3. Choledochorrhaphy
4. Bypassing the cyst

Without surgical treatment, the outcome is almost certain to be fatal. Of 232 cases reviewed by Tsardakas and Robnett,[2] 30 patients were treated medically and 29 of these died.

We are of the opinion that removal of the cystic dilatation with reconstruction of the normal anatomy by anastomosis of the biliary tree to the second portion of the duodenum is the treatment of choice. McWhorter,[6] in 1922, was the first to carry out this procedure. Our review[1] of 94 cases reveals that choledochocyst-duodenostomy was performed 44 times with 2 deaths. Twenty-nine of the 42 survivors were given follow-up examinations by the authors, nine developed various degrees of ascending cholangitis, 2 had attacks of vomiting and pain, and 4 revealed that the anastomosis had closed. This gave a morbidity of 31 per cent. Cholecyst-gastrostomy in our review was performed 8 times with three deaths and a mortality of 38 per cent. Among the 94 patients analyzed, choledochocyst-jejeunostomy was performed 17 times with 2 deaths, and 2 died within one year. Of 10 of the 13 remaining patients where follow-up was possible, two developed complications: the anastomosis closed in one and another developed diarrhea and steatorrhea.

Although choledochocyst-duodenostomy and choledochocyst-jejunostomy are simpler than removal of the cyst and anastomosis of the remaining biliary tree to the intestine, the pathological dilatation remains in the patient.

The objection to excision of the cyst in the past was the high mortality rate, 29.4 per cent in the review of 232 cases by Tsardakas and Robnett.[2] However, in our review of 94 newly analyzed cases, there were 2 deaths in 19 cases with a mortality of 15 per cent.

If one peruses the literature, as we have pointed out in our review,[1] the mortality rate drops with each new report and there is a tendency toward removal of the cyst as the treatment of choice. The drop in mortality can be accounted for by better overall surgical management, careful preoperative preparation, advances in anesthesia, and increased knowledge of electrolyte balance, blood transfusions, and antibiotics.

References

1. Pessagno, D. J., et al.: Congenital choledochal cyst, with a report of two and an analysis of 94 cases. Surg., Gynec. and Obst., *108*:1, 1959.
2. Tsardakas, E., and Robnett, A. H.: Congenital cystic dilatation of the common bile duct. Report of 3 cases, analysis of 57 cases and review of the literature. Arch. Surg., *72*:311, 1956.
3. Wheeler, W. I. De Courcey: An unusual case of obstruction to common duct (choledochocele?) Brit. J. Surg., *110:5559*, 1939.
4. Glove, W. M.: Recognition and treatment of congenital choledochal cyst. Arch. Surg., *75*:443, 1957.
5. Hertzler, J. H., and McGuire, C. J.: Congenital dilatation of the common bile duct. Report of 2 cases in children. Arch. Surg., *62*:275, 1951.
6. McWhorter, G. L.: Congenital cystic dilatation of the common bile duct. Arch. Surg., *8*:604, 1924.
7. Schurholz: Ein fall sogenannten idiopatischer choleduchuscyste. Arch. Klin. Chir., *118:* 91, 1921.
8. Seeliger, S.: Beitrag zue kenntnis der choledochuscysten. Beitr. klin. Chir., *99*:158, 1916.

Common Duct
Exploration
during Cholecystectomy

Introduction

The indications for exploration of the common bile duct in association with cholecystectomy have been enumerated so often that they may almost be described as being "classic." For those who feel that the indications have somewhat less tenure than those deserving the connotation "classic," we re-iterate here the reasons usually given for exploring the extrahepatic ducts operatively during cholecystectomy: presence or recent history of jaundice, acholic stools or dark urine, presence of a dilated common bile duct, palpation of stones, tumors or other abnormalities in the bile ducts or pancreas, and presence of small stones in the gallbladder which could traverse the cystic duct. To this list, some surgeons have added that an abnormal appearance of the ductal system on a cystic duct cholangiogram constitutes another indication for exploration.

The use of operative cholangiograms as a means of detecting unsuspected stones is sometimes controversial, and was presented in Current Surgical Management II (1960). Recently, the hallowed indications for operative exploration of the ducts have been threatened by those surgeons who feel that the chance of leaving unsuspected stones in the extrahepatic ducts after cholecystectomy is too great to omit this procedure when operating for stones in the gallbladder.

We must remind ourselves also that even when surgical exploration of the ducts has been done there may still be retained stones which have eluded even the experienced surgeon. It has been suggested that more frequent or even routine exploration will reduce the incidence of traumatic strictures of the duct. On the other hand, it also has been suggested that more frequent use of choledochotomy actually may increase the possibility of injury to the ducts. Certainly the "smaller than normal" duct, which is seen occasionally, particularly in cases of chronic pancreatitis or portal cirrhosis, is more susceptible to permanent deformity from operative exploration.

The following presentations are excellent and extremely interesting accounts of opposing points of view regarding management of the common duct during cholecystectomy. This is a problem which becomes more important with the passage of time, with the rapid trend to the "civilizing" of humans, with the increasing use of radiologic aids in operative diagnosis, and with the increasing numbers of surgeons operating on increasing numbers of patients with biliary tract disorders. The titles of the presentations themselves say a lot for the philosophy of each aspect of the controversy: "Leave the Common Duct Alone," and "The 'Compleat' Cholecystectomy."

S. R. F.

Leave the Common Duct Alone

Heneage Ogilvie

Guy's Hospital, London

The bacterial diseases have been pretty well abolished by the antibiotics. Acute and chronic middle ear diseases have become so rare, that otologists would be trooping round, cap in hand, singing, "Brother, can you spare a dime," had they not invented reconstructive operations on the middle ear to take their place.

A new group of diseases have appeared, which are due to the increasing subjection of the body to conditions for which it was not designed. These conditions can be summed up in one pathological entity—*civilisation*. The only normal things that a modern civilised man does during his earthly span is to eat fruit, to drink water, and to die. He is born by instruments and under the influence of drugs; he is suckled on a theory and out of a tin; he lives on food that is chemically, physically, thermally, and biologically wrong. He is deprived throughout life of all those stimuli that are the normal physiological call to function. He uses his brain too much, and his muscles not at all.

The diseases of civilisation fall into three groups: those due to dietary abnormalities, those due to stress, and those due to pathological prosperity. Gallstones fall into this last group. Prosperity varies from country to country and from time to time, but it is in the poorer countries that we find prosperity carried to pathological excess, because it is in them that we find the contrast between the favoured few and the miserable many most marked.

The great majority of gallstones are mixed stones, with a nucleus of pigment and bacteria, and concentric coatings of cholesterol and calcium bilirubinate. This structure is an argument in favour of Moynihan's aphorism that "Gallstones are tombstones erected to the memory of dead bacteria." Apart from this solitary and unsupported wisecrack, there is little to support the infective theory. I have not been impressed with the liability of those who have had typhoid fever, intestinal infections, or suppurative conditions in the region of the portal vein, or who have had septicaemia and recovered, to suffer subsequently from gallstones.

My experience has led me to believe that the common mixed stones are the price that modern man pays for security, comfort, and good living, just as hypertension, thyrotoxicosis, and coronary thrombosis are the price he pays for psychological stress, and cancer of the lung is the price he pays for living in an atmosphere of smoke.

My claim that gallstones are due to security and good living is founded on no more than personal observation, but observation made over many years and in many countries. In the University Hospital of East Africa, a hospital that serves the needs of about four million people, less than half a dozen cases of gallstones are seen every year. In the North Island of New Zealand, with a population of similar size, whose chief source of prosperity is dairy farming, operations for gallstones are the commonest of all surgical procedures, exceeding those for peptic ulcer by about six to one. In Iraq, gallstones are almost unknown among the Bedouins, but among the prosperous trading communities of Bagdad and Basra, they are very common. The Victorians described the typical gallstone patient as a fair, fat, fecund, flatulent female of forty. Today the influences of sex and pregnancies seem unimportant. The chief characteristics of the gallstone patient are that he is fat, good-tempered, and prosperous.

Today, in the seventh decade of the twentieth century, Anno Domini, gallstones are top priority because:

1. They are the leaders in a comparatively new class of diseases, those due to altered circumstances of life. They are comparatively new as a major problem, and they are likely to become more common as the world becomes more prosperous.

2. They affect an important social stratum in any community.

This statement will provoke criticism. It is a basic dogma of some political parties that the prosperous members of the community are parasites, who live in luxury by grinding the faces of the poor. Like most political dogmas, this view is at least half a century out of date. However, much legislation seeks to make all men equal in what they get and not in what they give; the best tend inevitably to rise to the top, the worst to sink to the bottom. The desires to get a little more comfort, a little more security than they experienced as children, and to give their own children a better start in life than they had themselves are the spur that drives men to scorn delights and live laborious days. The people who get gallstones are not the titled *tycoons* with their inherited wealth, but the man who started with a small shop and has built up a prosperous business, the *Trades Union leader* who has come to command hundreds of thousands, the *sheik* whose father fed his flocks on land where oil now flows, the *communist dictator*. They are all Very Important People. It is the V.I.P.'s who get gallstones. The possessors of gallstones are prosperous, and they deserve their prosperity. They are cheerful and kindly, and they deserve our help.

3. They have been treated with quite foolish levity in the past. Medical textbooks tell us that gallstones are often discovered accidentally during investigation of patients who have had no symptoms, and that they are found postmortem in those who have died of other diseases. They say that

symptoms can be treated by diet, chemotherapy, and antispasmodics, and that when the attack has subsided, it may never be repeated. These statements are perfectly true. But the writers do not tell us that even symptomless gallstones are often responsible for constant ill health, that medical treatment can only alleviate symptoms by giving the gallbladder no reason to contract, and that medical "cure" usually means incarceration of the gallbladder in a mass of fibrous tissue and bacteria that may flare up and become cancerous. While stones remain, many complications, most of them dangerous and some fatal, are still possible.

The chief sin of the medical writer is that he mentions surgery only as a dangerous alternative, to be avoided if possible. In 1930, that was a comfortable generalisation that could be handed out with a certain amount of justification to old ladies with gallstones. In 1930, patients died after abdominal operations—from anaesthetic complications, from haemorrhage, from shock, or from sepsis. All these dangers have vanished. People do not die after an operation for gallstones competently performed; they die of gallstones because operation has not been done.

4. We have at last come to realise that the disease passes through two phases. In the first phase, the stones are in the gallbladder only; in the second, they are also in the common duct. In the first phase they are a minor malady; in the second they are a dangerous disease. In the first phase, gallstones can be cured without question, and without risk, but in the second phase an operation is required that is always exacting, sometimes difficult, occasionally dangerous, and not always successful.

5. Their treatment must be done by first-class surgeons, or not at all. Any fool can remove a gallbladder. Most of them do. Many of them remove a lot of other things as well. In contrast to most of the disasters of incompetent surgery, the mistakes of the amateur cholecystectomist can seldom be remedied. The quality of the surgery of any region can be judged by the number of common ducts that are injured yearly. In most countries, that is the vital statistic that is never disclosed.

The common bile duct should be opened when it contains stones, and the stones should be removed, but a blank choledochotomy, like a blank laparotomy, should bring a blush to the cheek of a mature surgeon. Few would claim, as Moynihan did without a blush, to be able to feel a grain of gunpowder in the common duct. But every experienced operator should be able to say with considerable confidence whether a common bile duct contains stones or not, and if he cannot do so he should be gently diverted to a less dangerous branch of surgery. If he cannot do so after careful examination, he may have recourse to cholangiography, but the need for this refuge of the diagnostically destitute, should not arise more than once or twice a year.

He can base his confidence on five points:

1. Though there may have been repeated gallstone attacks, several of which have been followed by deep jaundice, there have been none of those periods of lemon-yellow discolouration accompanied by malaise and slight rigors, which signal the lodgement of a stone in the common duct.

2. The common duct, when inspected, does not exceed a third of an inch in diameter, or show that blue colour that suggests black contents.

3. When the duct is palpated between finger and thumb from the hilum to the bile papilla, no irregularities can be felt in its course.

4. Aspiration of the duct with a fine needle draws off clear yellow bile only, with no debris or solid flecks.

5. After the cystic duct is isolated prior to its junction with the common duct, its diameter is found to be less than that of any stone that can be felt in the gallbladder.

If he has satisfied himself on these five points, the surgeon can proceed to remove the gallbladder and to peritonealize its bed, feeling sure that none of those sequelae that may follow the wanton incision of the main common duct will afflict his patient. A stone so small that a careful surgeon cannot feel it should be able to slip unnoticed through the papilla into the duodenum.

When we have deemed it necessary to open the common bile duct, we should do as little as possible inside it. We should remove any stones it contains, but we should remember that the duct is possibly the most delicate passage in the body, the most resentful of injury, mechanical or chemical. Stones should be lifted out, coaxed out, or washed out, never pulled out or scraped out, and never, never torn out by using a strip of ribbon gauze as a mechanical excavator. After the stones have been removed, a gum-elastic olive-head bougie should be passed gently into the duodenum. It should never be introduced with force, for it may make a false passage, and it should not be too big, or it may tear the fibres of the sphincter.

The mistake most commonly made by an experienced surgeon, having opened the duct and removed what appear to be all the stones it contains, is to leave one stone behind. When the stones are multiple, he must be particularly careful before closure, to look for outlying stones that may have escaped removal. One place where a stone may easily be missed is a dilated ampulla, for a bougie may easily slip past it into the duodenum without encountering any obstruction. Another place is the liver itself. When there are many stones that have been causing intermittent obstruction for some time, the whole duct system is dilated by back pressure into a honeycomb system of cavities, of which the region of the hilum is the lowest point in the supine position. Stones tend to drop back into the hepatic ducts, or even to find their way back into the finer branches, where they cannot be felt, and from which they cannot be extracted. These stones are washed down into the main ducts when the flow of bile is restored and the patient starts to move about, and they may cause recurrent obstruction so long after the first operation that they are thought to have been formed in the ducts.

Operative Cholangiography

It is in cases where the surgeon, having removed a number of stones from the common duct, feels some doubt whether there may not be more, and in such cases only, that operative cholangiography is needed. An ectopic and solitary stone, when shown by this means, can often be removed while the duct is open.

Operative cholangiography has an almost irresistible appeal to the gadget-minded surgeon, the man who wants to be in the fashion, the man who loves to festoon the walls of the operating room with wet x-ray films, the man who needs to have his mind made up for him by some mechanical substitute for thought. It should not be necessary in more than one operation in fifty. Contrast media (usually compounds containing iodine) are highly irritating substances, as any surgeon who has been unfortunate enough to inject even small amounts into perivascular tissues knows well. They cannot do the mucous membranes lining the bile passages any good.

Stenosing choledochitis is a condition of diffuse fibrosis involving the whole of the extrahepatic biliary system, or sometimes the common duct only. The cause is obscure, but it is rarely seen in a patient who has not been operated on previously, and uncommonly in one whose common duct has not been opened. It seems in some way to be related to the trauma of exploration, and possibly to the injection of chemicals, particularly ether. It provides an additional reason why the common duct should not be explored lightheartedly.

Possibly related to stenosing choledochitis is the syndrome of papillary stenosis. Some years after a successful cholecystectomy (rarely less than six), attacks of common duct obstruction make their appearance, and gradually become more frequent and more severe. A tentative diagnosis of stone in the duct is made, but the long interval of freedom after the first operation does not fit the picture. At operation the common duct is found to be dilated to the diameter of a finger. No stones are found, but a bougie passed downward enters the duodenum with difficulty, and its point is tightly gripped in a tough collar.

The condition is cured by transduodenal division of the stenosed papilla, and of the duct for half an inch above it. Papillary stenosis is seldom seen except where the common bile duct has been explored, and it is probably the result of forcible dilation and rupture of the fibres of the sphincter of Oddi. The papilla should never be dilated to a diameter of more than seven millimetres. The sphincter of Oddi should never be cut except under direct vision. Various ingenious "oddi-tomes" and acorn-shaped biliary dilators of alarming size are to be found in every surgical museum. They have been presented by the ingenious but misguided surgeons who invented them. They should be left there, as a warning to gentler surgeons.

Two devices must be avoided in the surgery of the biliary tract; diathermy and the gallbladder bridge.

Diathermy, as a means of dividing vascular structures with a sparse fibrous stroma, and as a means of sealing vessels too small to ligate, is a permissible and even a valuable method. It may be used in making the abdominal incision, though the *meticulous* surgeon must wrestle with his conscience before he uses it for this purpose, and conscience usually wins. Diathermy has paved the way for advances in neurosurgery and urological surgery. On the whole, however, it has proved the canker that has dulled surgical conscience and blunted the fine edge of surgical technique, allowing the bad surgeon to undertake, and to perform after a fashion, operations that he should not be allowed to attempt. As a means of cauterising large slabs of tissue, such as the liver, to stop bleeding, and of removing organs or parts of organs, such as the gallbladder, by wholesale coagulation, it cannot be condemned too strongly. There is no finer *culture* medium known to bacteriological science than cooked liver.

The gallbladder bridge brings the duct region forward, but it also increases the tension in the anterior abdominal wall. It hyperextends the spine of an elderly and often plethoric individual to an extent that would be impossible without anaesthesia and relaxants, and it leads to shock at the time, and an intractable backache afterwards. If the ducts will not come to the surgeon, the surgeon must go to the ducts.

The best advice that an experienced surgeon can give to a less experienced one is: "Leave the common duct alone."

To fail to recognize that there may be a stone in the duct, and hence to fail to open the duct, is an unfortunate mistake, but a less serious one than to open the duct in case there may be something.

The surgeon who leaves an occasional stone behind, having looked for it carefully, will improve in time, but the habitual duct opener will remain through life a *dabbler* and a menace.

The "Compleat" Cholecystectomy

C. Frederick Kittle

The University of Kansas Medical Center, Kansas City, Kansas

Despite the frequency of operative procedures on the gallbladder and the many years that cholecystectomy has been done, the indications for common duct exploration continue to be arbitrary. The indications involve not only medical reasons, but also the technical ability and the philosophy of individual surgeons. Among leading surgeons these indications vary; this variability exists between different countries, between various parts of the same country, and indeed between surgeons of the same department or clinic. One of the perplexing and difficult problems confronting the surgeon who operates on the diseased gallbladder and biliary system is his management of the common duct—specifically, whether or not he should explore this structure.

Apart from the controversy regarding common duct exploration, do present results of cholecystectomy indicate that improvement is needed? Published articles and general experience attest that better results could be obtained and are desirable. About 10 per cent of patients[2] operated on for biliary tract disease have residual common duct stones or cystic duct remnants, often referred to as the "post-cholecystectomy syndrome," and future efforts should be directed at reducing this incidence.

Virtually all common duct stones in man are initially formed in the gallbladder. In patients with cholelithiasis there is a broad spectrum of pathology involving the size, number, type, and location of these calculi. In patients with the typical history of an obstructed common duct, or an obvious stone in the common duct by palpation, or a common duct much larger than acceptably normal, there is no question regarding exploration of the duct. In these patients the duct is explored without misgiving or hesitation. From this end of the spectrum, however, there is a gradual and variable transition to patients without choledocholithiasis. In this intermediate range the common duct only recently may have fallen heir to a calculus, so that its obstruction and dilatation are not yet apparent. The calculus (or calculi) may be too small to be detected by palpation of the common duct; it is also conceivable that a calculus may pass from the gallbladder into the common duct during the course of cholecystectomy without causing the usual indications for exploration. Conversely, the indications for common duct exploration may be present without choledocholithiasis.

What is a dilated common duct? Careful measurement with calipers at one specific anatomic point gives an average diameter of 7.6 mm. for the normal duct.[4] Variation occurs according to the size of the patient and his age. Generally, however, at operation the duct is estimated visually, often while it is being elevated or displaced. No one definite point has been accepted for measurement; a measuring device is seldom used; and the definition of dilatation is a subjective expression of the individual surgeon's estimate and judgment.

Operative Cholangiography

In the midst of varying recommendations for common duct exploration, the hesitancy to traumatize a duct unnecessarily (that is, a negative exploration), and the awareness of the large number of patients with overlooked common duct stones and residual cystic duct remnants, can a satisfactory solution to operative evaluation of the common duct be obtained? Routine operative cholangiography, whenever common duct exploration is not clearly indicated, provides thorough evaluation of the extrahepatic passages. A positive cholangiogram is a clear indication for common duct exploration. A negative cholangiogram permits the operating surgeon to leave the operating table free of any nagging doubt that a common duct stone may have been overlooked. A negative cholangiogram assures the operating surgeon of the most complete evaluation of the extrahepatic biliary passages now possible.

What are the advantages and disadvantages of common or cystic duct cholangiography? In numerous reported series routine cholangiography has been shown to detect unsuspected stones, abnormalities of the biliary passages, and whether reflux into the pancreas can occur.[3] All these are individually and variously important in reaching the goal of the best possible operative procedure and in reducing the number of patients requiring reoperation. Complications with this technique are minimal and incidental.

In a recent review of 4948 cholecystectomies, the indications for common duct exploration were reviewed and discussed. It was stated:[1]

> "We follow the policy of 'when in doubt explore.' In our experience a negative exploration of the common duct adds little if any to the morbidity or risk associated with cholecystectomy by itself."

Others have provided statistics supporting the latter viewpoint.

But—when in doubt? Surely, cholelithiasis or cholecystitis always invokes some doubt about common duct stones, and reassurance for the patient and surgeon can only come after the most thorough search possible.

There is little excuse for an incomplete operation in which a common duct stone is missed or the cystic duct is incompletely removed, and reoperation is eventually required.

Perhaps of equal importance surgically is the technical instruction to younger surgeons. If common duct exploration or operative cholangiography were expected, would it not increase the technical proficiency in this region? Would not cholecystectomy pass from the hands of the occasional surgeon to those well qualified to do the expected procedure? Common duct strictures usually occur in patients who have *not* had their ducts explored, and in whom the dissection has been hasty or haphazard. Improvements in technique by dissection of the common duct for exploration or visualization should assist in decreasing the incidence of these strictures.

Cholecystectomies and common duct stones become more frequent as life expectancy increases.[5] The advent of safe and relaxing anesthesia, the availability of operating room roentgenology, and the extension of surgical procedures to include prophylaxis encourage the acceptance of routine common duct evaluation.

For many years a time-honored question about biliary tract disease has been: "What are the indications for common duct exploration?" In discussing a cholecystectomy, why not ask, "Why was the common duct *not* explored or visualized?"

References

1. Appleman, R. M.: Cholelithiasis and choledocholithiasis: factors that influence relative incidence. Proc. Staff Meet. Mayo Clin., *39*:473, 1964.
2. Kornfield, H. J., and Allbritten, F. F., Jr.: The roles of choledochostomy and antibiotics in gallbladder surgery. Surg., Gynec., and Obst., *113*:277, 1961.
3. Swedberg, J.: Routine cholangiography at operation for gallstones. Acta chir. scandinav., *103*:175, 1952.
4. Wilhelm, M. C., and Smith, A. M.: Evaluation of the common duct at operation. Virginia Med. Monthly, *89*:219, 1962.
5. Zollinger, R. M., and Williams, R. D.: Cholecystectomy. J.A.M.A., *190*:145, 1964.

Method of Common Duct Drainage

Introduction

When a surgeon operates on a patient for cholecystolithiasis a number of alternatives in the technical aspects of the operation present themselves, and decisions usually are made more or less empirically. The controversial issue of whether to explore the extrahepatic bile ducts routinely in association with cholecystectomy is presented in the preceding section. Another question of management, when exploration of the common bile duct has been done, is whether the choledochotomy wound should be closed without drainage or with choledochostomy; this controversial issue was presented in Current Surgical Management II (1960). The next set of alternatives which is sometimes quite controversial relates to the method of bile duct drainage—for instance, should the surgeon use a short-arm or a long-limb T-tube? There are other means for decompressing the bile duct, including straight catheters through the wound of exploration or via the cystic duct, but the usual controversy is whether the distal limb of the T-tube should extend through the sphincter of Oddi into the duodenum.

As is so often the case, the controversy is more apparent than real, particularly when it is noted that those who advocate the use of the long-limb T-tube do so with specific indications for its use and not necessarily routinely. Furthermore, the underlying pathologic condition in the biliary-pancreatic system and the *method* of using either type of tube probably have more to do with the incidence of complications when choledochostomy has been done than does the mere selection of the type of tube.

Proponents of each method have good reasons for their viewpoints of management, based on extensive experience, as stated in the following presentations.

S. R. F.

Page 133

Short-Arm T-Tube for
Drainage of the Common Duct

Deward O. Ferris

Mayo Clinic and Mayo Graduate School of Medicine,
University of Minnesota

On most occasions, the common bile duct is opened for the purpose of searching for and removing calculi. After this is accomplished the surgeon is faced with several methods of closure of the duct.

Historical Aspects

Primary closure of the common duct is probably the oldest method, having been used by the German and French surgeons at the turn of the century.[4] American surgeons, however, have been reluctant to adopt the operation, but in some centers today the procedure is being used with increasing frequency.

Robson[7] of England is thought to be the first surgeon to write about employing catheter drainage of the common bile duct. In 1902 he described the introduction of an ordinary rubber catheter through an incision in the dilated common duct and directed upward toward the liver. This allowed bile to escape from the upper hepatic ducts and thereby decompressed the entire biliary tract. Some surgeons, however, considered it important to insert a second catheter directed in the opposite direction and extending through the distal common duct and papilla into the duodenum. McArthur[6] advocated this second catheter "for the purpose of administration of fluids, bile and nourishment." Most likely the idea of a single catheter with two limbs (T shape) arose from this use of a double tube. The first description of its use is generally attributed to Deaver[2] who, in his article entitled "Hepatic Drainage," described the T-tube and advocated its use in 1904. It is also interesting to note his warning that neither arm of the T-tube should be of such length that it might cause obstruction of the hepatic duct or of the pancreatic duct.

Since early times, therefore, the surgeon has had three choices: (1) primary closure, (2) drainage with a single catheter directed upward into

Page 135

the hepatic duct, and (3) drainage with two catheters, one of which extends through the distal portion of the common duct into the duodenum. Translated into today's terminology, the choice is (1) primary closure, (2) use of the short-arm T-tube, and (3) use of the long-arm T-tube. My choice is the use of the short-arm T-tube, and I have encountered no untoward results which could be attributed to its use.

General Considerations

The primary reason for draining the common duct after exploration is to maintain reduced intraluminal pressure until healing is complete. If the gallbladder has been removed at the same time, the bile duct must handle all of the bile at all times because the bile can no longer flow into the gallbladder and be concentrated and stored temporarily. During instrumental exploration of the bile ducts, the traumatized sphincter tends to stay in spasm for days, and is further stimulated to remain contracted if the intraluminal pressure is increased. The surface tension of bile is such that it tends to leak through the most minute hole, and leakage in sufficient quantity could cause bile peritonitis. At times, when cholangitis or pancreatitis is present, decompression of the bile ducts is important and must be maintained for a considerable time. In spite of what is thought to be an adequate exploration of the common duct, stones will be overlooked at times. In such cases the stones may cause obstruction, and the T-tube is a life-saving safety valve. It also affords an opportunity for introducing various chemicals in an attempt to dissolve or dislodge the remaining stone.

Use of Dilators

More and more attention has been given in recent years to partial obstruction of the sphincter of Oddi by spasm, fibrosis, and scarring. Several points should be kept in mind in the instrumental exploration of the sphincter and evaluation of this condition.

First, graduated dilators, such as the Bakes type, may be used to calibrate the diameter of the sphincter. In passing dilators of successively larger diameters, that is 3 mm., 4 mm., and so forth, one soon arrives at a size that will not pass with ease. The largest size that passes with ease is the caliber of the duct at the sphincter. Normally it is in the range of 3 to 7 mm.

Second, the dilators are used to dilate the sphincter of Oddi. Dilatation of this sphincter, like dilatation of other sphincters, is only temporary. Extreme dilatation may cause temporary lack of function of the sphincter, but it also may cause tearing and splitting of the structures with the possibility that excessive scar tissue may develop; then, when this contracts, it causes a degree of stenosis. Branch and co-workers,[1] in their investigation of the consequences of instrumental dilatation of the sphincter of Oddi in dogs, showed that scarring actually does occur after extensive dilatation, and that dilatation does not result in permanent enlargement. They concluded that no further dilatation should be carried out after patency has been ascertained. I have made it a practice not to pass a dilator of a diameter greater than 7 mm.

The third point regarding the use of dilators is to avoid creation of false passages. The use of a filiform-guided dilator[5] makes possible more accurate evaluation of the distal part of the common duct and sphincter of Oddi without risk of making a false passage and with minimal trauma.

If, in any case, the surgeon is not entirely satisfied that the sphincter of Oddi and the ampulla of Vater are normal, it is best to open the duodenum and explore from this approach as well.

Fibrosis of the sphincter, if demonstrated, requires correction by transduodenal biopsy and sphincterotomy.

Argument against Long-Arm T-Tube

The obstruction having been corrected, there is no reason to use a long-arm T-tube extending through the sphincter into the duodenum. In my opinion, its use in such cases, or in any case for that matter, creates an unnecessary risk of obstructing the pancreatic duct with resultant pancreatitis in a significant number of cases.[3]

Shortcomings of Simple Catheter

An indwelling catheter (or stint) in the bile ducts should be used only as a last resort, because it acts as a foreign body and tends to cause healing by secondary intention with increased laying-down of fibrous tissue and subsequent contracture or stricture formation. For instance, in repair of common duct stricture I prefer to carry out a primary end-to-end repair and place the drainage tube in such a manner that it does not traverse the site of anastomosis.

I wish only to decompress the main bile duct with as simple and safe a tube as possible. A simple catheter has two shortcomings: (1) if passed 8 to 10 cm. within the ducts it may obstruct one of the hepatic ducts; if directed in the opposite direction it may obstruct the pancreatic duct or both the common and pancreatic ducts, or it may enter the duodenum and not decompress the bile ducts at all, or (2) if passed only several centimeters into the extrahepatic ducts it may easily be completely dislodged from the duct, allowing free leakage of bile into the peritoneal cavity. Therefore, I employ the short-arm T-tube as a simple catheter drainage, but use the T-bar primarily to anchor the tube.

Technique

The arms of the T-tube should never be longer than 1.5 cm. The size of the tube should be one-half to two-thirds the diameter of the lumen

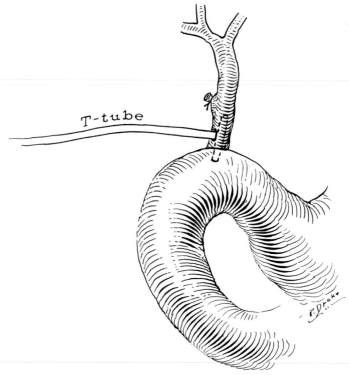

T-tube

Fig. 1. The short-arm T-tube. Note that it is placed in the upper portion of the common bile duct. The arms are 1.5 cm. long. Its size is half that of the duct.

of the common bile duct, to facilitate easy removal and also to allow passage of bile around it (Fig. 1). That most frequently employed is a No. 10 or a No. 12 F. Many surgeons think it highly desirable to cut a small piece out of the posterior part of the T-tube, just opposite the junction of the two tubes, to facilitate removal. If one uses a small tube, this is not at all necessary and, I must point out, this maneuver weakens the anchoring effect of the T-bar. Opinions differ as to the length of time the T-tube should remain in place. Ordinarily I do not leave it in place longer than 2 weeks, but on occasion I have permitted it to remain as long as 3 weeks. As long as all stones are removed and other forms of obstruction have been corrected, continued presence of the tube seems unnecessary. In general, the tube should not be removed prior to 10 to 12 days after insertion. This much time is required for the edema and spasm incident to instrumental exploration of the common bile duct to disappear. Likewise, this much time allows development of a fairly adequate tract through which bile may drain to the surface of the skin, should leakage occur from the opening in the common duct from which the tube is removed. Incidentally, there is no need to keep the patient in the hospital until the T-tube is removed.

My choice of method for closure of the common duct is the simplest, safest tube drainage for a relatively short period of time, that is, the short-arm T-tube.

References

1. Branch, C. D., Bailey, O. T., and Zollinger, R.: Consequences of instrumental dilation of the papilla of Vater: an experimental study. Arch. Surg., *38:*358, 1939.
2. Deaver, J. B.: Hepatic drainage. Brit. M. J., 2:821, 1904.
3. Diffenbaugh, W. G., and Strohl, E. L.: Acute hemorrhagic pancreatitis following biliary-tract surgical procedures. Tr. West. S. A., *63:*195, 1955.
4. Edwards, L. W., and Herrington, J. L., Jr.: Closure of the common bile duct following its exploration. Ann. Surg., *137:*189, 1953.
5. Ferris, D. O.: A new dilator of the common bile duct. Proc. Staff Meet. Mayo Clin., *33:*344, 1958.
6. McArthur, L. L.: Further advances in the therapeutic use of the bile tracts. New York J. Med., *45:*168, 1912.
7. Robson, A. W. M.: The surgical treatment of obstruction in the common bile-duct by concretion: with especial reference to the operation of choledochotomy as modified by the author. Illustrated by 60 cases. Lancet, *1:*1023, 1902.

Long-Limb T-Tube:
Its Current Place in Biliary Surgery

Kenneth W. Warren *and* William M. McDonald

Lahey Clinic Foundation, Boston, Massachusetts

Background and Indications for Use

Cattell's development of the long-limb T-tube was a direct response to the problem of maintaining patency following transcholedochal dilatation of a fibrotic contraction of the sphincter of Oddi and after transduodenal sphincterotomy.[2] Later this T-tube was used successfully as an internal splint in end-to-end repair of traumatic strictures of the bile duct.

At the present time, its uses are diverse and include the following:

1. As a splint in end-to-end repair of benign biliary strictures.

2. As a splint after dilatation of the sphincter of Oddi or advanced duodenal sphincterotomy.

3. As a cannula in the management of inoperable malignant tumors of the common bile duct or hepatic ducts and the periampullary area.

4. As an external vent from the common bile duct after the difficult extraction of an impacted stone at the papilla of Vater.

5. As a splint to delineate the position of and protect the intrapancreatic segment of the bile duct at the time of gastrectomy for a low-lying or extensive duodenal ulcer.

In Repair of Benign Biliary Strictures

End-to-end repair of benign strictures of the bile ducts is employed less frequently at this clinic when the caliber of the distal duct is small in relation to that of the proximal duct; but when end-to-end repair is decided on under these circumstances, the long-limb T-tube has an important place. A similar long-limb T-tube is frequently used when an extrahepatic bile duct is anastomosed to the duodenum or to the jejunum. Although in the latter instance the length of the distal limb of the tube may be shorter than the usual long-limb T-tube, the principle underlying the application is the same. A tube, or splint, which passes through the anastomosis, not only allows the decompression of the proximal bile ducts and the passage of bile through the tube into the intestinal tract, but also maintains the caliber of the fibrotic ring of the anastomosis until the scar tissue has matured. This maturation takes time and is often delayed by infection characterized by cholangitis, which usually accompanies bile duct strictures. It is important that the splint remain in place for a sufficient interval. Otherwise, the immature scar tissue may contract, causing an eventual obliteration of the anastomosis. A long-limb T-tube is far less likely to be displaced inadvertently than the more commonly used short-limb T-tube.

To Maintain Patency of the Sphincter of Oddi

Although this tube was designed to maintain patency of the sphincter of Oddi following dilatation of a fibrous contraction, this approach is rarely used at the Lahey Clinic now. Currently transduodenal sphincterotomy is preferred. Transduodenal sphincterotomy with retrograde dilatation

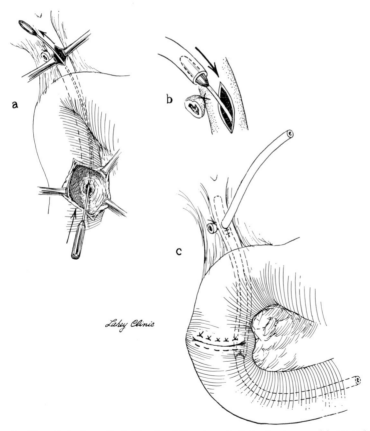

Fig. 1. Use of the long-limb T-tube following choledochostomy with transduodenal sphincterotomy. *a,* Bakes dilator through the papilla of Vater after sphincterotomy; *b,* method of insertion of long-limb T-tube; *c,* long-limb T-tube in place.

of the pancreatic ducts is favored by us as the initial surgical treatment of the early stages of chronic relapsing pancreatitis (Fig. 1). Although we do not believe that use of a long-limb T-tube is an essential part of this operation, we can find no objections to its use as a means of decompressing the bile ducts, provided the caliber of the tube traversing the sphincter is significantly smaller than the caliber of the sphincter of Oddi. When postoperative pancreatitis follows such a procedure, the period of copious biliary drainage through the external vent of the T-tube is shortened because bile flows through the lumen of the tube into the duodenum. Therefore, although initially the tube was used to ensure patency of the dilated or divided sphincter, a condition not considered essential after transduodenal sphincterotomy, it is valuable in allowing passage of bile into the duodenal lumen in the early postoperative phase.

Considerable criticism of the long-limb T-tube as an etiologic factor in postoperative pancreatitis has been recorded by other authors.[7] An extensive experience with postoperative pancreatitis at this clinic indicates that the incidence of this complication is no greater after use of the long-limb T-tube. It occurs most frequently after operations on the common bile duct, duodenum, and pancreas, and it may occur nevertheless after any operation, including gynecologic and neurosurgical procedures. It has been a sequel to adrenalectomy and, especially, to excision of parathyroid adenomas. In a recent report, Cattell and Braasch showed that the incidence of postoperative pancreatitis was identical following operations on the common bile duct regardless of whether a short- or long-limb T-tube was used.[3]

In Malignant Disease of the Extrahepatic Biliary Ducts

Because the long-limb T-tube is unlikely to be inadvertently displaced by the patient, there is a definite place for it in the palliative treatment of malignant diseases arising in or involving the distal extrahepatic bile ducts and periampullary area. If the condition is not amenable to radical resection by pancreatoduodenectomy, and if it is possible to pass a Bakes dilator and the long limb of a T-tube through the strictured area into the duodenum without creating a false passage, successful palliation of biliary obstruction can be obtained for a considerable length of time (Fig. 2). Inadvertent displacement of the tube by the patient must be prevented because usually further extension of the malignant process makes replacement impossible.

When choledochojejunostomy is used to bypass a malignant process involving a distal common bile duct, considerable palliation can be obtained if it is possible to introduce a proximal limb of the T-tube into the hepatic duct and a distal limb into the distal common bile duct, with the external vent brought out through the choledochojejunostomy anastomosis to lie in the lumen of the jejunum. A long-limb T-tube can be modified to suit this procedure.

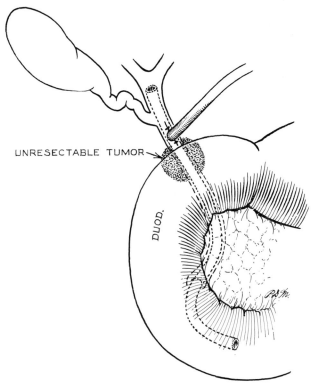

Fig. 2. Use of the long-limb T-tube to bypass an inoperable tumor in the periampullary area.

After Extraction of an Impacted Stone From the Papilla of Vater

Extraction of an impacted stone from the papilla may be extremely difficult, requiring extensive manipulations around the sphincter area and very often a transduodenal approach. Edema of the adjacent structures following these manipulations is not uncommon, and a long-limb T-tube frequently will bypass this swelling successfully and allow the drainage of bile into the duodenal lumen. The patient can be discharged from the hospital before all the swelling has resolved, because it is possible to clamp the external vent safely without fear of bile extravasation.

To Protect the Common Bile Duct During Gastrectomy

We use the long-limb T-tube during the performance of gastric resection for duodenal ulcers that have penetrated posteriorly or are of such a size that the integrity of the common bile duct may be endangered during the mobilization and closing of the duodenal stump (Fig. 3). With a long-limb T-tube or Bakes dilator inserted as a splint in the lumen of the bile duct, not only is the surgeon assured of the location of the common

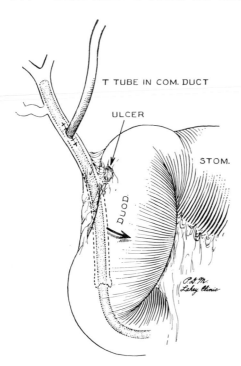

T TUBE IN COM. DUCT

ULCER

STOM.

DUOD.

Fig. 3. With the long-limb T-tube in place the surgeon is assured of the location of the common bile duct when performing gastric resection for a difficult duodenal ulcer which has penetrated posteriorly. (From Ann. Surg., *159*:1003, 1964.)

bile duct during performance of the operation, but also safe closure of the duodenal stump is facilitated. Use of this type of T-tube after the completion of such difficult and traumatic dissection allows decompression of the proximal biliary system and also of the afferent loop of the jejunum during the postoperative period.

Objections to the Long-Limb T-Tube

Surgeons have objected to use of the long-limb T-tube after limited trials because of a seemingly greater incidence of postoperative pancreatitis. It is most important, before condemning the procedure, to ascertain whether the T-tube has been used correctly and whether the damaging impression is the result of improper application. The T-tube should fit loosely within the lumen of the common bile duct and the ostium of the papilla of Vater; it should not be a close-fitting tube.

Is It Necessary?

Use of this type of T-tube is indicated most definitely in the end-to-end repair of traumatic strictures of the extrahepatic bile ducts. Its use in these patients is most important if the surgeon believes that the splint should remain in place through the anastomotic site for a period of six to eight months. The inadvertent dislodgment of a short-limb T-tube by the patient's body movement is a common occurrence despite all practical precautions, while the chance of the spontaneous dislodgment of a long-limb T-tube is remote. If it is possible to bypass an inoperable carcinoma of the distal bile duct by means of a T-tube, it is likewise most important that the tube not be displaced accidentally; a long-limb T-tube gives a greater guarantee of stability.

Maintenance of the patency of the sphincter of Oddi following an adequate sphincterotomy is unnecessary. However, in patients who have required considerable surgical manipulation of the head of the pancreas and the distal common bile duct, considerable swelling or even acute pancreatitis may result, and the bile duct may thus become compressed. Proximal decompression of the extrahepatic bile ducts by a short-limb T-tube may result in a long-lasting biliary drainage through the external vent until such time as the edema or pancreatitis has resolved. A long-limb T-tube inserted through the lumen of the distal common bile duct and papilla may allow closure of the external vent after a shorter interval and thereby decrease the length of hospitalization.

Is It Dangerous?

It is extremely difficult to evaluate an added factor in procedures which in themselves may lead to postoperative complications such as pancreatitis. The manual dilatation of the sphincter of Oddi, transduodenal sphincterotomy, calibration of the sphincter of Oddi in which no fibrosis is demonstrable, and the technically difficult gastrectomy are such procedures. It is true that postoperative pancreatitis has been seen after the use of long-limb T-tubes, but the incidence of this complication was highest when the tube was used as part of the procedure of transduodenal sphincterotomy and retrograde dilatation of the ducts of Wirsung. This operation is most commonly used in the surgical management of the early stages of chronic relapsing pancreatitis. These same operative procedures also induce postoperative pancreatitis when a short-limb T-tube is used or when no T-tube is used.

In 1961 Cattell and Braasch evaluated the use of the long-limb T-tube in 535 patients operated on at the Lahey Clinic.[3] Pancreatitis developed in five patients (0.9 per cent); two of the five died as a result. Choledochostomy with the insertion of a long-limb T-tube was performed on 205 patients, and no case of pancreatitis developed. Transduodenal sphincterotomy performed on 174 patients resulted in 2 fatal cases of pancreatitis, and end-to-end bile duct anastomosis in 156 patients produced 3 nonfatal cases of pancreatitis. These same authors reviewed 637 patients in whom either no T-tube or a standard short-limb T-tube was used. In 415 patients who had choledochostomy, pancreatitis developed in 2, in 1 of whom it was fatal. Of 53 patients who had end-to-end anastomosis, none developed postoperative pancreatitis, and of 169 patients who had hepaticojejunostomy for stricture, pancreatitis developed in 2 patients. Postoperative pancreatitis occurred in 0.6 per cent of the total number of patients, with only 1 death.

In 1954 Warren reported 892 patients who had a gastric resection, in 7 of whom pancreatitis developed postoperatively.[8] Bartlett and Quinby reported that pancreatitis developed postoperatively in 8 of 963 patients who had a choledochostomy.[1] Marshall and Bland reviewed 235 patients who had a choledochostomy, and found that pancreatitis developed post-operatively in 3 of these patients.[6] A long-limb T-tube was not used in any of a total of 2090 patients reported in these three series, but in 18 patients (0.9 per cent) pancreatitis developed postoperatively.

Proper Use of the Long-Limb T-Tube

The long-limb T-tube should not lie snugly within the ducts; its caliber should be significantly smaller than that of the sphincter of Oddi, thereby eliminating or reducing the chance of occluding the ostium of the pancreatic duct. The incidence of postoperative pancreatitis at the Lahey Clinic after use of a T-tube of proper size is approximately 1 per cent, and is comparable to the incidence seen after similar procedures on the bile duct or the stomach when a short-limb or no T-tube is used. The patient in whom postoperative pancreatitis develops fits no rigid pattern. The complication may occur after any procedure, and especially after major manipulation of the sphincter of Oddi or difficult operations on the duodenum or common bile duct. Indeed, it may occur after any operative procedure, and has been noted after transurethral resection of the prostate gland[5] and after gynecologic operations on organs that are not anatomically related to the pancreas.[4] Awareness of the possibility that such a condition can occur allows successful treatment to be undertaken early in the course of the illness.

Extrabiliary Uses of the Long-Limb T-Tube

Apart from its conventional uses in surgery of the bile duct and pancreas, we have found the long-limb T-tube to have considerable value as a gastrostomy tube for feeding the debilitated patient. The long limb, which is to lie proximally in the stomach, is tied. The T-tube is inserted into the lumen of the stomach through a small aperture, with the proximal and distal limbs in their correct positions. The stomach wall is then closed about the tube with a purse-string suture and reinforcing interrupted black silk sutures. This area is then buttressed against the anterior abdominal wall. A gastrostomy can thereby be created without producing a tunnel from the muscular and mucosal layers. In the same fashion, a feeding jejunostomy can be made.

In the presence of serious metabolic disturbance, a state not infrequently accompanying biliary and pancreatic fistulas, fluids such as sterile glucose and saline solution can be administered through a long-limb T-tube, with the proximal limb in the hepatic duct and the distal limb traversing the sphincter of Oddi, after surgical correction of the fistulas. Some fluid may reflux into the intrahepatic bile ducts, but cholangiograms taken with the long-limb T-tube in place show this to be unlikely.

Conclusion

The long-limb T-tube is probably valuable in situations in which it is currently used, but has especial merit when used in patients having end-to-end anastomosis for repair of benign strictures of the bile duct. A lack of the proper understanding of its use may make this type of T-tube potentially hazardous, but if care is taken that its caliber is significantly smaller than the lumen of the common bile duct and the ostium of the papilla of Vater, the chance of its being associated with postoperative pancreatitis is no greater than when a standard T-tube or no T-tube is used. Postoperative pancreatitis following biliary tract, pancreatic, or gastric surgery is related to the difficulty of the operation rather than to the employment of a particular type of T-tube.

References

1. Bartlett, M. K., and Quinby, W. C., Jr.: Surgery of biliary tract; mortality and complications of cholecystectomy and choledochostomy for chronic cholecystitis. New England J. Med., 254:154, 1956.
2. Cattell, R. B.: New type of T-tube for surgery of biliary tract. Lahey Clin. Bull., 4:197, 1946.
3. Cattell, R. B., and Braasch, J. W.: An evaluation of the long T-tube. Ann. Surg., 154: 252, 1961.
4. Ferris, D. O., Lynn, T. E., and Cain, J. C.: Fatal postoperative pancreatitis. Ann. Surg., 146:263, 1957.
5. Levine, S. R., Cambill, E. E., and Greene, L. F.: Acute pancreatitis following transurethral prostatic resection: report of six cases. J. Urol., 88:657, 1962.
6. Marshall, J. F., and Bland, R. W.: Operations upon the common bile duct for stones. Ann. Surg., 149:793, 1959.
7. Thompson, J. A., Howard, J. M., and Vowles, K. D.: Acute pancreatitis following choledochotomy. Surg., Gynec. and Obst., 105:706, 1957.
8. Warren, K. W.: Pancreatic considerations in gastric surgery. J.A.M.A., 154:803, 1954.

Acute Pancreatitis

Introduction

In recent years the treatment of acute pancreatitis in its initial stages for the most part has been nonsurgical and directed toward the relief of pain, the lowering of intraductal pressure, the control of pancreatic secretion, the neutralization of proteolytic enzymes, the restoration of electrolyte and blood volume losses, and the prevention of secondary infection. Surgical treatment has been avoided, except in the presence of a worsening acute cholecystitis or a rapidly increasing jaundice, presumably the result of a common duct stone impacted in the ampulla of Vater. If suppuration occurs, drainage of any resultant abscess is accomplished, and in rare instances, an attempt will be made to control a persistent and worsening process by emergency drainage of a necrotic pancreas. The prognosis in these patients, however, is extremely poor.

In contrast, cholecystostomy, either with or without drainage of the lesser sac, has been practiced by some as an acceptable adjunct for the treatment of acute pancreatitis after adequate replacement of blood volume and correction of gross chemical imbalances. Such an approach has some theoretical value if one is concerned about the possibility of continued perfusion of the pancreatic ductal system with activated pancreatic enzymes. On the other hand, the originator of this concept and one of our essayists (D. E.) continues to advocate nonoperative management for acute pancreatitis, and reports an overall mortality of 7.2 per cent in 334 patients treated at the Ohio State University Hospitals during a 15-year period.

Notwithstanding the many advances in the understanding and treatment of acute pancreatitis, the overall country-wide mortality in these patients continues at a high level. In turn, some surgeons have challenged the routine nonoperative management of acute pancreatitis, and one of our essayists (H. R. B.), points out that in one instance the diagnosis even had not been suspected in some 40 per cent of patients suffering from a fatal pancreatitis. In addition, we are reminded that several common surgical problems, including perforated duodenal ulcer, mesenteric vascular occlusion, and other acute abdominal catastrophes, may simulate acute inflammation of the pancreas and frequently lead to an elevation of the serum and peritoneal amylase. All would agree that under such circumstances, nonoperative treatment might prove to be fatal; however, it is difficult to evaluate the overall significance of such misdiagnoses or their occurrence, since this kind of data is seldom included in the usual clinical report. Finally, the author supporting early laparotomy suggests that removal of gallstones or correction of other surgical abnormalities of the pancreaticobiliary tree should reduce the incidence and associated risk of recurrent attacks of pancreatitis. The results of the reported cases are quite similar to those reported by Elliott.

The final essayist is advocating early and even emergency transduodenal sphincteroplasty and internal decompression of the pancreatic duct for those patients in whom the disease has failed to subside in the usual fashion and for patients with pancreatitis who have undergone operation because of an erroneous diagnosis. This approach is also suggested for those unfortunate patients who develop a full-blown pancreatitis after operation on the biliary tract.

The arguments pro and con for these varied approaches are well presented in the papers immediately following.

E. H. E.

Nonoperative
Management of Acute Pancreatitis

Dan W. Elliott

The Ohio State University Hospitals

The nonoperative management of acute pancreatitis appears to be growing in favor. This course of action depends on three basic concepts:

1. Acute pancreatitis is a self-limited sterile inflammation from which most patients will completely recover, if they are adequately supported through the first few critical days.

2. An accurate diagnosis can be made without operation in the vast majority of cases, with the aid of amylase determinations.

3. Beyond confirming the diagnosis, emergency operation offers no therapy capable of modifying the natural course of the acute attack.

The basic soundness of these concepts seems to be supported by the experience with acute pancreatitis at the Ohio State University Hospitals during the past 15 years. Here the initial treatment has been almost uniformly nonoperative. These cases have been reviewed to provide up-to-date figures indicating the results of such treatment.

Differential Diagnosis

Acute pancreatitis should be suspected whenever there has been an abrupt onset of upper abdominal pain. This pain is rarely absent, except in patients too old or feeble to communicate with the examining physician; in these patients, only upper abdominal tenderness and a sudden worsening in appearance raises the correct suspicion.

An upper abdominal location for the acute process is confirmed by tenderness and rigidity in the anterior abdominal wall. Otherwise there are no important or characteristic physical findings. There is usually a marked leukocytosis, but only slight fever, and no shock. Many other acute surgical lesions of the abdomen could present this picture, and indeed acute pancreatitis is frequently misdiagnosed as perforated ulcer, acute cholecystitis, intestinal obstruction, or myocardial infarction.

The key to modern diagnosis is the serum amylase determination. The amylase is elevated after such an attack in almost every patient during the first 24 hours, and in many patients up to 48 hours. After that time the serum amylase returns to normal, even if the pancreatitis grows worse. Because of these rapid changes in the circulating blood levels, a serum amylase should be drawn at once, day or night, from every patient presenting with upper abdominal pain. The determination should be carried out as soon as possible. If no laboratory help is available, the tube of blood may be stored in the refrigerator overnight with little change in its amylase level. If that same blood had been allowed to circulate in the patient until morning, its diagnostic amylase elevation might have disappeared!

In contrast to serum, a diagnostic elevation of amylase often persists in the peritoneal fluid and in the urine for three to seven days after the onset of the acute attack. Urine amylase is easily obtained and is a reliable indicator of increased amylase production, provided that amylase excretion is expressed in *units per hour*. This calculation eliminates the variations in urine flow and concentration. Usually the upper limit of normal for amylase excretion per hour in the urine is easy to remember, since it is exactly the same as the upper limit of normal for amylase in the serum, expressed in milligrams per cent.[3]

When abdominal pain is combined with a high amylase in any fluid, acute pancreatitis will be responsible in about nine cases out of ten.[1] In the tenth, some other important surgical lesion requiring early operation is likely to be present, and this possibility must be excluded. Perforated ulcers, mesenteric infarction, intestinal obstruction, and many other lesions producing abdominal pain have all been reported to elevate the amylase in any body fluid. These elevations may be just as high as those seen in acute pancreatitis. Therefore, two additional steps are required: x-rays of the chest and abdomen, and a diagnostic paracentesis.

X-rays are of value principally to exclude the presence of free air, which would indicate a perforated viscus. The film should also exclude the possibility of a mechanical small bowel obstruction, although this may be a little more difficult. X-rays may reveal some helpful signs characteristic of pancreatitis, but none of these are truly specific: (1) a small left pleural effusion; (2) paralytic ileus with a "sentinal loop" of dilated jejunum near the pancreas; (3) dilated transverse colon; or (4) radiopaque stones in the gallbladder or pancreas.

The diagnostic paracentesis is far more specific. This measure should be employed in every patient not responding well to treatment, or for whom an emergency operation is being seriously considered. Fortunately, almost all of the nonpancreatic surgical lesions associated with a high serum amylase produce ascitic fluid in abundance. The fluid can be aspirated with greatest ease from the abdominal quadrant that is most rigid and tender. In acute pancreatitis, this fluid is pale yellow and never more jaundiced than the patient's serum, has a high amylase level, no odor, and no bacteria in a stained smear. In contrast, the gastrointestinal lesions requiring early operation produce an ascitic fluid which is totally inconsistent with a diagnosis of acute pancreatitis. For instance, the presence of bile indicates a perforation. Hemorrhagic fluid or a foul odor suggests gangrenous bowel. Bacteria in the stained smear indicates intestinal obstruction, compromised bowel, or a localized abscess. If the ascitic fluid shows any of these findings, emergency operation is usually indicated without regard for any amylase elevations.

Nonoperative Treatment

Most physicians would like to fit the treatment of acute pancreatitis to the severity of the individual attack. There are certain signs that clearly warn of a serious illness ahead: (1) rapid pulse, (2) distended or rigid abdomen, (3) mental aberrations, (4) dusky cyanosis of the extremities, (5) unstable blood pressure, or (6) tetany with a low serum calcium. If any of these is present, treatment must be both prompt and vigorous. However, it is a mistake to await these morbid signs before beginning serious therapy, because of the completely unpredictable course of the disease. Early in an attack, young adults may appear only mildly ill and yet progress to extreme toxicity, shock, and death within 24 hours. Fortunately, within the same period, about 40 per cent of the patients will be free of pain and definitely improving.[1] At the onset it is impossible to tell which course the individual patient will follow. The amylase level provides no clue. Therefore, "overtreatment" should be the rule for the milder cases, in order to anticipate the needs of the 60 per cent who will become seriously ill.

Good nonoperative treatment has one important characteristic: its various measures all add up to excellent preparation for an operation, if that should become necessary at any time. The general principles followed in treatment may be outlined as follows:

1. *The injured part should be placed at rest.* In the pancreas, this is done by suppressing all three stimuli for secretion. The vagus nerve and two hormones are involved. One of these, pancreozymin, is released when fat contacts the upper jejunum; therefore, complete starvation will prevent its release. The other hormone, secretin, may be released as long as gastric acid enters the duodenum. To prevent this acidity, gastric suction should be employed. This also helps to combat the accompanying paralytic ileus. Nervous stimuli to secretion are carried mostly by the vagus nerve and may be blocked by atropine, given by hypodermic, usually in a dose of 0.4 mg. every 4 to 6 hours.

2. *Pain must be relieved,* and the initial pain of pancreatitis can be extreme. Block of the splanchnic nerves with procaine has been advocated, and this procedure does effectively relieve pain. However, bilateral blockade is usually necessary, and this is frequently accompanied by a falling blood pressure. Hypotension must be avoided at all costs in acute pancreatitis, since it will make even a mild case much, much worse. It is preferable to

use adequate quantities of the milder synthetic narcotics, such as meperidine or anileridine. With adequate decompression of the stomach, only small quantities of narcotics are usually necessary after the first few hours. Morphine should be avoided because of its tendency to produce spasm and paralysis in the smooth muscles of the upper gastrointestinal tract.

3. *The blood volume requires special support.* Rapidly progressive dehydration is the rule in acute pancreatitis, manifested by a rising pulse rate, a diminishing urine flow, and a dusky cyanosis of the peripheral extremities. These signs are accompanied by a progressive loss in circulating blood volume. There is a greater loss of plasma than of red cells, resulting in the typical rising hematocrit. In more than 40 patients the successive changes in blood volume have been actually measured by radioactive iodinated albumin techniques.[2] Among the more severe cases the average loss in blood volume after 24 hours of illness was 1500 cc. Patients with tachycardia and abdominal distention or rigidity regularly developed this deficit, although it was not found in the milder cases with no serious abdominal changes.

Where does the missing blood volume go? Operation or autopsy early in the course of an attack will demonstrate huge quantities of edema fluid, rich in plasma proteins, loculated in and around the pancreas, in the free ascitic fluid, in the mesentery, and within the lumen of the distended bowel. Calculations based on actual measurement of the water and protein within these tissues indicates that the entrapped edema is sufficient to account for the deficiency of circulating plasma usually observed.

Just as in third degree burns of the skin, this entrapment of plasma takes place in the first 48 hours of illness. Therefore, in all but the mildest attacks, generous quantities of plasma or whole blood should be administered. Now that safe and inexpensive plasma is commercially available,* this is probably the agent of choice. A minimum of 1000 to 1500 cc. usually is required in the first 48 hours. More should be used if necessary to slow the pulse, stabilize the blood pressure, and obtain a good urinary output.

4. *Complications should be anticipated.* Among the most serious are secondary infections. Gastric aspiration and immobilization for four to five days account for a high rate of septic pneumonias. Necrotic tissue in the pancreas or a collection of juice in the lesser sac is extremely vulnerable to secondary infection. Because of these dangers, prophylactic antibiotics are probably worthwhile. Penicillin, in combination with streptomycin, has been used most frequently.

Gastrointestinal hemorrhage from stress ulceration is a common and serious threat. Hemorrhage into the lesser sac behind the stomach has also occurred in the more serious cases. Therefore, a falling prothrombin level and its hemorrhagic tendencies should be minimized by the parenteral administration of vitamin K.

Symptoms of hypocalcemia sometimes appear in these patients. This may be corrected by the addition of calcium gluconate to the intravenous

* Plasminate or Albumisol

solutions ordinarily required. Before calcium is given, however, a serum calcium determination should be obtained. An occasional patient may have developed his acute pancreatitis secondary to an underlying parathyroid adenoma. The principal means for identifying such a situation is an elevation in the serum calcium, which otherwise will be depressed during an attack of acute pancreatitis.

5. *Cortisone should be used rarely.* There is considerable rationale for the addition of cortisone in large doses to this therapeutic regime, since pancreatitis is an acute, sterile, self-limited inflammatory process of unknown cause. (These are the characteristics supposed to favor cortisone treatment.) Animal experiments indicate that cortisone can limit pancreatic inflammation, and help combat shock.[5] However, there are at least two specific drawbacks to its regular use: when cortisone is given for other diseases, chronic inflammation in the pancreas is often produced. In addition, cortisone increases the likelihood of serious gastrointestinal hemorrhage from stress ulcer, and this is a strong argument against its administration. In summary, the use of cortisone should probably be restricted to those patients not responding to conventional therapy, in whom shock has developed despite adequate colloids, or in whom there is some other good reason to suspect acute adrenal insufficiency. The place for trypsin inhibitors in clinical treatment remains entirely problematic and experimental.[4]

This program of treatment is analagous to preparation of the patient for operation. There should be a slow but steady and continuing improvement in his clinical appearance. Of particular importance are improvements in color, breathing, pulse rate, and urinary flow. These should all be evident within four to eight hours, and abdominal pain, distention, and rigidity should not progress. When these favorable changes are not obtained within 8 to 12 hours, the diagnosis of acute pancreatitis should be seriously questioned, and the possibility of operation considered. Under these circumstances, diagnostic paracentesis can be extremely helpful. If diagnostic fluid was not obtained in an earlier effort, this procedure should now be repeated.

Conditions Justifying Emergency Operation

Early emergency operation is justified for: (1) a doubtful diagnosis, (2) acute cholecystitis accompanying acute pancreatitis, or (3) an acutely enlarging pancreatic abscess or pseudocyst. If pancreatitis is confirmed at operation, only the very minimum procedures should be performed to obtain good drainage of the biliary tree and the pancreas.

Convalescence

In the very mild cases gastric suction can be discontinued after 24 hours, but in the majority three to five days of suction are required. Feeding must begin with caution, since stimulation to the pancreas is now introduced. A bland ulcer diet should be used to avoid peaks of gastric acid and, therefore, pancreatic stimulation. Atropine-like drugs should be continued in oral form. Coffee and caffeine-containing colas must be avoided because of their acid-stimulating potentials.

Since approximately 60 per cent of all patients recovering from an attack of acute pancreatitis will have demonstrable gallstones, these should now be searched for. An oral cholecystogram should be performed. Even if only faint visualization is achieved, this may be enough to demonstrate gallstones in these patients. However, complete nonvisualization of the gallbladder cannot be taken as evidence of biliary disease until four weeks after the pancreatitis begins to subside. At this time the oral cholecystogram should be repeated. Early in convalescence a barium contrast examination of the stomach should also be obtained to rule out a gathering pseudocyst, lesser sac abscess, or undue swelling in the head of the pancreas.

If x-ray study reveals gallstones, an elective operation for their removal should be performed. The operation should always include a careful evaluation of the common bile duct, either by exploration or by a completely satisfactory operative cholangiogram. This procedure may be carried out electively as soon as the patient is up and about, eating a bland diet, and having normal bowel movements. Once gallstones are demonstrated there is no need to send the patient home from the hospital to await further subsidence of pancreatitis. This delay only invites a recurrent attack. These elective biliary operations are usually performed between the seventh and fifteenth days after the onset of the acute attack. By this time the tremendous edema of the pancreatitis has largely subsided, and good exposure of the common duct is not too difficult to achieve.

Results of Initial Nonoperative Management

At the University Hospital 334 patients have been seen with a diagnosis of primary or idiopathic acute pancreatitis during the years 1947 to 1963, a total of 15 years. During this period a primary effort at nonoperative management was undertaken in all of these cases. For inclusion in this series a patient had to have abdominal pain together with an elevated amylase in the serum, urine, or peritoneal fluid, or else pancreatitis demonstrated at operation (2 cases) or at autopsy (3 cases). The average severity of pancreatitis encountered in this series may be judged from the fact that 60 per cent required gastric suction for more than 48 hours. Biliary tract disease was demonstrated by x-ray, operation, or autopsy in 62 per cent; a definite history of alcoholism was elicited in 20 per cent, and no primary cause for the attack of pancreatitis could be found in the remaining 18 per cent. Emergency operation was avoided whenever possible, and only 17 patients or 5 per cent of the entire group had an operation performed during the first week of illness. On the other hand, good-risk patients with proved

TABLE 1.   TREATMENT OF ACUTE PANCREATITIS

	Number	Deaths	Mortality Rate (Per Cent)
Emergency operation	17	6	35
Elective operation	89	1	1.2
No operation	228	17	7.5
Totals	334	24	7.2

gallstones, pancreatic masses, or other indications for laparotomy had elective operations performed without hesitation early in convalescence. The combined overall results of this approach to acute pancreatitis are indicated in Table 1.

The very high operative mortality for emergency surgery is not hard to understand. These operations were performed rarely, for only the most urgent reasons, and usually in patients not responding well to nonoperative management. In contrast elective operations were performed in 26 per cent of the entire series, and on carefully selected patients after suitable preparation. The operation almost always involved the common bile duct and included cholecystectomy, unless the gallbladder had been previously removed. The mortality rate of 1.2 per cent seems acceptable, and is comparable to that reported for similar operations done without any antecedent pancreatitis. The rate of postoperative complications was 12 per cent and, surprisingly enough, almost never included postoperative pancreatitis. The overall mortality rate for the entire series was 7.2 per cent, including all the operations performed. This figure may be the only significant statistic in the table, but it does seem to support the general efficacy of nonoperative management.

Close scrutiny of the 24 deaths in this series was undertaken to find any measures that might have improved the overall record. These cases have been examined particularly with reference to whether emergency operation could have been performed, and might have been helpful. The results are listed in Table 2. There were clear-cut contraindications to any operation in 14 of the 24 cases. In four younger patients, shock was unremitting from hospital admission and precluded operation. The majority of the deaths, however, occurred in older patients with seriously disabling diseases before the pancreatitis appeared, or who avoided medical attention until the appearance of such serious complications as oliguria or bronchopneumonia. As a result these patients were extremely unwelcome candidates for any type of surgery.

There were no contraindications to operation among the remaining ten patients who died. Emergency operations were performed in six (to establish the diagnosis in two, and to drain acute pseudocysts in four). No operation was performed in the remaining four deaths. In retrospect, one of these patients would clearly have benefited from emergency drainage of a rapidly enlarging pseudocyst. In the remaining three, the possible benefits of early

TABLE 2. WOULD EMERGENCY OPERATION HAVE HELPED IN THE 24 PATIENTS WHO LATER DIED?

Contraindications to Operation	Cases
Unremitting shock from admission	4
Serious illness before pancreatitis diagnosed	
Advanced uremia, oliguria	4
CVA with paralysis	3
Severe generalized arthritis	1
Pneumonia at admission	2
None of these contraindications	
Emergency operation performed	6
No operation	4
Total	24

operation are not so evident. Therefore, it appears that the most frequent causes for death in acute pancreatitis are not amenable to the emergency operations that can be performed today.

Summary

Nonoperative management of acute pancreatitis seems to be the best initial treatment because:

1. Pancreatitis is an acute sterile chemical inflammation which, in most patients, will run a brief self-limited course.

2. The diagnosis can be accurately established with amylase determinations, and without operation, provided special care is used to rule out extrapancreatic causes for amylase elevation.

3. Nonoperative therapy is normally very effective, and provides good preparation for operation, should it become necessary.

4. Emergency operation can do very little to alter the natural course of the acute inflammation, and therefore should be reserved for specific indications: (a) an uncertain diagnosis, (b) an accompanying acute cholecystitis, or (c) pancreatic cyst formation.

5. Elective operation for proved gallstones may be carried out during the second or third week after pancreatitis in selected patients with technical ease and good safety.

The general experience with acute pancreatitis at the University Hospital during the past 15 years totals 334 cases, with a 7.2 per cent overall mortality, and appears to support these principles.

References

1. Elliott, D. W., and Williams, R. D.: A re-evaluation of serum amylase determinations. Arch. Surg., 83:130, 1961.

2. Elliott, D. W.: Treatment of acute pancreatitis with albumin and whole blood. A.M.A. Arch. Surg., 75:573, 1957.
3. Gambill, E. D., and Mason, H. L., One-hour value for urinary amylase in 96 patients with pancreatitis. J.A.M.A., 186:24, 1963.
4. Nemir, P., Jr., Hoferichter, J., and Drabkin, D. L.: The protective effect of proteinase inhibitor in acute necrotizing pancreatitis. Ann. Surg., 158:655, 1963.
5. Stewart, W. R. C., Elliott, D. W., and Zollinger, R. M.: Cortisone in the treatment of experimental acute pancreatitis. S. Forum, 9:537, 1958.

Early Laparotomy to Confirm
Diagnosis of Acute Pancreatitis

Harvey R. Bernard

Washington University School of Medicine, St. Louis, Missouri

As a consequence of experiences in hospitals in St. Louis* over the past 13 years, it is evident that all patients, ill because of severe, sudden, upper abdominal pain and shock, with or without an increase in pancreatic ferments in the body fluids, should be regarded as acute operative surgical problems until proved otherwise by their response to preoperative preparation.

The data indicate that exact pathologic definition of acute illnesses of the pancreas and surrounding organs is impossible without direct observation of them. Indirect attempts at such definition are presumptive at best, and may result in danger to the patient if false positive results are obtained in the presence of other illnesses that require aggressive operative treatment. A complete understanding of the physiologic implications of pancreatitis, and eventual evolution of effective methods for its prevention and cure must necessarily be based on exact knowledge of the pathologic process.

Advantages of "Early" Laparotomy in the Diagnosis of Acute Pancreatitis

Direct observation of the pancreas through early laparotomy permits exact definition of the pathologic changes; it affords an opportunity for the diagnosis of other related or unrelated surgical illnesses; and it permits the institution of direct surgical measures when indicated.

Problems Associated with Attempts at Diagnosis by Indirect Means

The formulation of accurate diagnoses prior to direct examination by autopsy or laparotomy has proved difficult as judged by analysis of our records.

* Barnes Hospital and St. Louis City Hospital

The difficulty in diagnosing acute pancreatitis was directly correlated with the seriousness of the illness. In a group of 26 who died of their disease, the nature of the illness, antemortem, was suspected only 58 per cent of the time, owing to variations in the presenting signs and symptoms and the association of pancreatitis with other illnesses. The symptom complex was not uniform. Many times these illnesses were very complicated diagnostic problems (e.g., comatose patients, patients admitted because of acute tubular necrosis, and patients struck by sudden intra-abdominal catastrophes following operations on other regions, such as the genitourinary tract). In 30 per cent of these patients (8 of 26), the serum amylase levels at the time they were drawn were found to be less than 500 Somogyi units/100 ml. Whatever the reason, the levels of serum amylase obtained in these patients were generally lower than those found in patients who suffered much less serious illnesses.

The same group of physicians and surgeons experienced equal difficulty in making an accurate assessment of the severity of pancreatitis in another group of patients so diagnosed, principally because of elevation of the serum amylase to 1000 Somogyi units/100 ml. or greater. Although severe pancreatitis was universally thought to exist, no evidence of pancreatitis remained in 86 per cent of 50 such patients at the time operations were performed (0 to 8 weeks after the onset of their illness). In several instances, during operations performed within a few days of the onset of the illness and at a time when the serum amylase was still elevated, the pancreas was found to be normal to outward appearance and, in one instance, microscopically as well. Although these patients were not as seriously ill and the pancreatic disease less far advanced, the serum amylase was usually found to be high, many times over 2000 to 3000 Somogyi units/100 ml.

Many authors suggest that examination of the peritoneal fluid obviates many of the problems caused by the lack of sensitivity of the serum amylase tests because of prolongation of amylase elevation within ascites. Rarely has this been of value in our experience, usually because it was not possible to obtain fluid at a significant period in the patient's illness. Study of the amylase levels in the urine has not been of practical value in the treatment of our patients.

Observations on patients operated on at increasingly shorter intervals after attacks of abdominal pain, thought to be caused by pancreatitis, have indicated that acute diseases of the biliary tract are frequently the most significant part of the illness and pancreatic inflammations relatively minor. It has been possible to predict with increasing accuracy the degree of technical difficulty to be expected by observing the rapidity with which hypovolemia may be repaired and the time required for resolution of pain, muscle spasm, fever, and leukocytosis. In the usual patient it is possible to select a safe time for early laparotomy based solely on the response of the patient to treatment.

The serum amylase test has thus proved unreliable because of false negative and weak positive reactions. In addition, false positive reactions have also been observed. These are especially important although not frequent. In the initial series of patients at the Barnes and St. Louis City Hospitals, thought to have severe pancreatitis because of elevation of the serum amylase, seven remediable surgical lesions were found. These illnesses, which were all associated with serum amylase values of 750 Somogyi units/100 ml. or greater, included perforated duodenal ulcer, acute cholecystitis, impacted stones at the ampulla of Vater, volvulus of the small intestine, and mesenteric occlusion. Surgeons at neighboring hospitals have since described similar findings in patients who suffered from ruptured abdominal and splenic aneurysms. Many of these illnesses demand immediate surgical operation. To delay is to doom the patient to additional hardship if not certain death.

For a few of the patients suffering from acute pancreatitis, early, exact diagnosis by laparotomy permits the institution of definitive measures for treatment of the illness or for prevention of recurrences. Our more recent experiences include a cancer of the body of the pancreas masquerading as acute pancreatitis, a small tumor of the ampulla of Vater associated with hemorrhagic pancreatitis, several patients with accompanying acute cholecystitis, and patients with stones impacted at the ampulla of Vater, one of whom returned to the hospital suffering from a second attack of pancreatitis within one week of the first from which he had recovered quickly. He died within 24 hours of the second attack from hemorrhagic pancreatitis.

The frequency with which accompanying biliary tract abnormalities will be found associated with pancreatitis will differ from hospital to hospital, and this must be considered in formulating the course of action within a given institution. One may expect to find biliary stones in 80 to 90 per cent of the patients suffering from acute pancreatitis at the Barnes Hospital. The incidence of stones as the associated factor will be less in other hospitals, e.g., some veterans' hospitals encounter acute alcoholic pancreatitis much more frequently; hospitals that care for Negro patients, especially those with a high proportion of men, find pancreatitis associated with gallstones rarely, because of the infrequent occurrence of gallstones in Negro men between the ages of 20 and 50.

Surgical measures at present will not cure all forms of pancreatitis. Despite this, surgical measures are presently the only definitive ones for the treatment and prevention of pancreatitis through removal of the inciting causes or diversion of the pancreatic or biliary tracts. Because of the severe implications of recurrent attacks of pancreatitis, it seems reasonable to recommend the early removal of gallstones and other inciting factors. There is evidence that the removal of stones is effective in preventing recurrent attacks of acute pancreatitis.

Results of Treatment

The methods used to treat pancreatitis at the Barnes Hospital have come about by evolution rather than by decree. The process is still underway.

Gradually the surgeons and internists have become less timid about operating on patients with inflammatory disease of the pancreas, and have learned more and more about the pathologic anatomy of pancreatitis at an earlier and earlier stage. In the early study made at the Barnes and St. Louis City Hospitals (1949 to 1954) the mortality risk of operation was 7 per cent (5 in 67). In the Barnes Hospital between 1957 and 1959, 2 in 22 died (9 per cent), and from 1957 to 1962, 1 in 22 (5 per cent). With one exception, these deaths occurred in patients nearly moribund during desperate attempts to preserve life. In the last 5 years, 40 per cent of the patients were operated upon immediately; an additional 30 per cent within ten days of the acute attack, and another 30 per cent after two weeks. The only death occurred in a 72 year old man, who was operated on for a presumptive diagnosis of perforation of a gastric ulcer diagnosed previously by x-ray examination.

How Should "Early" Operative Management Be Employed?

Early operation does not necessarily mean emergency operation. The exact timing of it must be determined by the illness, which varies from patient to patient. This is especially pertinent since great variations in the external manifestations of this illness have, in our experience, been characteristic of it.

How may accurate diagnoses be obtained in order to assess various forms of treatment; how may remediable lesions be treated expeditiously in order to prevent the overlooking of intra-abdominal surgical catastrophes not associated with pancreatitis; and how may future attacks of pancreatitis be prevented while an increase in risk to the patient is avoided, especially in a patient who truly has simple catarrh of the pancreas? The solution to these problems may be found through active, careful study of all the patient's signs and symptoms before and during treatment, which is designed to prepare the patient for a surgical operation in a rapid and effective way. This should include the relief of pain, continuous gastric suction, and the treatment of complicating hypovolemia or extracellular fluid volume deficit, with appropriate sodium-containing solutions. All reasonable diagnostic tests should then be performed, and the patient's response to the treatment carefully evaluated.

Most patients will respond rapidly, so that their general condition is quickly improved and the severity of their symptoms reduced. These patients should be permitted to continue their improvement while the biliary tract is studied by both oral and intravenous cholecystography, cholangiography, and other diagnostic measures. Those who are considered likely to suffer from stones in the biliary tract are operated on after this decision is made, and as soon as the patient's circumstances warrant it. The degree of technical difficulty expected and the surgical risk attendant on such an operation may be assessed rather accurately by careful observation of the patient as the illness progresses. Persistence of fever, elevation of the white blood count, slow decrease in the serum amylase level, the continued presence of abdominal spasm, and an indefinite mass indicate that serious inflammation, in and about the pancreas, continues, and increased technical difficulties should be expected. The rapid regression of fever, leukocytosis, and abdominal spasm, leaving a residual mass confined to the area occupied by the gallbladder, indicate a much less serious technical problem and the likelihood that the primary problem is acute cholecystitis with lithiasis.

In all patients, an attempt should be made to remove gallstones or other surgical abnormalities of the pancreaticobiliary system as early as possible, consistent with the general condition of the patient, in an attempt to prevent recurrence of the pancreatitis. Those patients who do not show rapid improvement with the treatment outlined and those patients who suffer recurrence of pain, shock, or other signs of intra-abdominal catastrophe are operated upon forthwith. The continuing loss of extracellular fluid and shock in these patients denote the presence of catastrophic surgical illnesses. The type of surgical procedure performed should be decided upon after an exact assessment of the problem is made at the time of operation.

It is believed that in this way the principle of helping the most and injuring the fewest may be achieved.

Summary

Early laparotomy should be considered seriously in the treatment of patients thought to be suffering from acute pancreatitis. The risk of this form of treatment is not great. A diagnostic accuracy is achieved which is not possible by indirect means. Early laparotomy also permits the diagnosis of other surgical illnesses and the institution of direct surgical measures when indicated.

References

1. Bernard, H. R., Criscione, J. R., and Moyer, C. A.: The pathologic significance of the serum amylase concentration. Arch. Surg., 70:311, 1959.
2. Bowers, R. F., and Greenfield, J.: Choledochojejunostomy—its role in the treatment of pancreatitis. Ann. Surg., 134:99, 1951.
3. Howard, J. M., and Ehrlich, E. W.: The etiology of pancreatitis: a review of clinical experience. Ann. Surg., 152:135, 1960.
4. Kaden, V. E., and Howard, J. M.: Clinical studies of the natural history of acute pancreatitis. Arch. Surg., 73:269, 1956.
5. Lieber, M. M.: The incidence of gallstones and their correlation with other diseases. Ann. Surg., 135:394, 1952.
6. Raker, J. W., and Bartlett, M. K.: Acute pancreatitis: the fate of the patient surviving one or more acute attacks. New England J. Med., 249:751, 1953.
7. Sanchez-Ubeda, R. L., Rousselot, M., and Gianelli, S.: The significance of pancreatitis accompanying acute cholecystitis. Ann. Surg., 144:44, 1956.

Emergency Operation for Internal Decompression: Role of Pancreatic Duct Exploration in Acute Pancreatitis

E. W. Salzman *and* G. L. Nardi

Harvard Medical School

Evaluation of Conservative Treatment

There is a need for re-evaluation of the accepted conservative treatment of acute pancreatitis.

In most patients, management of the acute attack by intubation, antispasmodics, fluid and colloid replacement, and symptomatic therapy leads to rapid subsidence of symptoms and resolution of the pathologic process. When indicated, definitive surgical treatment can be offered in a later quiescent interval.

An appreciable number of patients, however, do not respond well to such a conservative program. Death is not uncommon in fulminating hemorrhagic pancreatitis, and not a few fatalities occur in patients whose downhill course is leisurely enough to permit new therapeutic maneuvers if such were available.

Failures of treatment also exist in the small but troublesome group of patients in whom the disease pursues a persistent, smouldering course without signs of abatement.

Other patients may respond initially to the conventional program, but eventually develop recurring attacks which require more specific therapy at a later date, when irreversible damage has occurred and treatment is more difficult.

In these persistent cases, the disease may go on to formation of an abscess or pseudocyst, or to pancreatic insufficiency, and these patients too must be considered failures of a conservative program.

A fourth group in whom conventional therapy has been particularly disappointing is that group in which pancreatitis develops postoperatively, most often after surgical manipulation of the common bile duct.

Case for Emergency Decompression

In patients suffering from these difficult and challenging forms of acute pancreatitis, we have begun to assess the value of pancreatic duct decompression by sphincteroplasty and exploration of the pancreatic duct during the acute or subacute phase of their illness. This operation has proved its worth during the quiescent interval phase of recurrent pancreatitis.[1, 2, 5, 6] An extension of its use to selected patients during the acute attack of the disease has appeared to be a logical next step.

In the past three years we have encountered six patients in whom acute pancreatitis has failed to subside in the usual fashion. Instead the disease has smouldered and sputtered, with persistent pain, tenderness, and ileus for many weeks.[7] All six patients have undergone transduodenal sphincteroplasty and exploration of the pancreatic duct. In each case, the diagnosis of acute pancreatitis was confirmed at laparotomy by the presence of retroperitoneal edema and fat necrosis.

One patient had been ill without remission for eleven weeks. He was operated on in desperation and proved to have stenosis of the orifice of

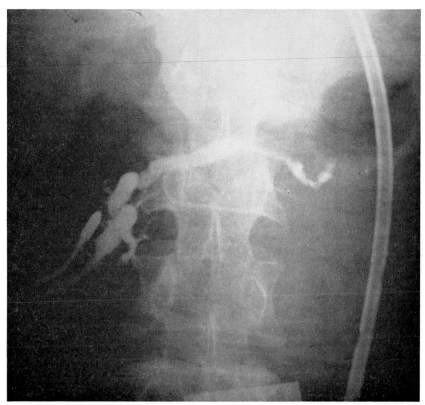

Fig. 1. Operative pancreatogram from the first patient mentioned in the text. A Bakes dilator lies in the common bile duct and a catheter in the dilated duct of Wirsung. (From Salzman and Bartlett.[7])

the duct of Wirsung, which was relieved by operation. Another, equally ill, had a stone lodged 1 cm. within the pancreatic duct.

Two others had common duct stones impacted at the papilla of Vater; the remaining two had evidence of recent passage of a common duct stone. Following operation, all patients had prompt subsidence of their disease. There was a rapid resolution of signs of peritonitis and a quick return of blood chemistries to normal. No complication resulted from the operative procedure, which included pancreatography (Fig. 1).

Prerequisites for Success

The success of this form of treatment appears to depend on selection of patients in whom disease is the result of obstruction of the pancreatic duct, which can be relieved by operation. We believe that the safety of the procedure in the face of active, acute pancreatitis lies in achieving free drainage of the pancreatic duct.

In the past, reports of operative intervention during the acute phase of pancreatitis have been discouraging, but it is likely that these gloomy results have occurred because operation had been employed as the last resort in a moribund patient, or because an operative procedure had been selected which did not correct the basic problem and thus only added an operative insult in an already sick patient. The procedure recommended here, on the other hand, has proved its value in relieving the basic pathology of the disease in a previous large experience with interval cases, and in a small series of patients with the acute disease.

Decompression for Other Forms of Acute Pancreatitis

This being so, it seems reasonable to evaluate this approach in other appropriate forms of acute pancreatitis. In addition to the persistent, stubborn, protracted case in whom the value of the operation has been demonstrated in the foregoing discussion, pancreatic duct decompression by sphincteroplasty with exploration of the pancreatic duct should be considered in patients who develop postoperative pancreatitis following manipulation of the common bile duct. In such patients, the etiology of their acute illness seems clearly to be the development of edema or hemorrhage at the lower end of the common duct, with consequent obstruction of the pancreatic duct. In these circumstances, pancreatic duct decompression should be effective if employed before the disease has progressed to massive pancreatic necrosis.

The procedure also may be indicated in patients with pancreatitis who undergo operation because of an erroneous diagnosis of some other disease. In such patients, performance of pancreatic duct decompression when technically feasible may avoid a useless and perhaps harmful operative insult, while at the same time shortening the ultimate course of the illness. Assessment of the true value of such an approach will depend on confirmation of its safety in subsequent patients.

We do not at present advocate operative intervention in the usual case of acute pancreatitis responsive to conventional treatment: the risk of operation in acutely ill patients may ultimately prove greater than in the interval phase of the disease (although our experience to date does not support this caution). Neither do we propose this operation in overwhelming fulminant cases, in patients who are moribund from pancreatic necrosis on admission to hospital, and in whom one could not expect pancreatic duct decompression to reverse the march of events.

However, in selected patients such as the ones mentioned above, the procedure described here appears to offer promise.

References

1. Bartlett, M. K., and Nardi, G. L.: Treatment of recurrent pancreatitis by transduodenal sphincterotomy and exploration of the pancreatic duct. New England J. Med., 262: 643, 1960.
2. Bartlett, M. K., and McDermott, W. V., Jr.: Exploration of the pancreatic duct for pancreatitis. Surg., Gynec. and Obst., 104:377, 1957.
3. Doubilet, H., and Mulholland, J. H.: Eight year study of pancreatitis and sphincterotomy. J.A.M.A., 160:521, 1956.
4. Jones, S. A., Smith, L. L., and Gregory, G.: Sphincteroplasty for recurrent pancreatitis. Ann. Surg., 147:180, 1958.
5. Nardi, G. L.: Current concepts in therapy: pancreatitis. New England J. Med., 268: 1065, 1963.
6. Nardi, G. L.: Technique of sphincteroplasty in recurrent pancreatitis. Surg., Gynec. and Obst. 110:639, 1960.
7. Salzman, E. W., and Bartlett, M. K.: Pancreatic duct exploration in selected cases of acute pancreatitis. Ann. Surg., 158:859, 1963.

Chronic Calcific
Pancreatitis

Introduction

The treatment of chronic recurrent pancreatitis continues to be controversial as evidenced by the stand taken by the contributors to this important section. Prior authors (see Volume I of Current Surgical Management) advocated surgical procedures designed to correct a disturbed dynamics of flow in the gland. These included division of the sphincter of Oddi and choledochojejunostomy to overcome partial or complete obstruction, spasm, or stricture of the sphincter or compression of the ductal system. In addition, these methods were designed to prevent further regurgitation of bile into the pancreatic duct by means of a common channel. One author, recognizing the importance of intrapancreatic obstruction as a secondary cause of recurrent attacks of pancreatitis, supported retrograde drainage of the proximally obstructed pancreatic ductal system following distal or caudal pancreatectomy, splenectomy, and Roux-en-Y pancreaticojejunostomy.

Doubilet has now modified this approach to conserve all pancreatic tissue and to avoid splenectomy by means of a "split" pancreaticojejunostomy, which is described in detail. Puestow would consider either of these latter techniques as inadequate, since additional strictures or duct obstructions frequently exist beyond the proximal stricture located in the head of the pancreas. In turn, a longitudinal pancreaticojejunostomy or fillet operation is proposed. The third contribution to this section discusses the possible role of total pancreatectomy as a last ditch approach to this problem.

E.H.E.

"Split" Pancreaticojejunostomy
for Obstruction of the Pancreatic Duct*

Henry Doubilet†

New York University School of Medicine

Development of Operation

We believe that, basically, recurrent pancreatitis results from the reflux of concentrated bile into the pancreatic duct. Therefore, the sphincter of Oddi is sectioned to destroy the common passageway and thus prevent further entrance of bile into the pancreatic duct. We have found, in over 700 patients, that sphincterotomy is an effective procedure in the treatment of recurrent pancreatitis.[1] However, it cannot be successful if the pancreatic duct is obstructed by stricture or stone.

Accordingly, in 1947, we developed the technique of operative pancreatography to demonstrate the patency of the pancreatic duct.[2, 3] If the pancreatic duct is found to be obstructed, further ancillary procedures are necessary to overcome the obstruction. Other surgeons, such as Whipple,[4] Zollinger,[5] Longmire,[6] Puestow,[7] and Partington,[8] have performed various procedures such as duodenopancreatectomy, caudal pancreatectomy, pancreaticojejunostomy after caudal pancreatectomy, or the "fillet" operation, which consists of freeing the tail of the pancreas and inserting it into the jejunum after splitting the duct open longitudinally. More recently, the operation used frequently has been to split the duct lengthwise for a variable distance, remove as many stones as possible, and with the pancreas in situ, anastomose the jejunum longitudinally to the capsule of the pancreas.

* Supported by U. S. Public Health Service Grant AM–01221, National Institutes of Health
† Deceased.

Basic Principles

We have performed, on 44 patients, an operation which we call the "split" pancreaticojejunostomy.[9] The operation is based on the following principles:

1. *To render the operation technically simple and safe.* No tissue is removed, the pancreas is left in its bed, and the spleen is not removed.

2. *To conserve all pancreatic tissue.* It has been demonstrated that after sphincterotomy and proper dietary treatment, the human acinar tissue regenerates in two to four years and produces a normal amount of pancreatic juice.[1]

3. *To prevent the development of diabetes.* In man, the major concentration of islet tissue resides in the tail of the pancreas. Observations on patients in whom the tail was excised showed that a number of them developed diabetes, if it was not present at the time of operation.

4. *To perform a mucosa-mucosal pancreaticojejunal anastomosis over a tube, to prevent subsequent stricture.* Observations on patients who had an onlay type of pancreaticojejunostomy, without a mucosa-mucosal anastomosis, demonstrated that stricture of the anastomosis was a common finding (Fig. 1).

5. *To localize, by means of operative pancreatography, the optimum point of transection of the pancreas.* If pancreatography, performed through a tube inserted into the duct of Wirsung after sphincterotomy, is unsuccessful owing to complete obstruction in the head of the pancreas, the pancreas is split at a point just to the left of the spine, and pancreatographic studies are completed through tubes inserted into each side of the transected duct.

Surgical Procedure

After the gallbladder is removed, a cholangiogram is performed through the cystic duct. Following this, a balloon tube is inserted through the cystic and common bile duct into the duodenum.[10] The duodenum is then opened between the second and third portions on the anteromedial aspect, for a distance of 1.5 cm., and the end of the balloon tube pulled out until the balloon lies in the ampulla. The balloon is then blown up and the ampulla pulled out through the small opening in the duodenum. Three traction sutures are placed to control the papilla (Fig. 2). A piece of plastic tubing is attached to the end of the balloon tube, which is deflated, and pulled back through the cystic duct, carrying with it the plastic tube. A sphincterotome is attached to the end of the plastic tube (Fig. 3) and pulled into position, with one jaw inside the ampulla.[11] The instrument is then closed, performing a sphincterotomy. The incision is no longer than 8 mm. The pancreatic duct opening is found in the posterior wall of the sectioned ampulla, which is held open by the traction sutures (Fig. 4). A plastic tube is inserted into the pancreatic duct for a distance of 3 cm., and a pancreatogram performed.

If no obstruction is found, the tube and the traction sutures are removed, the duodenum closed, and the cystic duct tied off, completing the operation.

If the pancreatic duct is found to be obstructed, the pancreas is exposed by the division of the gastrocolic omentum, and two traction sutures placed

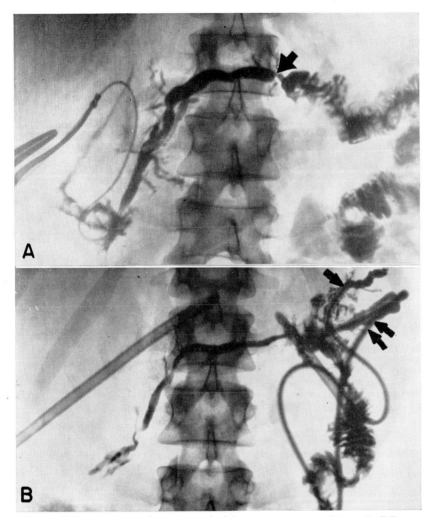

Fig. 1. Stricture of an onlay pancreaticojejunostomy corrected by a "split" pancreaticojejunostomy. *A,* One year after the original operation, a pancreatogram through a tube placed in the duct of Wirsung after sphincterotomy showed almost complete obstruction of the anastomosis proximally (arrow). The caudal duct was completely obstructed. *B,* After excising the anastomosis and performing a "split" pancreaticojejunostomy, a postoperative pancreatogram showed one tube in the distal pancreatic duct (one arrow) and one in the proximal duct (two arrows). The patient is without symptoms and fully employed three years after operation.

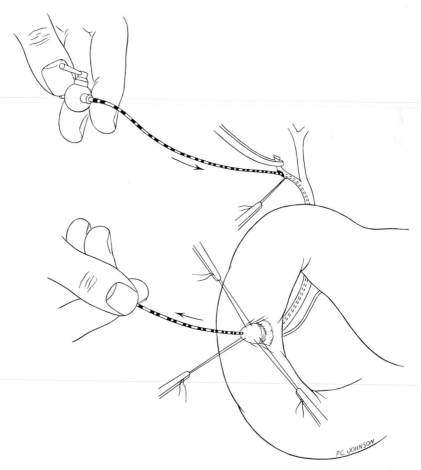

Fig. 2. The balloon tube has been passed through the cystic and common ducts into the duodenum, and pulled out through a small incision in the duodenum. The papilla is pulled out by inflating the balloon in the ampulla. Note three traction sutures.

in the body at the proper point, depending on the findings of the pancreatogram (Fig. 5A). The pancreas is then transected intracapsularly with minimal danger. The openings of the transected pancreatic duct are found, and the ducts cleaned of stones and strictures as much as possible. Occasionally some stones are left in the head of the pancreas. A small French catheter is inserted into each of the opened ends and fixed in place with a suture passing through the pancreatic duct wall (Fig. 5B). A defunctionalized Roux-Y loop of jejunum is then brought up through the mesocolon, the end of it closed, and three sutures placed in such a way as to catch the jejunum and each side of the transected pancreas on the posterior edge (Fig. 6A). With the jejunum pressed firmly between the sectioned ends of the pancreas, the sutures are tied, thus closing the posterior part of the capsule (Fig. 6B). A longitudinal incision, about 2 cm. long and including only the serosa and muscle, is then made in the jejunum. A fine mosquito

clamp is pushed through the mucosa at the upper end of the incision and
passed from the inside through the wall of the jejunum opposite the right
pancreatic duct opening, between two sutures, each of which passes through
the whole thickness of the jejunal wall and through the pancreatic duct wall
(Fig. 7A). The end of the catheter is then seized and pulled through the
jejunum. By tying these sutures, a mucosa-to-mucosa anastomosis is made
over an inlying tube (Fig. 7B). The tube is brought out through the jejunal
wall so that it lies for a distance of 2 cm. between the mucosa and serosa,
thus forming a tunnel. This procedure is repeated on the left side (Fig. 8A).
Then, the anterior part of the capsule of the pancreas, on each side, is
sutured to the jejunum (Fig. 8B), completing the anastomosis. The tubes
are brought out through a stab wound on the left side of the abdomen and

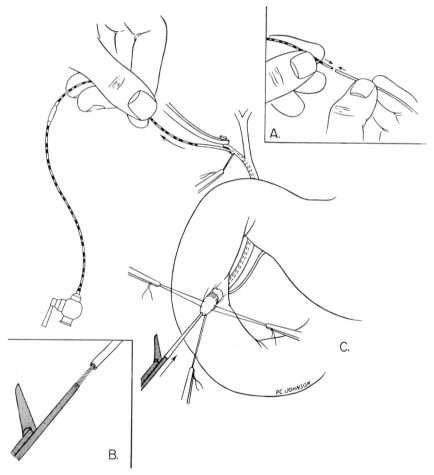

Fig. 3. *A*, A plastic tube, attached to the end of the balloon tube is pulled back
through the cystic duct. *B*, The sphincterotome, attached to the end of the plastic tube, is
being pulled inside the ampulla, *C*.

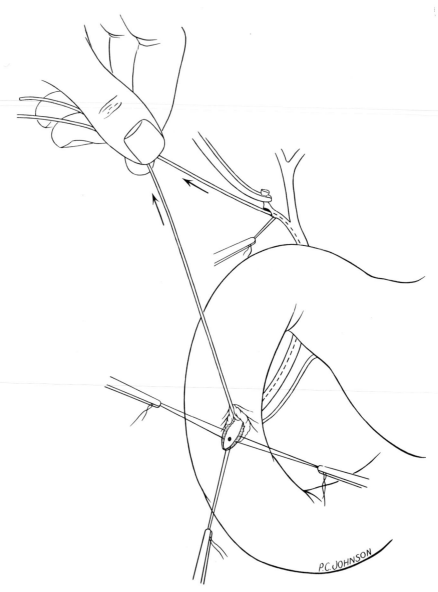

Fig. 4. After sphincterotomy, the ampulla is held up and open by the plastic tube and three traction sutures. The opening of the pancreatic duct is easily found for intubation.

kept in place for two months to permit healing of the anastomosis without stricture.

Autopsy on a patient who died 4 years after operation, from cirrhosis of the liver, confirmed our belief that such procedure would tend to prevent stricture of anastomosis (Fig. 9A, B).

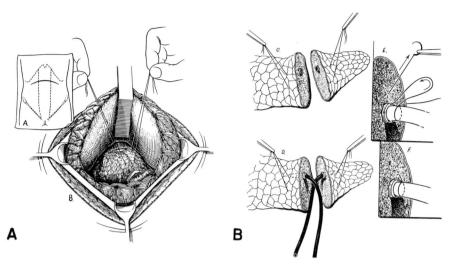

Fig. 5. *A,* The body of the pancreas is exposed through the gastrocolic omentum and held up by two heavy traction sutures. *B,* After completely transecting the pancreas intracapsularly, its ducts are cleaned out and intubated. The tubes are held in position by a single suture.

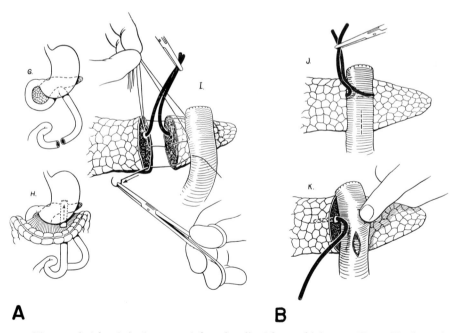

Fig. 6. *A,* After bringing up a defunctionalized loop of jejunum (Roux-Y) through the mesocolon, three sutures are placed as shown. *B,* After pushing the jejunum between the sectioned parts, the sutures are tied, closing the posterior part of the pancreatic capsule. A seromuscular incision is made in the jejunum.

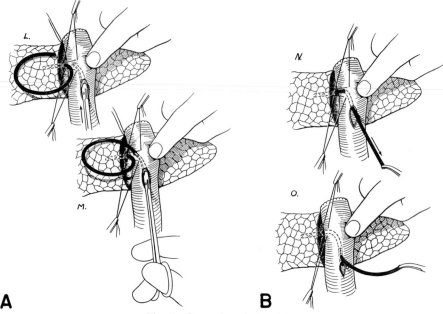

Fig. 7. *Legend on facing page.*

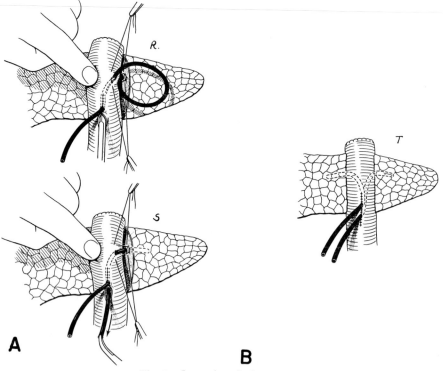

Fig. 8. *Legend on facing page.*

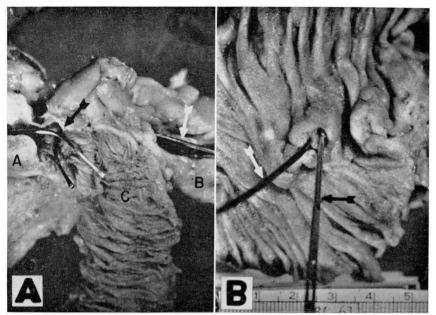

Fig. 9. Autopsy findings in a patient who died four years after "split" pancreatico-jejunostomy. *A*, The jejunum (C) is seen anastomosed to both the proximal (A) and the distal part (B) of the pancreas. A probe is seen lying in the open mucosa-lined proximal anastomosis (black arrow). Another probe passes from the caudal duct into the jejunum (white arrow). *B*, The sectioned sphincter is seen lying open in the posterior wall of the duodenum, with probes inserted into the common duct (black arrow) and pancreatic duct (white arrow).

Results of Treatment

Two illustrative cases are presented:

P.H. (University Hospital) was a 46 year old male who suffered four attacks of severe upper abdominal pain in the spring of 1959. Exploration at another hospital in July, 1959, revealed acute pancreatitis with a retroperitoneal hematoma and thickened gallbladder. The abdomen was closed without any further surgery. Because of constant pain, a cholecystectomy and transduodenal sphincterotomy (without pancreatogram) were performed on January 20, 1960. Three weeks postoperatively, pain recurred, and was persistent. Following admission to this hospital on June 19, 1960, a "split" pancreaticojejunostomy was performed on June 20, 1960. A pancreatographic study through the inlying tubes clearly demonstrated a stricture in the head of the pancreas (arrow) (Fig. 10). Since the operation, the patient has remained well on a fat-free and alcohol-free diet. Epigastric pain recurs only when he drinks alcohol. He is fully employed. He was last seen on October 24, 1963.

Fig. 7. *A*, Two sutures are placed between the jejunal wall and the pancreatic duct. A mosquito clamp is forced through the mucosa at the upper end of the jejunal incision, and passed from the inside through the right side of the jejunal wall between the two sutures. *B*, The end of the tube is grasped and pulled out. The two sutures are tied, producing a mucosa-mucosal anastomosis. An intramural tunnel is created in the jejunal wall.

Fig. 8. *A*, A procedure similar to that shown in Figure 7 is carried out on the left side. *B*, The capsule of the pancreas is then sutured to the jejunum anteriorly.

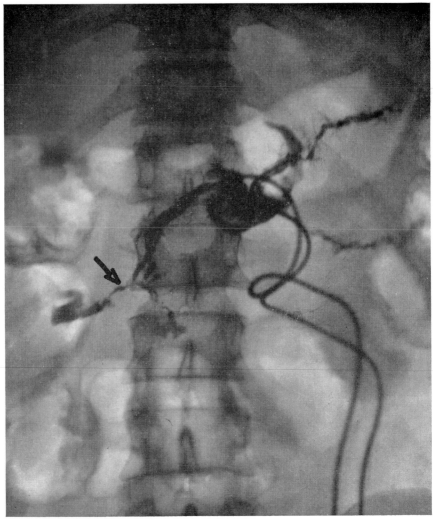

Fig. 10. Case 1. Postoperative pancreatogram after "split" pancreaticojejunostomy, showing partial obstruction of the pancreatic duct in the head of the pancreas (arrow).

E.S. (Bellevue Hospital), an alcoholic for 14 years, was a 36 year old male first admitted to Bellevue Hospital on October 13, 1956, with acute pancreatitis (serum amylase, 670 mg. per cent). He responded well to conservative management, but was readmitted three months later with epigastric pain radiating to the back, accompanied by nausea and vomiting. An operation consisting of cholecystectomy and transduodenal sphincterotomy was performed on January 17, 1957. At that time, the pancreas was found to be hard and nodular; pancreatographic study demonstrated stricture of the duct in the tail. As a result of dietary indiscretions and alcoholic intake, he was readmitted with acute attacks in January and May 1958. Persistent pain, while hospitalized under adequate treatment, indicated that there was obstruction of the pancreatic duct. On May 27, 1958, a "split" pancreaticojejunostomy was performed. Operative pancreatograms, taken after strictures were broken down and tubes inserted, showed puddling of the dye in the tail, due to stricture

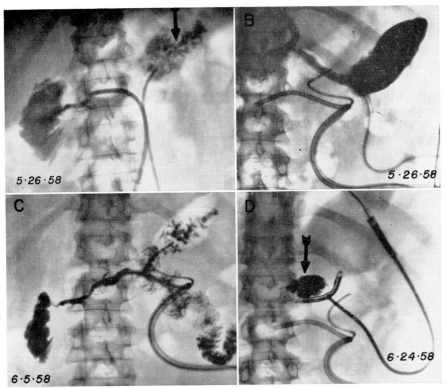

Fig. 11. Case 2. Operative pancreatogram, *A*, taken through the sectioned ends of the pancreas, shows stricture (arrow) in the tail, and dilatation of the duct behind the stricture. Injection through a small T-tube inserted retroperitoneally above the pancreas, demonstrates a large pseudocyst behind the spleen, *B*. Postoperative studies, *C*, show an open proximal duct, and a caudal duct decompressed by the tube passing through the stricture. A cystogram taken one month after operation, *D*, shows complete disappearance of the pseudocyst. The small amount of dye seen (arrow) is due to excessive pressure of injection.

(Fig. 11A). A needle, inserted into a boggy retroperitoneal area above the pancreas, revealed the presence of clear pancreatic juice. When injection was made through a small T-tube inserted in this space, a large pseudocyst lying behind the spleen was noted (Fig. 11B). Postoperative studies (Fig. 11C) showed the tubes lying in position proximally and distally. The T-tube lying in the retroperitoneal space did not drain. A study one month after operation showed complete disappearance of the pseudocyst because free drainage from the tail of the pancreas had been established (Fig. 11D).[12] He has had complete relief of pain, but has not regained his normal weight. He has not modified his diet or alcoholic intake despite advice, and has not taken the prescribed Viokase. Stools are frequent and foul-smelling, particularly after an alcoholic spree.

Discussion

Although some surgeons cannot resist the temptation to cut the Gordian knot by removing stones and strictures in one fell swoop by cephalic duodenopancreatectomy, or by total pancreatectomy, we feel that such ablative procedures for a benign condition, are not justified. The ideal of complete retention of all pancreatic tissue by the operation of "split" pancreaticojejunostomy cannot always be attained. Decision as to the proper procedure should be deferred until the pancreas is split and pancreatographic studies made. It may be necessary to do a caudal pancreaticojejunostomy, because the tail of the pancreas may have an obliterated duct or be completely absent due to the necrotizing process of the disease. These problems may be approached rationally by the step-by-step procedure we have outlined above.

References

1. Doubilet, H., and Mulholland, J. H.: Eight-year study of pancreatitis and sphincterotomy. J.A.M.A., *160:*521, 1956.
2. Doubilet, H., and Mulholland, J. H.: Intubation of the pancreatic duct in the human. Proc. Soc. Exper. Biol. and Med., 76:113, 1951.
3. Doubilet, H., Poppel, M. H., and Mulholland, J. H.: Pancreatography. Radiology, *64:*325, 1955.
4. Whipple, A. O.: Radical surgery for certain cases of pancreatic fibrosis associated with calcareous deposits. Ann. Surg., *124:*991, 1946.
5. Zollinger, R. M., Keith, L. M., Jr., and Ellison, E. H.: Pancreatitis. New England J. Med., *251:*497, 1954.
6. Longmire, W. P., Jordan, P. H., and Briggs, J. D.: Experience with resection of the pancreas in the treatment of chronic relapsing pancreatitis. Ann. Surg., *144:*681, 1956.
7. Puestow, C. B., and Gillesby, W. J.: Retrograde drainage of the pancreas for chronic relapsing pancreatitis. Arch. Surg., 76:898, 1958.
8. Partington, P. F., and Rochelle, R. E. L.: Modified Puestow procedure for retrograde drainage of the pancreatic duct. Ann. Surg., *152:*1037, 1960.
9. Doubilet, H.: Treatment of pancreatitis by sphincterotomy. Am. Surgeon, *24:*3, 1958.
10. Doubilet, H.: A new instrument to facilitate transduodenal sphincterotomy. Surg., Gynec. and Obst., *98:*643, 1954.
11. Doubilet, H.: Section of sphincter of Oddi. S. Clin. North America, *36:*865, 1956.
12. Doubilet, H.: Pancreatic pseudocysts. Surgery, *41:*3, 1957.

Longitudinal Pancreaticojejunostomy

Charles B. Puestow *and* William J. Gillesby

University of Illinois College of Medicine

Disadvantages of Other Procedures

The surgical treatment of chronic relapsing pancreatitis should be directed first to the correction of any primary disease, such as biliary tract disease or peptic ulcer, to which pancreatitis may be secondary. A primary disease frequently exists in women, but is less commonly found in men. If no primary disease exists, surgery should be directed to the pancreas itself. Various operations designed to divide nerve pathways and relieve pancreatic pain have usually given unsatisfactory results. In addition to failing to relieve pain on a permanent basis, they also fail to attack the cause of chronic relapsing pancreatitis, which in the majority of our patients has consisted of partial or complete pancreatic duct obstruction. We have found in most of our patients that a long stricture exists from the ampulla of Vater into the head of the pancreas for a distance of one or more centimeters. Multiple strictures usually exist beyond the primary stricture at intervals, with dilated areas between, creating a "chain-of-lakes" effect. It has been our experience that all such strictures must be opened and adequate drainage of all pockets established to relieve the pain and permit restoration of pancreatic function.

Because of the long proximal stricture and multiple additional strictures, we do not believe that transduodenal sphincterotomy will establish adequate pancreatic drainage. Some surgeons have recommended that a transduodenal sphincterotomy be performed and a catheter be inserted into the pancreatic duct for decompression and to obtain pancreatograms. Such drainage will give only temporary decompression, and when the catheter has been removed the strictures will recur. Furthermore, the mortality of sphincterotomy alone, as reported in the literature, is greater than the mortality we have experienced in longitudinal pancreaticojejunostomy. Needle pancreatograms have been recommended prior to pancreatic drainage to demonstrate the condition of the ducts. If these are obtained, one must drain the pancreas or run the risk of possible acute hemorrhagic pancreatitis or pancreatic fistula. Where the disease is obvious, we do not believe pancreatograms to be essential and are of the opinion that they create an additional hazard.

The Operation

Longitudinal pancreaticojejunostomy has proved to be a satisfactory operation. It consists of an incision into the anterior surface of the pancreas and into the pancreatic duct extending from the most distal to the most proximal pocket in the pancreas. It is essential that total drainage of all pockets be established into a defunctionalized limb of jejunum. The duct need not be opened into the duodenum, but no undrained pockets should remain in the head.

Occasionally extensive fibrosis will be found in portions of the gland, and no ducts can be located. When this situation exists, three or four parallel longitudinal incisions should be made into the pancreas, and should extend through at least two-thirds of the thickness of the gland.

When all pockets have been opened or the gland has been incised as outlined above, the jejunum is divided 12 to 15 inches below the ligament of Treitz, and the distal limb sutured to the pancreas in such a manner that all incised portions of the pancreas will drain into the bowel. The proximal divided end of the jejunum is then sutured to the distal limb of jejunum, creating a Roux-en-Y anastomosis.

Author's Technique

We utilize two main principles in establishing a longitudinal pancreaticojejunostomy. The decision as to the technique to be used is made after the pancreas has been exposed and examined. If the pancreas is found to be short, broad, and thick, and the tail is not in contact with the hilus of the spleen, splenectomy may not be necessary. The anterior surface of the pancreas can be incised to open all pockets (Fig. 1A). The defunctionalized limb of jejunum can then be sutured to the surface of the pancreas well beyond the edges of the incision (Fig. 1B). The tail and body of the pancreas need not be inserted into the lumen of the bowel, but satisfactory drainage can be obtained by a side-to-side anastomosis between the pancreas and the defunctionalized jejunum.

If the pancreas is not shortened and if the tail is in apposition to the spleen, we believe a more satisfactory operation can be performed by removing the spleen and mobilizing the pancreas from the left to right (Fig. 2) as far as the superior mesenteric vessels. By incising the tail of the pancreas, the dilated ducts will be encountered. By passing a probe into the duct, the anterior surface of the pancreas and the anterior wall of the duct can be incised until an intervening stricture is reached. When this is incised the next pocket is entered. The incision is extended to the right until all pockets have been opened. Frequently a large pocket is

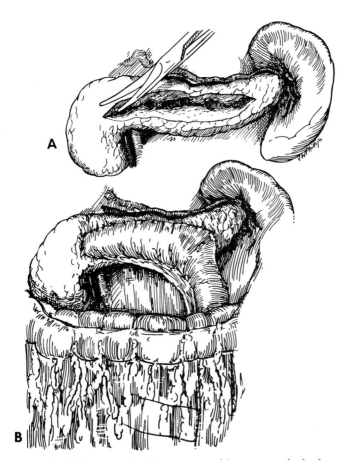

Fig. 1. Longitudinal pancreaticojejunostomy without removal of spleen.

encountered well into the head of the gland and must be opened. We do not consider it necessary to pass a probe through the ampulla of Vater. After adequate drainage has been established, a defunctionalized limb of jejunum is brought through the transverse mesocolon, and the tail and body of the pancreas inserted into its open end (Fig. 2). The bowel is passed over the pancreas to the right for a sufficient distance to suture the serosa of the bowel to the surface of the pancreas well beyond all incised portions. We prefer to use interrupted cotton sutures for this anastomosis. The jejunojejunostomy is then performed.

Principles of Treatment

Dictums in surgery are hazardous. We believe there are some which are essential to the success of the longitudinal pancreaticojejunostomy.

1. All pockets in the "chain-of-lakes" must be opened.

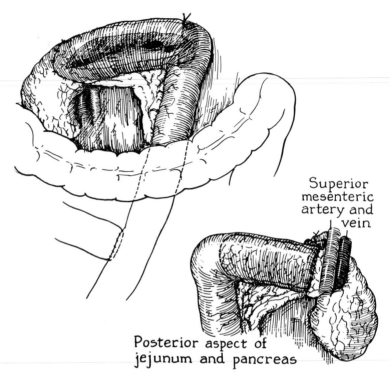

Superior
mesenteric
artery and
vein

Posterior aspect of
jejunum and pancreas

Fig. 2. Anterior and posterior view of completed longitudinal pancreaticojejunostomy where spleen has been removed.

2. The pancreas must always be anastomosed to a defunctionalized limb of jejunum and never to the bowel in continuity.

3. The defunctionalized limb of jejunum should always be brought to the pancreas through the transverse mesocolon. If it is brought anterior to the colon, tension may exist on the pancreaticojejunal anastomosis, and this can result in separation and leakage.

4. One should not anastomose the mucosa of the bowel to the duct wall. A mucosa-to-mucosa anastomosis does not permit the small ducts of the incised pancreas to drain into the bowel. The serosa of the bowel should be sutured to the outer surface of the pancreas one-half to one centimeter beyond the incised edges.

Results

The results of longitudinal pancreaticojejunostomy have been very gratifying. If complete drainage has been established, the patient volunteers when he comes out of the anesthesia that his pain has been relieved. If adequate drainage has not been established, the patient states that his pain is still present. The rapid relief of narcotic addiction is quite remarkable in many of these patients. If the use of opiates has existed for a number of years, many of these patients request no further drug within a few days after operation. We have also shown by roentgenograms that calcification of the pancreas has diminished or disappeared after longitudinal pancreaticojejunostomy. There is a gradual reduction in the calcium over a period of years. If a patient with chronic relapsing pancreatitis has developed diabetes, this operation seldom improves this disease; however, proper medical management can control it. After operation there is a gradual return of pancreatic function manifested by a gain in weight, a return of the consistency of the stools to normal, and an apparent restoration of normal digestive functions.

Total Pancreatectomy for
Chronic Calcific Pancreatitis*

William J. Schulte *and* Edwin H. Ellison

Marquette University School of Medicine

Factors Influencing Choice of Treatment

When one considers any form of surgical treatment for chronic calcific pancreatitis, he must accept the fact that he is dealing with a severe
and progressive disease in a patient who, more likely than not, finds it
difficult to cooperate with his physician, i.e., he continues his dietary
indiscretion and high intake of alcohol. Pain progresses to the point where
the patient refuses to eat, as this exaggerates his discomfort. Narcotics
are employed with increasing frequency and addiction may occur, thus
compounding the difficulties. The progressive calcific fibrosis destroys the
acinar tissue with its exocrine function, and the islet cells with their endocrine metabolic function. The end result may be a recalcitrant patient,
severely incapacitated by pain, suffering from steatorrhea, malnutrition,
and diabetes mellitus.[1] Not infrequently these patients have an associated
alcoholic cirrhosis or have had several operations for pancreatitis, including
diagnostic explorations, operations on the biliary tract with sphincterotomy,
and possibly drainage of the pancreatic ductal system by one or more
methods. As one might suspect, these operations do not always control the
symptoms or the progressive unrelenting course of chronic calcific pancreatitis, suggesting the need for more drastic forms of treatment including
the possibility of total pancreatectomy, which is quite capable of leaving
the patient with as severe a problem postoperatively as the disease for
which he was being treated. Following a discussion of this possibility, an
experience with one such patient subjected to total pancreatectomy with
the mistaken belief that he also harbored a pancreatic malignancy will be
presented.

* Aided in part by USPHS Grant C-4150-5

Page 188

Criteria For the Selection of Patients

Now that the operative mortality for total pancreatectomy has been lowered to more acceptable levels, particularly if the disease is benign, the selection of patients who possibly would benefit by having a pancreatectomy for chronic calcific pancreatitis becomes of increasing importance. Longmire[2] has suggested that this approach might be considered under the following circumstances: (1) failure to obtain an elevated serum amylase with an attack of pain when formerly this was possible; (2) the presence of pancreatic calcifications, diabetes, and severe weight loss; (3) bulky, fatty, and more frequent stools; (4) failure to obtain a positive secretin test; and (5) the finding of a fibrotic calcified pancreas with many small pseudocysts at laparotomy. Howard[3] has proposed similar criteria, i.e., patients with severe progressive disease and with unrelenting pain and inability to eat because of the pain, and who are not relieved by the usual methods of analgesia, including nerve blocks, and in the presence of severe nutritional debility. A profile of pancreatic function tests advocated by Shay and Sunn[4] would be useful in selecting those patients with severe pancreatic insufficiency. These tests include: (1) a provocative serum enzyme test in which both pancreozymin and secretin are used; (2) the starch tolerance test on iodine; and (3) I^{131}-labeled triolein excretion test in the stool.

Results of Treatment

Experience with a patient who has had a total pancreatectomy for chronic calcific pancreatitis illustrates some of the problems to be encountered. The fact that the preoperative diagnosis was carcinoma of the pancreas does not alter the postoperative results.

Case History

F.G., a 60 year old white male entered the Milwaukee County General Hospital on January 15, 1960, through the Medical Outpatient Clinic, where he had been studied for six months because of increasing abdominal pain, a 36-pound weight loss, nausea, and some constipation.

X-ray studies of the upper gastrointestinal tract just before admission showed a deformity in the proximal descending duodenum suggesting the presence of a tumor mass. An intravenous cholangiogram showed good visualization of the gallbladder and a deformity of the lower common duct.

The past history was significant in that the patient had suffered four minor strokes and had a residual left hemiparesis, although he was then ambulatory and was able to take care of himself. There was no history of melena, jaundice, or diarrhea. The patient steadfastly denied heavy drinking, but the family reported a high alcoholic consumption over the preceding 10-year period.

Clinical Findings: The patient was well developed and thin, with an obvious left hemiparesis, but was in no acute distress. The liver was palpable three fingerbreadths below the right costal margin and was nontender with a soft edge. There were no other palpable masses at that time. The blood pressure was 118/80; the pulse was 84 and regular.

On the first hospital day the patient complained of right flank pain, and the presence of a renal calculus was considered by several examiners. On the third hospital day the patient was jaundiced, and he continued to complain of right flank pain. The total bilirubin at this time was 2.8 mg. per cent, and the alkaline phosphatase was 10.7 King-Armstrong units. He was seen by the surgical service on the eighth hospital day, and it was reported that a vague mass was palpable deep in the right upper quadrant. Because of the jaundice, pain, weight loss, and an abdominal mass, the patient was highly suspect for a malignancy of the pancreas, and abdominal exploration was recommended.

Preoperative laboratory studies included a glucose tolerance test which showed a positive diabetic curve. The prothrombin was 100 per cent; the total protein was 6.39 Gm./100 cc. and the A/G ratio was 3.6/2.79. The serum amylase was 107 Somogyi units.

Operative Findings: At operation on the seventeenth hospital day, the pancreas was found to be hard and fibrotic throughout and a large irregular mass was palpated in the head of the pancreas. Although frozen section studies of multiple needle biopsies showed only a chronic granulomatous reaction, the surgeon still thought that he was dealing with a pancreatic tumor and elected to do a total pancreatectomy with subtotal gastrectomy, duodenectomy, and splenectomy.

Postoperative Course: Postoperatively the patient had a mild febrile course, demonstrating on one occasion a small infiltrate in the right lower lung field. During the first 72 hours the insulin requirements were gauged by the urinary glucose level, but on the fourth postoperative day the patient was started on 15 units of NPH in the morning plus regular insulin gauged by urinary glucose. By the seventh postoperative day this was increased to 20 units of NPH, but following an episode of hypoglycemia the insulin dosage was again reduced to 15 units of NPH without any regular insulin. Prior to discharge the NPH dosage was again increased to 20 units, and the blood sugar was ranging between 130 and 140 mgs. per cent. A diabetic diet of 3000 calories and oral pancreatin tablets ground into a powder was well tolerated.

The patient's preoperative weight was 136 pounds, with a height of 5 feet 9½ inches. On the nineteenth hospital day his body weight had fallen to 127 pounds, and he continued to lose weight until his discharge from the hospital to the convalescent unit, at which time his weight was 119 pounds. One month after discharge to his home, his weight had increased to 122 pounds, and the diabetes was well controlled with 20 units of NPH daily.

Readmission: Ten weeks later the patient was readmitted to the hospital because of vomiting, weakness, and nausea. He was disoriented, confused, and had the odor of alcohol on his breath. His pulse was 110, blood pressure 118/40 mm. Hg, his respirations were the Kussmaul type at a rate of 20 per minute, and his rectal temperature was 97.4°.

The skin was warm and dry with a decreased tissue turgor. The remainder of the physical examination was essentially unremarkable. His urine at this time tested 4+ for sugar, and was strongly positive for acetone. After 12 hours the patient had received some 240 units of regular insulin along with 20 units of NPH insulin, 90 mEq. of potassium, and 8000 cc. of saline intravenously. The urinary output had approximated 900 cc. He remained lethargic at this time, but was otherwise improved. The pulse slowed and the respirations returned to a more normal character. Three days later his acidosis was well controlled and he responded as usual. At this time the family admitted that the patient had shown considerable indiscretion and had been drinking alcoholic beverages to excess.

Since a radioactive triolein study showed considerable impairment of fat absorption, the powdered pancreatin was discontinued, and treatment with Viokase, 3 tbsp. with each meal, was instituted. Because of blood sugars in the range of 400 mg. per cent, the NPH insulin was increased to 35 units. Since the wife was unable to make certain that he followed his diet or that he received his insulin, it was decided that the patient should be placed in a nursing home.

At approximately 18 months following surgery, because of continued problems with an elevated blood sugar, the NPH insulin dosage was raised to 45 units. The patient's weight at that time was 124 pounds and he was having two bulky, floating stools per day. In the past four years the patient has had five more admissions to the hospital because of reactions to insulin. He has, however, been free of abdominal pain and has maintained his weight at 124 pounds.

Discussion

This patient is a good example of some of the problems that one encounters following a total pancreatectomy. Perhaps they are even more severe, since we are dealing with an individual who was suffering from a chronic brain syndrome of both arteriosclerotic and ethanolic origin. Even though he has not regained his preoperative weight, he is pain-free and able to maintain an acceptable nutritional status. On the other hand, the diabetes has been quite difficult to control, with severe insulin reactions occurring on a number of occasions. This is the one problem that has led some authors to wonder about the efficacy of a total pancreatectomy for chronic pancreatitis.[2, 5] Others have suggested a 95 per cent resection, leaving a rim of pancreas along the duodenum or a small section of the tail, thus preserving some islet cells.[3, 6, 7] It is theorized that the diabetes should be less of a problem in the presence of some endogenous insulin. As yet, however, sufficient experience is lacking to answer this question.

Although our patient's weight is 12 pounds less than his preoperative weight, his nutritional status is satisfactory for a person of his age and limited activity. Longmire reported that six of his eight patients regained either their ideal or preoperative weights, while the remaining two patients were below their preoperative weights, although the patients were doing well.[2] McLaughlin reported a case of total pancreatectomy for calcific pancreatitis in whom no pancreatic replacement has been given; the patient is maintained on a very high caloric intake and has had very few nutritional problems.[8]

Summary

A patient who had total resection of a chronic calcific and fibrotic pancreas is presented. He represents some of the problems encountered postoperatively, including a severe and a very labile diabetes and some change in nutritional status; he has, however, been free of pain and his jaundice has completely cleared without recurrence.

This experience, together with reported experiences of others, suggests that total pancreatectomy might be justified for severe or chronic recurrent pancreatitis in the presence of severe, unrelenting abdominal pain in patients with good evidence of pancreatic insufficiency, i.e., steatorrhea, weight loss, and abnormal pancreozymin and secretin tests.

A possible solution to the severe diabetes is to perform only a 95 per cent resection, thus preserving the islet cells in a section of pancreas attached to the duodenum. A final judgment on this approach has not yet been possible.

References

1. Ellison, E. H., and Carey, L.: The Pancreas. *In* Davis, L. (Ed.): Christopher's Textbook of Surgery. Philadelphia, W. B. Saunders Co., 1963.
2. Longmire, W. P., Jordan, P. M., and Briggs, J. D., Experience with resection of the pancreas in the treatment of chronic relapsing pancreatitis, Ann. Surg., *144*:681, 1956.
3. Howard, J. M., and Jordan, G. L.: Surgical Diseases of the Pancreas. Philadelphia, J. B. Lippincott, 1960, Chapter 24.
4. Shay, H., Sunn, D. C. H., Chey, W. W., and O'Leary, D.: Pancreatic function profile for the diagnosis of chronic pancreatic disease. Am. J. Digest Dis., *6*:142, 1961.
5. Howard, J. M., and Ehrlich, E. W.: A clinical study of alcoholic pancreatitis. Surg. Gynec. and Obst., *113*:167, 1961.
6. Child, C. G., III, and Kahn, D. R.: Current status of therapy of pancreatitis. J.A.M.A., *179*:363, 1962.
7. Warren, K. W., and Veidenheimer, M.: Pathological considerations in the choice of operation for chronic relapsing pancreatitis. New England J. Med., *260*:323, 1962.
8. McLaughlin, E. F., and Harris, J. S. C.: Total pancreatectomy for recurrent calcareous pancreatitis. Ann. Surg., *136*:1024, 1952.

Operative
Treatment of
the Zollinger-
Ellison Syndrome

Introduction

Nearly 10 years have passed since the proposal that a fulminating ulcer diathesis could result from an ulcerogenic or gastrin-like hormone arising in non-beta islet cell tumors of the pancreas. Since that time, 260 such cases have been reported in the world literature or brought to our attention, and a potent gastric secretogogue has indeed been isolated from many of these tumors and their metastases.[1]

The surgeon faced with treating one of these problem cases might, on the one hand, direct his attention toward removal of the tumor to eliminate the source of the ulcerogenic hormone, or he may elect to resect the end-organ, the stomach. The several factors that influence this decision are important, and should be kept in mind by the reader while he evaluates the approaches advocated by Oberhelman and by Howe, Elliott, and Zollinger.

First of all, three-fifths of the cases reportedly are malignant, and 44 per cent of the total patients present with metastatic disease when first diagnosed. Solitary and benign adenomas occur in less than one-third, and multiple microadenomata are present in one-fifth of the total cases.

Three-fifths of the reported cases are dead, and the majority (70 per cent) of these were operated on for gastric hypersecretion, or islet cell tumors of the pancreas, or both. For the most part, death occurred following complications from recurrent peptic ulceration, and resulted from either misdiagnosis, residual tumor, or an inadequate ulcer operation. Finally, the persistence of symptoms for over 10 years in several patients with malignant islet cell tumors suggests the possibility that malignant change may occur in a benign ulcerogenic tumor.

The contributors to this section use well these observations to support their points of view, i.e., excision of tumor and total gastrectomy.

E. H. E.

Reference

1. Ellison, E. H., and Wilson, S. D.: The Zollinger-Ellison syndrome: re-appraisal and evaluation of 260 registered cases. Ann. Surg., *160:*512, 1964.

Total Gastrectomy for
the Ulcerogenic Tumor

Colin Howe, Dan W. Elliott, and Robert M. Zollinger

Ohio State University

Introduction

Clinical reports,[6] as well as bio-assay studies,[1] have confirmed the association of non-beta islet cell tumors of the pancreas with a fulminating ulcer diathesis or enteritis. The clinical syndrome is being recognized more frequently, and a wide range of surgical procedures have been used in the treatment. In the original report of two cases,[5] total gastrectomy was advised as the most logical, and overall, the safest procedure for the control of the fulminating ulcer diathesis. A third patient discussed in that report survived four years after removal of an islet cell pancreatic tumor in 1948 without total gastrectomy, although a previous vagotomy and posterior gastroenterostomy had resulted in recurrent ulceration. Despite this solitary early success with local treatment of the pancreatic tumor, subsequent experience with these tumors as well as study of the reported cases tends to strengthen the original recommendation that total gastrectomy should be considered in the initial management of these patients.

Although the syndrome is well known, it is still uncommon and remains a rarity in the experience of many surgeons. The majority of reports reflect this, since they consist either of a solitary case or of groups that never reach double figures. It is difficult, therefore, for the individual surgeon to assess the effectiveness of different types of treatment in a small group of personal cases. In order to provide more information about treatment, 186 cases have been collected for analysis: 145 from publications, 35 by personal communication, and 6 from personal experience. The natural history and the effects of the ulcerogenic tumor of the pancreas have been studied, and the results of the various forms of treatment have been compared. With these as a guide, the indications will be presented for total gastrectomy and for the occasional use of other procedures.

The ulcerogenic tumor presents two separate but interlinked problems. First and most lethal are those due to peptic ulceration, and second are

Page 195

those due to growth of the tumor itself. Peptic ulceration and its complications caused death in 85 per cent of the 93 patients who succumbed. The remaining 15 per cent died as a result of enteritis with hypokalemia, or of cachexia due to tumor growth. Death is therefore most commonly due to the effects of the gigantic acid hypersecretion regularly found in these patients. Digestion of previous gastrojejunal anastomoses with perforation, abscess formation, and massive hemorrhage were commonly reported. Enteritis, with diarrhea and its consequent fluid and electrolyte depletion, was reported in nearly half the cases,[3, 4] and this also is caused by the excessive production of acid.[2] If this hyperacidity can be controlled, long survival usually can be anticipated.

The hypersecretion is the result of a potent gastric secretagogue elaborated by the tumor and its metatases, which is probably gastrin.[1] Even microscopic deposits of tumor are capable of stimulating the acid-secreting parietal cells of the stomach, which multiply and produce a tremendously hyperplastic gastric mucosa. Very large quantities of acid may be produced by the smallest residual gastric pouch left after operation.

There are two alternative courses of treatment. Either the primary source of gastrin can be removed by total excision of the tumor, or its target organ, the gastric parietal cell, can be removed by total gastrectomy.

Argument against Excision of Tumor Alone

To attempt a cure by excision of the ulcerogenic tumor alone is a gamble, and the chances of a successful outcome are governed by the following figures:

1. Sixty-two per cent of all the tumors reported were malignant and

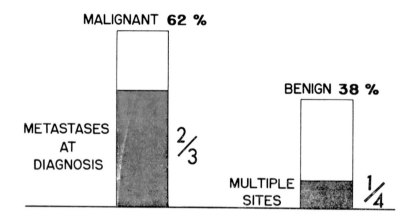

Fig. 1. Incidence of malignant tumor and metastasis in 186 patients with ulcerogenic tumor of pancreas.

two thirds of these (or 40 per cent of all the tumors) metastasized at the time of operation (Fig. 1).

2. One quarter of the benign tumors (or 10 per cent of all the tumors) arose from multiple sites throughout the pancreas. Based on these figures, the theoretical chance of curing acid hypersecretion simply by excision of the ulcerogenic tumor is therefore somewhere about 50 per cent, or one in two. Two additional facts make the primary tumor difficult to excise at operation: (a) in 12 per cent the tumor was not found in the pancreas at all, but in ectopic sites of which the duodenal wall was the most common; and (b) in 6 per cent, no primary tumor could be found, even at autopsy, despite the presence of multiple metastases.

The Case for Total Gastrectomy

Total gastrectomy on the other hand, will certainly prevent any recurrence of ulceration and any other effects of gastric hypersecretion whether or not the primary tumor has been removed. However, the operation has a bad reputation for morbidity and mortality. Most surgeons are therefore reluctant to employ it in this condition for a variety of reasons. First, the patients are often young; second, it appears an unnecessarily radical operation to treat peptic ulceration; and third, many of the patients at laparotomy are found to have widespread hepatic or nodal metastases. An analysis of the results of surgical treatment, however, shows that the best results follow total gastrectomy.

One hundred thirty-two patients were reported as having had some type of surgical treatment. The follow-up period was necessarily variable, and extended only to the time of the published report in most cases. This interval varied between one month and ten years, but in the majority it was less than one year. In 103 of these patients a variety of surgical procedures were performed in which some portion of the acid-secreting gastric mucosa was preserved (Fig. 2). The operations performed were divided into three groups: first, the excision of the pancreatic tumor without any gastric procedure, 37 cases; second, excision of the tumor with subtotal gastrectomy and vagotomy, 47 cases; and third, subtotal gastrectomy with only biopsy of the tumor, 11 cases.

In the first group of 37 cases, excision of the ulcerogenic tumor without gastric resection resulted in a recurrent ulcer or death rate of 49 per cent. The addition of subtotal gastrectomy or some other standard ulcer operation to excision of the tumor, as in the second group, did not significantly improve these results. Death or further ulcer symptoms followed in just over half or 51 per cent of the 47 patients so treated. In the 11 cases treated by gastric resection and only biopsy of the tumor, either death or recurrent ulcer occurred in 73 per cent. Judged by these results, subtotal gastric resection alone would appear to have a very limited place in the treatment of this condition.

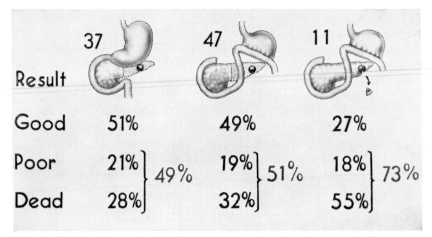

Fig. 2.   Results of operation in 95 of the 103 patients in whom gastric tissue was retained. In the remaining 8 patients, surgery was supplemented by other forms of treatment (see text).

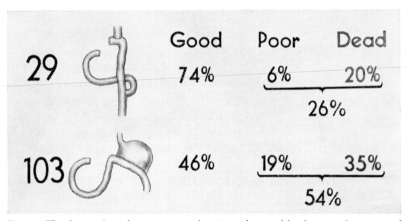

Fig. 3.   Total vs. subtotal gastrectomy in 132 patients with ulcerogenic tumor of the pancreas.

Eight other cases were treated in a variety of ways. These included the use of cytotoxic drugs, specific alpha-cell toxins, or interstitial irradiation of the pancreatic tumor. Five of these patients also had a course of deep x-ray therapy to the gastric remnant in an attempt to control the gastric hypersecretion, but only two survived for any significant period after such treatment.

It is striking that the 50 per cent recurrence and death rate actually observed in this brief follow-up period is precisely the rate that was predicted from the proportion of tumors exhibiting metastases or a multifocal origin. Since gastrin is elaborated in any residual tumor, however small, as well as in its metastases, such deposits continue to stimulate acid secretion by the gastric remnant. Any operation that preserves such acid-secreting gastric tissue is a calculated risk, since a source of potential danger is left behind in at least one-half of the patients having a proved ulcerogenic tumor.

Compare with this the results in the 29 patients who had a total gastrectomy (Fig. 3). The mortality following this operation was 20 per cent, and two patients or 6 per cent had continuing symptoms following operation for a total of 26 per cent. Satisfactory results were therefore produced in three-fourths of these patients, even though in one-half, metastatic tumor was known to be present at the time of operation.

Surgical Approach

When a patient is strongly suspected, on clinical grounds or from laboratory investigation, of having an ulcerogenic tumor, detection depends on thorough and complete examination of the pancreas. However, laparotomy usually is performed after previous surgery for ulcer. Therefore, examination of the abdomen should first exclude the more mundane causes for recurrent ulceration, such as an inadequate gastric resection, an intact vagus nerve, an entero-enterostomy, a retained antrum, or extensive calcific pancreatitis.[6] If none of these abnormalities is found, the pancreas should be examined throughout its length. The head is mobilized by using the Kocher maneuver, which allows thorough digital palpation. This will also make it easier to open the duodenum and inspect or feel the interior for ectopic nodules of tumor. These are usually found on the medial wall of the duodenum adjacent to the pancreas.

The pancreatic body and tail are approached through the lesser peritoneal sac by separating the omentum from the transverse colon and retracting the stomach upwards and the colon downwards. The pancreas and spleen are then mobilized to allow thorough examination and palpation of the body and tail. If no definite tumor is located, but the index of suspicion remains high, the pancreatic body and tail should be excised for multiple sectioning and microscopic examination. This is logical, since the majority of ulcerogenic tumors are found in the body and tail of the pancreas, and many of them are microscopic in size. If after such a thorough search no tumor is found, the operation may be completed by an adequate subtotal gastric resection.

Alternative Procedures

If a tumor is found, alternative procedures are possible, and the decision between them is often difficult. Biopsy and immediate microscopic examination should be performed first to determine the nature of the tumor. The pathologist's answer may be inconclusive. Sometimes a "pancreatic carcinoid" is suggested, but the endocrine pattern suggests the ulcerogenic adenoma, and is quite distinct from the usual adenocarcinoma of the pancreas. When a definite pathological diagnosis of malignancy is made, when there is obvious nodal involvement or metastasis, recurrence of a previously treated pancreatic tumor, or multiple tumors in the pancreas, total gastrectomy should be carried out whatever the age of the patient. Metastases, far from being a contraindication to total gastrectomy, are a positive indication in this disease, since recurrent ulceration will occur long before death from this slow-growing tumor. These indications for total gastrectomy hold true whether or not the patient has had previous ulcer surgery.

If definite microscopic proof is available that the lesion is benign, and complete exploration of the pancreas and interior of the duodenum has excluded the presence of other metastatic tissue, excision of the tumor alone may be used, as long as the risk of recurrent ulceration is clearly understood. The addition of any further gastric resection short of total gastrectomy, or of any other standard procedure for ulcer, is futile and will not improve the prognosis.

Statistics alone cannot adequately set the scene in which most of the 29 total gastrectomies were performed. Elective total gastrectomy as a primary procedure was rare. The majority were performed under emergency conditions and in poor-risk patients. Uncontrollable hemorrhage or perforation due to acid digestion of a recent gastrojejunal anastomosis was the usual reason for the operation. A 74 per cent salvage rate for an operation performed under these circumstances is therefore good, and certainly better than the results of any other procedure. If employed earlier in the disease by choice and not "de rigeur," total gastrectomy might yield even better results.

This radical operation is not necessarily synonymous with chronic ill health. One of the original patients recorded in 1955 is still alive 10 years after total gastrectomy. She has regained her normal weight and leads a normal life, and she has had two children since her operation; all this despite the presence of metastatic islet cell tumor at the original operation.

Summary

One hundred eighty-six cases of ulcerogenic tumor of the pancreas have been analyzed to determine the early results of surgical treatment. By far the most common cause of death was the ulcer diathesis and its complications, since the tumor and its metastases contain large amounts of gastrin which continually stimulate acid production. At operation, excision of the tumor alone was followed by death or recurrent ulceration in one-half of the cases treated. This is to be expected, since one-half of these tumors have metastases or a multifocal origin. These results were not improved by the addition of vagotomy or subtotal gastrectomy. Whether or not all of the tumor could be removed, total gastrectomy was followed by the best results, since it is the only certain way of controlling the ulcer diathesis.

References

1. Gregory, R. A., Tracy, H. J., French, J. M., and Sircus, W.: Extraction of a gastrin-like substance from a pancreatic tumor in a case of Zollinger-Ellison syndrome. Lancet, *1*:1045, 1960.
2. Parker, P. E., Soergel, K., and Ellison, E. H.: Effects of excessive hydrochloric acid on the gastrointestinal tract. Surg. Forum, *XIV*:333, 1963.
3. Priest, W. M., and Alexander, M. K.: Islet-cell tumor of the pancreas with peptic ulceration, diarrhea, and hypokalemia. Lancet, 2:1145, 1957.
4. Verner, J. V., and Morrisson, A. B.: Islet-cell tumor and a syndrome of refractory watery diarrhea and hypokalemia. Am. J. Med., *25*:374, 1958.
5. Zollinger, R. M., and Ellison, E. H.: Primary peptic ulcerations of the jejunum associated with islet-cell tumors of the pancreas. Ann. Surg., *142*:709, 1955.
6. Zollinger, R. M., Elliott, D. W., Endahl, G., Grant, G. N., Goswitz, J. T., and Taft, D. A.: Origin of the ulcerogenic hormone and endocrine induced ulcer. Ann. Surg., *156*:570, 1962.

Excision of Ulcerogenic Tumor

Harry A. Oberhelman, Jr.

Stanford University School of Medicine

Background

The lethal effect of non–insulin-producing islet cell tumors of the pancreas and duodenum, associated with enormous gastric hypersecretion, is usually by virtue of the progressive peptic disease and its complications, or from overwhelming diarrhea, rather than from tumor invasion or metastasis. It has been variously estimated that 50 to 75 per cent of ulcerogenic tumors are malignant, as evidenced by lymphatic invasion or distant metastases. That these tumors produce a potent gastric secretory hormone has been verified by Gregory,[1] who first extracted a gastrin-like substance from non-beta islet cell tumors and their metastases. Therefore, it would seem logical to direct our therapeutic efforts at removing the tumor, not only to control the hypersecretion of gastric juice, but also to rid the patient of a potentially fatal malignant tumor. However, conflicting opinions regarding the management of this syndrome currently exist because of the origin and location of the tumor, the difficulties in establishing an accurate diagnosis at the time of operation, and the hesitancy to subject patients to total pancreatectomy.

Personal experience with 13 patients during the past six years suggests that local or radical excision of the tumor will satisfactorily control the ulcerogenic syndrome in the absence of distant metastases.

Location of Ulcerogenic Tumors

Following the report of Zollinger and Ellison,[2] in 1955, on ulcerogenic tumors of the pancreas, I called attention to the occurrence of similar tumors in the duodenum associated with intractable peptic ulcer or diarrhea.[3] It is of interest that 9 of the 13 patients in our series were found to have duodenal tumors without pancreatic involvement. The tumors are commonly located in the submucosa of the second portion of the duodenum proximal to the ampulla of Vater. They are usually solitary unless associated with multiple endocrine adenomatosis, in which case they may be distributed throughout the duodenum and proximal jejunum. They have all been less than 10 mm. in diameter, often making diagnosis at operation difficult. Only 33 per cent have been considered malignant in contrast to those occurring in the pancreas proper, where 50 to 75 per cent are cancerous and 25 per cent multiple.

The origin of ulcerogenic tumors remains obscure, although those located in the pancreas are presumably of islet cell derivation. That duodenal adenomata are derived from pancreatic islet cells or their progenitors is largely presumptive, based on similarities in histologic appearance. The possibility exists that these tumors originate from cellular rests of the duodenum or conceivably from enterochromaffin cells, since not infrequently they assume a carcinoid-like appearance.

Nature of the Disease

In contrast to pancreatic adenomas, islet cell tumors of the duodenum occur predominantly in males, with the onset of ulcer symptoms usually in the fourth or fifth decades of life. Peptic ulceration frequently is located in the second or third portions of the duodenum, and in the jejunum as well as the esophagus, stomach, and duodenal bulb. Recurrent ulceration occurs despite adequate medical and surgical therapy. The ulcerogenic syndrome is characterized by the excessive amounts of gastric secretion, ranging from 100 to 300 mEq. of free HCl in the 12-hour, overnight secretion test. Since most patients have previously undergone one or more operative procedures for ulcer, gastric hypersecretion usually does not approach the high levels of those patients with intact stomachs. Recently, Marks[4] has emphasized the importance of the ratio of basal secretion to the maximal acid output in response to the augmented histamine test in establishing the diagnosis of ulcerogenic tumors. The ratio is usually always greater than 60 per cent compared to those patients with ordinary peptic ulcer disease, in whom the ratio is usually less than 35 per cent.

Watery diarrhea or steatorrhea frequently results in hypokalemia, owing to loss of potassium by the bowel. Nocturnal diarrhea is a characteristic feature of these patients. Although the exact mechanism responsible for diarrhea remains unknown, it is thought to be due to hyperperistalsis and impaired digestion of food resulting from the inactivation of pancreatic and intestinal enzymes by the enormous quantities of hydrochloric acid produced. In support of this concept, Parker, Soergel, and Ellison[5] have recently shown that the prolonged administration of excessive amounts of hydrochloric acid into the stomach of dogs results in watery diarrhea, weight loss, and jejunal ulceration. When removal of the adenoma abolishes gastric hypersecretion, diarrhea or steatorrhea ceases.

In about 25 per cent of patients, one or more glands of endocrine origin in addition to the pancreas or duodenum are involved. These may include the parathyroids, adrenals, pituitary, and thyroid. A smaller number of patients exhibit multiple endocrine adenomatosis first recognized by Erdheim in 1903.[6] Subsequently, Wermer[7] emphasized the frequent association of polyglandular involvement and intractable peptic ulcer disease, and emphasized the genetic aspects in the etiology of this syndrome, including the cause of the peptic ulceration. Our experience indicates involvement of the parathyroid as most common. Consequently, routine serum calcium and phosphorus determinations are obtained in all ulcer patients. Conversely, all patients with hyperparathyroidism and ulcer disease are suspected of having pancreatic involvement as well.

Diagnosis at Operation

Accurate diagnosis at operation requires adequate exposure of both duodenum and pancreas, so that careful visualization and palpation can be accomplished. In the absence of pancreatic involvement, a biopsy of the pancreas is performed and examined by frozen section. Islet cell hyperplasia of varying degrees is characteristic of this syndrome. In addition, the duodenum or duodenal stump in previously operated patients is opened, permitting more accurate palpation of the duodenal wall by the insertion of one finger into the lumen. It is also helpful to excise and examine by frozen section any enlarged or suspicious regional lymph nodes. Continuous measurement of gastric secretion by nasogastric suction for free acid during operation has shown that gastric hypersecretion persists despite general anesthesia in the presence of an ulcerogenic tumor. The secretion of acid by the gastric glands in the usual patient with peptic ulcer is of vagal origin and abolished by general anesthesia. Following removal of the tumor, secretion gradually decreases and ceases within 30 minutes or so. It is readily apparent that this measurement will prove most useful when therapy is directed to the primary lesion in assuring complete removal.

One cannot underestimate the importance of a careful and complete exploration, for it has resulted in the avoidance of extensive operative procedures on the stomach, such as total gastrectomy with its disturbing mortality and morbidity.

Rationale of Therapy

Intelligent surgical therapy depends primarily on the findings at operation. If an adenoma is found in the wall of the duodenum without evidence of lymph node or distant metastasis, treatment by local excision is justified. In those patients in whom the diagnosis of malignant duodenal tumor is made on the basis of lymph node involvement without distant spread, a partial pancreaticoduodenectomy is the treatment of choice. In our experience, local or radical excision of ulcerogenic duodenal tumors has resulted in a reduction of gastric secretion to normal levels, with healing of the ulcer in eight of nine patients. There was one postoperative death in the series. The follow-up has ranged from one to six years. Total gastrectomy, as suggested by some authors, is reserved for those patients with distant metastases.

If an adenoma cannot be found in the duodenum or pancreas by the usual methods of exploration, the first portion of the duodenum or duodenal stump following a previous gastric resection is excised down to the level of the ampulla of Vater. This permits a more careful examination of the duodenum for suspicious nodules by the surgeon and pathologist. This will enhance the chances for establishing a diagnosis when the index of suspicion is high.

When the tumor is found in the pancreas proper, local excision, or partial or total pancreatectomy should be considered. In view of the incidence of malignancy and multiplicity of lesions, the more radical approaches are justified. If distant metastases are present, total gastrectomy becomes necessary to control the fulminating ulcer diathesis. The relatively high incidence of malignancy of ulcerogenic tumors and their apparent slow rate of growth favor a direct attack upon the lesion to control the hypersecretion of gastric juice as well as to effect a tumor cure.

Total pancreatectomy can be achieved with no greater mortality than total gastrectomy in these patients. The dreaded sequelae after pancreatectomy can be adequately managed in respect to both the resulting diabetes and the pancreatic exocrine deficiency. In our experience these patients have been able to maintain their normal weights without difficulty. Substitution therapy consists of Viokase, a pancreatic supplement, vitamin B_{12}, and insulin. Serious and debilitating postgastrectomy syndromes are thus avoided by this approach.

Summary

Excisional therapy for ulcerogenic tumors of the pancreas and duodenum, without distant spread, are recommended for the following reasons:

1. Local or radical removal of duodenal adenomas associated with fulminating peptic ulceration will abolish gastric hypersecretion and permit healing of the ulcer, or eliminate intractable diarrhea, at the same time removing a potentially malignant or malignant tumor.

2. Excisional therapy for pancreatic tumors similarly eliminates the tumor and ulcer diathesis in the absence of distant metastases.

3. The mortality and postoperative morbidity do not exceed that following total gastrectomy, a procedure that leaves the primary tumor, often malignant, untreated.

References

1. Gregory, R. A., Tracy, H. J., French, J. M., and Sircus, W.: Extraction of a gastrin-like substance from a pancreatic tumor in a case of Zollinger-Ellison syndrome. Lancet, *1:*1045, 1960.
2. Zollinger, R. M., and Ellison, E. H.: Primary peptic ulceration of the jejunum associated with islet cell tumor of the pancreas. Ann. Surg., *142:*709, 1955.
3. Oberhelman, H. A., Jr., Nelsen, T. S., Johnson, A. N., and Dragstedt, L. R., II.: Ulcerogenic tumors of the duodenum. Ann. Surg., *153:*214, 1961.
4. Marks, I. N.: The augmented histamine test. Gastroenterology, *41:*599, 1961.
5. Parker, P. E., Soergel, K., and Ellison, E. H.: Effects of excessive hydrochloric acid on the canine gastrointestinal tract. Surg. Forum., Vol. XIV, 1963.
6. Erdheim, J.: Zur Normalen und Pathologischen Histologie der Glandula Thyreoidea, Parthyreoidea, and Hypophyses. Beitr. path. Anat., *33:*158, 1903.
7. Wermer. P.: Genetic aspects of adenomatosis of endocrine glands. Am. J. Med., *16:* 363, 1954.

Acute
Suppurative Parotitis

Introduction

The fact that acute suppurative parotitis still occurs occasionally in seriously ill surgical patients, and is attended by and portends an alarming incidence of mortality, suggests that the management of this condition be reviewed. As is the situation in many instances in which one specific mode of therapy is recommended to the exclusion of others, controversy exists; on the other hand, when a serious illness requires several or all the weapons available, little or no controversy is apparent. In the instance of acute suppurative parotitis, and particularly since the introduction of specific antibiotic drugs, there is more and more agreement regarding therapy: No one questions the need for prompt and effective drug therapy, or for surgical drainage on proper indication. There is, however, real variance in concepts of the effects and proper place of irradiation in the management of the disease, and these are sharply outlined here.

S. R. F.

Irradiation in Treatment
of Acute Suppurative Parotitis

James E. Bell

Marquette University School of Medicine

Acute suppurative parotitis still represents a considerable therapeutic challenge. In the 85 cases treated at our hospital during the last ten years the mortality rate was 45 per cent. Although parotitis often was not the sole cause of death, there were many cases in which it seemed to play an important role in the patient's demise.

Staphylococcus aureus is the organism most frequently implicated in this process.[2] The route of infection is ordinarily through retrograde flow of mouth bacteria into the salivary duct. Factors contributing to the onset of parotitis are dehydration, which diminishes the flow of saliva; oral infection, which provides organisms in good quantity; and general debility, which lowers the systemic response to infection. Another item that warrants acknowledgement in etiology is antibiotic therapy. This alters the normal mouth flora and allows the staphylococcus to flourish as in staphylococcal pseudomembranous enterocolitis.

Our initial treatment is three pronged: correct the dehydration, administer specific antibiotics, and irradiate the parotid. If these fail or fluctuation develops surgical drainage is considered important.

Although it is not possible to administer a specific antibiotic until sensitivity studies are done, it is possible to select a drug that is efficacious against the most resistant hospital strains of staphylococcus. Naturally a culture should be obtained prior to the institution of this type of therapy. There is no doubt that specific antibiotic therapy is of extreme importance in the treatment of this condition.

Irradiation May Have a Specific Antibacterial Action and Should be Employed Promptly in All Cases

Irradiation of the parotid is started as soon as the diagnosis is established. A dose of 100r/air is given per day up to a total of 9 days.

Currently there is a controversy concerning the use of radiation in acute parotitis. Its use has been condemned as a "therapeutic anachronism."[3] This unacceptable condemnation is based on the following acceptable facts. The dose has no effect on staphylococci in vitro. The dose given has no immediate effect on a normal parotid gland. There is no clinical study that warrants the conclusion that irradiation is unequivocally effective.

The original observations that irradiation seemed to benefit inflammatory conditions occurred in the preantibiotic era. Although improvement in mortality and morbidity occurred, there were parallel improvements in general patient care. Studies done at that time and since do not prove that irradiation is ineffective.

The lack of a good thesis as to why irradiation should be effective disturbs the modern physician. There is at least some evidence that irradiation is effective in control of staphylococcal infection in experimental animals.[1] Although the effect has been observed, the mechanism continues to be obscure. Kahn advances a theory of "antilocalization" caused by irradiation. To carry this theory to man would be to suggest that irradiation allows more effective natural drainage, better antibiotic access, and greater host resistance. All of these are, of course, highly speculative. We do need studies to see the in vivo enhancement of antibiotic effectiveness by irradiation.

We favor the use of small doses of ionizing radiation in the treatment of acute parotitis. There is no evidence that it is harmful. Even specific antibiotic therapy has not proved 100 per cent effective. There is still a high mortality rate associated with this disease. There is no room for a complacent acceptance of any presently employed treatment scheme.

References

1. Kahn, R. L.: Irradiation and tissue immunity. J. Inf. Dis., *10*:107, 1962.
2. Krippaehne, W. W., Hunt, T. K., and Dunphy, J. E.: Acute suppurative parotitis. Ann. Surg., *156*:251, 1962.
3. Spratt, J. P.: The etiology and therapy of acute pyogenic parotitis. Surg., Gynec. and Obst., *112*:391, 1961.

Antibiotics and Hydration in the Management of Acute Suppurative Parotitis

Wayne W. Glas *and* Alfred Lui

Wayne County General Hospital, Eloise, Michigan

Acute suppurative parotitis was first given clinical recognition in the early part of the nineteenth century.[5, 12] Historically, the first mode of therapy in this disease was surgical incision and drainage of the lesion. Subsequently, deep x-ray therapy was used. More recently, the introduction of antibiotics has provided an additional and more effective means of treating this disease.

There has been considerable controversy regarding the most effective treatment of acute suppurative parotitis. Our experience indicates that early in the disease process certain antibacterial agents are very effective in its control. When the disease has progressed to necrosis, we believe antibiotics should supplement incision and drainage.

Incidence

Acute suppurative parotitis is primarily a problem in patients who are elderly (usually 70 years old or older).[6, 7] An important factor in the occurrence of this disease is that other serious diseases are almost always present.[7] In the opinion of most investigators, acute suppurative parotitis has remained a smoldering problem and continues to be a relatively infrequent but recurrent problem on most large surgical services. Because of the age group involved, it is imperative that this condition be recognized and treated as early as possible.

Signs and Symptoms

The early diagnosis of acute suppurative parotitis usually presents some difficulty, particularly after surgery and in the elderly or confused patients in whom it most commonly occurs. The infection is usually characterized, in its early stages, by pain and swelling in one or both of the parotid glands. There is almost always marked pain and tenderness upon palpation, followed by erythema of the overlying skin in 12 to 24 hours. There is associated fever and leukocytosis.[3]

Later in the disease, if the lesion has progressed without recognition, or if the disease has developed rapidly with necrosis, pressure over the swollen parotid area will usually produce purulent material at the orifice of the parotid duct.[3]

Etiology

Although other organisms have been recovered from infected parotid glands,[3] the offending organism is most frequently Staphylococcus aureus.[1, 3] It is almost universally agreed that ascending infection by way of the parotid duct is the usual cause of acute suppurative parotitis.[2, 7] Other avenues of infection, such as the blood stream or the lymphatics,[3] have been noted, but only rarely, and never in our own personal experience. Important factors that contribute to the development of acute suppurative parotitis are dehydration, drug-induced dryness of the mouth, poor oral hygiene, avitaminosis, and general malnutrition and debility.[3, 6] In our experience, 19 of 28 patients (68 per cent) with acute suppurative parotitis were dehydrated when the disease was first noted. In addition, 2 of these patients had been receiving anticholinergic drugs.

Antibiotic Prophylaxis

So-called "prophylactic antibiotics" have been ineffective in the prevention of acute suppurative parotitis;[6, 9] indeed, it has been suggested that the prophylactic administration of antibiotics should be considered as a cause of this lesion.[11] In our experience, acute suppurative parotitis occurred in 12 of 28 patients while antibiotics were being administered for the treatment of other infections. In 10 of these instances, the antibiotics used were proved to be ineffective against the organisms that caused the acute suppurative parotitis.[6]

Diagnosis and Treatment

We believe that cultures of the parotid duct should be obtained as soon as a diagnosis of acute suppurative parotitis is considered. Material for smear and culture usually can be obtained by moderate pressure applied over the affected gland. Early in the disease this material may not be purulent, but since the disease usually originates in the duct, the material will contain the responsible organism.

If the smear and culture reveal the presence of Staphylococcus aureus, the patient should be given, immediately and in substantial dosage, an antibiotic that is effective against this pathogen. There are now several antibiotics that are effective against the staphylococci. At the same time, any factors that might contribute to the disease should be corrected immediately. Such measures include adequate hydration, the restoration of salivation, the discontinuance of anticholinergic drugs, and the greatest possible improvement of oral hygiene.

Once the diagnosis of acute suppurative parotitis has been established and aggressive nonoperative management is decided on, it is imperative that the patient be followed closely for the next 24 to 48 hours. Fluctuation of the gland, which indicates that the disease is advancing, may appear rapidly.[6, 9, 11] Should there be no improvement despite treatment with an appropriate antibacterial agent, incision and drainage is indicated even when fluctuation is absent.[4, 9]

We See No Place for X-ray Therapy

In our experience, deep x-ray therapy has not been as effective in the treatment of acute suppurative parotitis as has the use of effective antibiotics. Although other investigators have reported a remarkable improvement in the symptomatology of this condition,[7, 8] we have not been sufficiently fortunate to observe such improvement. Indeed, the actual mechanism by which x-rays are supposed to control the infection is unknown.[8] Furthermore, it does not seem reasonable to us to use deep x-ray therapy in the treatment of a bacterial infection of the parotid gland when it is not used to treat similar infections of other organs or organ systems. It is our opinion that those patients who responded to x-ray therapy would have done as well had only the conservative measures outlined above been used, such as local heat, hydration, discontinuance of anticholinergic drugs, and improvement of oral hygiene.

Conclusion

We are convinced that appropriate antibiotic therapy and associated supportive care, such as hydration and restoration of salivation, in conjunction with surgical incision and drainage when needed, constitute the treatment of choice in acute suppurative parotitis. In none of our patients who have been treated in this manner has any mortality occurred from the uncontrolled disease.[6]

References

1. Altemeier, W. A.: Acute secondary parotitis. Surgery, *20*:191, 1946.
2. Berndt, A. L., and Buck, R.: Pathogenesis of acute suppurative parotitis: an experimental study. Am. J. M. Sc., *182*:639, 1931.
3. Binder, L. S.: Postoperative parotitis. Anesth. and Analg., *40*:475, 1961.
4. Blair, V. P., and Padgett, E. C.: Pyogenic infection of parotid glands and ducts. Arch. Surg., *7*:1, 1923.
5. Brodie, B. C.: Inflammation of the parotid gland and salivary fistulae. Lancet, *1*:450, 1834. Cited by Gustafson in Surgery, *29*:786, 1951.
6. Carlson, R. G., and Glas, W. W.: Acute suppurative parotitis: twenty-eight cases at a county hospital. Arch. Surg., *86*:659, 1963.
7. Gustafson, J. R.: Acute suppurative parotitis. Surgery, *29*:786, 1951.
8. Hodges, F. M.: Roentgen therapy of certain infections. Am. J. Roentgenol., *35*:145, 1936.
9. Krippaehne, W. W., Hunt, T. K., and Dunphy, J. E.: Acute suppurative parotitis: a study of 161 cases. Ann. Surg., *156*:251, 1962.
10. Lampe, I.: Personal Communication. November, 1963.
11. Petersdorf, R. G., Forsyth, B. R., and Bernanke, D.: Staphylococcal parotitis. New England J. Med. *259*:1250, 1958.
12. Report of Hôtel Dieu. Lancet, *2*:540–541, 1829. Cited by Gustafson in Surgery, *29*:786, 1951.

Treatment of
Acute Suppurative Parotitis:
Role of Surgical Drainage

Thomas K. Hunt, William W. Krippaehne, *and* J. Englebert Dunphy
University of Oregon Medical School

The basic treatment of localized bacterial infection is firmly established. Type-specific antibiotics, correction of systemic inadequacies or deficiencies, rest, and prompt adequate drainage when suppuration has occurred are well tested principles. There is nothing sufficiently unique about acute suppurative parotitis to nullify any of these principles or to make any other type of therapy particularly advantageous. However, we cannot overemphasize the value of well timed, adequate incision and drainage.

Pathogenesis

Under stress, dehydration, and starvation, the parotid secretion thickens and the sodium chloride content drops.[4] Particularly if oral sepsis is present (lack of intake, nasogastric tube, dental caries, etc.), the bacteria that frequently inhabit the distal end of the duct ascend it.[1] Microscopically, the first changes seen are aggregates of white cells and bacteria within the ducts. These changes probably antedate clinical signs. Local abscesses form within the ducts and the duct walls are subsequently destroyed. The now parenchymal abscesses enlarge and coalesce. Unless drainage is established at this point, the abscesses may spread down the neck deep to the cervical fascia, or may penetrate and spontaneously drain into the external ear or on to the face. In some cases severe edema may spread down the neck and seriously endanger the airway. Visible abscesses are rarely present by the second day of clinical infection, but are almost always present by the fifth day in a patient whose parotitis has not responded to antibiotic therapy. Fluctuation is a very late sign, and its absence should in no way delay a decision to incise and drain.

Many bacterial studies have shown staphylococcus to be the most common pathogen in parotitis.[2, 3] Quite commonly, streptococcus, pneumococcus, or gram-negative bacteria may coexist with the staphylococci. Patients already receiving antibiotics specific for the staphylococci in the environment may occasionally develop parotitis that is not due to staphylococci. Parotitis occurring during antibiotic therapy is always caused by an organism that is not sensitive to the currently or recently used antibiotics.

Review of Cases

We have reviewed 212 cases of parotitis occurring in the University of Oregon Hospitals from 1940 through 1963. The mortality figures expressed are gross rates and include all deaths occurring within 20 days of onset of parotitis. By this time, the disease has either subsided or become chronic and no longer vitally influences the patient's course. Many of these deaths occurred in patients either clinically cured or apparently recovering from parotitis, but these were nevertheless included. It is estimated that approximately 15 per cent of these patients would have died even without parotitis.

Results of Therapy

Incision and Drainage

It is universally accepted that, in the course of a localized bacterial infection, when suppuration and abscess formation have occurred the infectious process is usually beyond cure by antibiotics alone. Incision and drainage at this point is the most effective treatment. Parotitis is not an exception.

Determination of the precise indications for timely drainage is difficult since there are no reliable clinical signs. It is apparent, however, from analysis of the findings at operation that parotitis follows a predictable course in terms of the time of suppuration. In this study, surgical drainage was accomplished 66 times in 62 patients. When incision was done in the first two days after onset, there was commonly edema and necrosis. In no instance were more than a few drops of pus obtained. On the third day, small amounts of purulent exudate were usually found. Of nine drainages done on the fourth day, six released 3 to 7 cc. of pus and three disclosed none. Four incisions were done on the fifth day; in three gross purulence was noted. Thirty-two glands were incised from the sixth day on. Of these, only three contained no pus, and in many of the remainder, it seemed obvious that incision and drainage should have been accomplished earlier.

Although no death has been directly related to the incision and drainage procedure itself, the gross mortality rate following drainage was approximately 30 per cent. This is higher than in the groups receiving type-specific antibiotics alone. However, this group represents patients seen late in the course of the disease, patients in whom abscess formation occurred despite antibiotic therapy, and patients who received nonspecific antibiotics. In many instances, incision and drainage represented the last chance to obtain control of the infection. In most of the patients who died following incision and drainage, the parotitis was resolving at the time of death. Despite the unfavorable prognosis of the patients in whom incision and drainage must be done, in many cases incision and drainage of a parotid abscess has brought about an acute reversal of the rapid downhill course and has led eventually to recovery.[3]

Such a high percentage of patients responds quickly and completely to antibiotics alone that there is little justification for incision and drainage prior to a test period with antibiotics. Earlier drainage may be indicated when the disease has been present long enough to indicate the obvious presence of suppuration, or when edema and toxicity are progressing so rapidly that the airway or the life of the patient is threatened.

Antibiotics

The lowest mortality rate in this series of patients was found in those treated with specific antibiotics. Seventy-four patients were given known specific antibiotics. Fourteen of these died, a mortality rate of 19 per cent. Of the remaining 138 patients, 47 died, a mortality rate of 34 per cent. The larger group represents patients receiving either no antibiotics or antibiotics not known to be type-specific by reason of deficiencies in culture or sensitivity data. The difference between the group of patients treated with known type-specific antibiotics and the group treated with antibiotics of unknown specificity is statistically significant within the 5 per cent level (chi square 5.4). In these hospitals, parotitis was almost invariably caused by staphylococci, strains of which were found to be 100 per cent susceptible to Staphcillin, 81 per cent susceptible to Albamycin, and 65 per cent susceptible to Chloromycetin. When patients receiving one or more of these drugs were removed from the group receiving antibiotics of unknown specificity on the grounds that these antibiotics were probably specific, the difference between the two groups became statistically significant at the 2 per cent level.

Many of our patients have responded quickly and completely to the early institution of specific antibiotic therapy as the only major treatment.

Parotitis is characteristically a disease of the aged and severely ill. It is rarely seen, even in the presence of staphylococcal oral sepsis, if the patient is not severely and systemically ill. Under these circumstances, it is often symptomatic of a generalized susceptibility to infection, and there is excellent reason to suspect that if unchecked, the infection will soon invade other areas, particularly the lungs. The role of systemic treatment with specific antibiotics and replacement of systemic deficiencies then becomes doubly important.

Even with the early use of specific antibiotics, however, incision and drainage may be necessary at a later date. As discussed above, it is possible that significant microabscess formation can occur before clinical symptoms appear. Of 33 patients given specific antibiotics within the first two days of parotitis, 11 required incision and drainage for suppuration. Neither do antibiotics prevent parotitis, as many have noted. Approximately one-third of the patients in this series developed parotitis while being treated with antibiotics.

Irradiation Is Principally a Palliative Measure

In the entire group of 212 patients, 120 received irradiation. Of those receiving irradiation, 40 died, and of 92 not irradiated, 21 died. Most patients under 30 years of age were in the nonirradiation group. When all patients under 30 are removed, the irradiated group becomes 119 patients with 40 deaths (33 per cent). The nonirradiated group becomes 78 patients with 21 deaths (27 per cent). There was no selection factor detectable in patients over 30 years of age. When the irradiated patients who also received antibiotics or surgical drainage are compared with their corresponding groups, again no difference in mortality is found except as accounted for by specific antibiotics. It appears quite clear that although irradiation given within the first 24 hours may be effective in reducing pain and swelling, it is of secondary importance to antibiotics and surgical drainage in terms of survival.

Recommendations for Treatment

As soon as the diagnosis of acute parotitis is made, smears and cultures should be obtained by expressing exudate from one or the other of the parotid ducts. Immediate attention should be directed to improvement of oral hygiene, hydration, and nutrition. If there is considerable pain and the disease is less than 24 hours old, irradiation of the gland in small doses is a reasonable procedure.

The early use of type-specific antibiotics is essential. If the patient is gravely ill, however, he should be treated immediately with an antibiotic known to be effective against the staphylococci most commonly encountered in the hospital. Changes can then be made as sensitivity data become available. If the disease responds promptly, no further therapy may be needed. If, despite these measures, the disease persists or progresses, incision and drainage should be considered as early as the third day. If there is moderate improvement or lack of progression, the drainage may be delayed for a day or two longer. Usually incision and drainage should not be delayed beyond the fifth day unless steady regression is occurring.

If parotitis is treated optimally, it rarely should be the cause of death.

References

1. Crile, G., Jr., and Manning, W. R.: Postoperative parotitis. Am. J. Surg., *50:*664, 1940.
2. Krippaehne, W. W., Hunt, T. K., and Dunphy, J. E.: Acute suppurative parotitis. Ann. Surg., *156:*251, 1962.
3. Petersdorf, R. G., Forsyth, B. R., and Bernanke, D.: Staphylococcal parotitis. New England J. Med., *259:*1250, 1958.
4. Spratt, J. S.: The etiology and therapy of acute pyogenic parotitis. Surg., Gynec. and Obst., *112:*391, 1961.

Esophageal

Hiatal Hernia

Introduction

In Current Surgical Management II (1960) there was presented a controversy as to whether hiatal hernias should be repaired transabdominally, transthoracically, or by gastropexy. This controversy has not found a universal solution; we now appreciate that increasing attention is being paid to the acid-peptic aspect of the symptomatology of hiatus hernia. The question now is whether good anatomic repair of these hiatal hernias, by any route, is sufficiently satisfactory, or whether the addition of measures such as vagotomy with a drainage procedure yields further benefits and fewer recurrences of symptoms, or, on the other hand, yields further complications. Should a physiologic approach be added to the purely anatomic approach to the problem? A good anatomic operation based on basic principles of hernia repair is necessary in either type of operative management; a difficulty with hiatal hernia is that good fascia for repair is not available as in other hernias—of the abdominal wall, for instance. Perhaps this is one of the reasons why recurrences, or recurrence of symptoms, after hiatal hernioplasty prompt a search for adjunctive or newer methods of management. The following two presentations succinctly describe the anatomic approach and the physiologic approach respectively.

S. R. F.

The Transthoracic Approach
in the Surgical Management
of Esophageal Hiatal Hernia

Donald B. Effler

The Cleveland Clinic Foundation

Hernia of the celomic cavity is generally regarded as within the surgeon's province. Medical treatment, in the strict sense, is virtually unknown for protrusion of the inguinal canal, the femoral canal, and the umbilicus. The need for mechanical support for surgical reconstruction of the weakened area is self-evident.

The outstanding exception to the above thesis concerns herniation through the esophageal hiatus. This form of celomic herniation, regardless of its size, is only apparent by radiographic visualization. Although the adult male may diagnose his inguinal hernia by direct inspection or palpation, the patient with symptomatic hiatal hernia is aware of his condition only by its symptoms or complications. The fact that hiatal hernia cannot be diagnosed by direct inspection, explains to a large extent why this form of celomic hernia has remained in the province of medical therapists. Another reason why patients with symptomatic and complicated forms of hiatal hernia are treated medically is related to past surgical failure, from poorly conceived or poorly executed operative procedures. A surgeon who has been schooled in technique and fundamentals of surgery may have a remarkable "blind spot" when he attempts to repair this particular rupture. The strongest arguments against surgical treatment of hiatal hernia have been the poor results that follow inadequate operations.

Abdominal vs. Transthoracic Approach

It is unfortunate that qualified surgeons interested in the problems related to esophageal hiatal hernia dissipate their energies in arguments over operative approach. Experienced surgeons dealing with this subject usually have fixed opinions and are not going to change as long as they obtain de-

Page 223

sired results. If the surgical mission is accomplished with minimal risk and with reasonable permanency, then the basic approach is a detail of secondary importance.

Thus, instead of arguing about basic approach, surgical energies should be combined to restore esophageal hiatal hernia to the province of the surgeon, and to remind all who practice medicine that this entity is no more than one form of celomic rupture.

This author prefers the transthoracic approach to the repair of hiatal hernia. Experience in The Cleveland Clinic Foundation with more than 600 operations since 1948 offers convincing evidence that it may be applied to every form of hiatal hernia, including those with acquired short esophagus. Basically the transthoracic approach offers excellent exposure to the structures utilized in the repair of esophageal hiatal hernia. The crura of the diaphragm are readily exposed, the phrenoesophageal ligament is directly accessible, and the esophagogastric junction and its related vagi are amenable to sharp dissection under direct vision with minimal retraction required. An associated factor of obesity is of little importance as far as the transthoracic approach is concerned, since there are virtually no fat depots in the thoracic cavity; exceptions to this would be the pericardial fat pad and the anterior mediastinum which are in no way related to this area of surgical endeavor.

Perhaps the most common argument against the transthoracic approach is the surgeon's inability to perform complementary intra-abdominal procedures. This is not a valid objection. The surgical treatment of symptomatic or complicated forms of hiatal hernia requires a specific operation and should not be offered or planned as part of a surgical "blue-plate special."

Selection of Subjects for Surgical Management

The radiographic demonstration of a hiatal hernia is not in itself an indication for surgery.

This entity is encountered frequently in routine clinical examination and after the patient disclaims any symptoms that may be attributable to the herniation. The lack of symptoms is frequently explained by the absence of reflux esophagitis or relative gastric achlorhydria. It has been my observation that some of the poorest results in surgical management of hiatal hernia have followed operations upon asymptomatic patients; asymptomatic as far as the hiatal hernia was concerned. As surgeons, we must remind ourselves constantly that it is difficult to improve a situation that is both benign and asymptomatic.

Considering those patients who demonstrate hiatal hernia and who have symptoms clearly attributable to this entity, the question of therapy, medical vs. surgical, arises. For the symptomatic hiatal hernia a trial of medical therapy is reasonable with two provisos: it should be clearly stated

—that medical therapy is in no way curative, and that curative surgery is available if the patient wearies of his medical regimen. Failure to acquaint the hiatal hernia patient with these basic facts of medical life accounts for the growing prosperity among those who sell nonprescription proprietary medications for heartburn.

Barring obvious medical contraindications to elective surgery, the patient with symptomatic hiatal hernia should be considered for elective surgery if (1) he is dissatisfied with the medical regimen or (2) finds that it is not compatible with his way of life. The basic symptoms attributable to hiatal hernia are heartburn and reflux, which occur after meals and in recumbency. If the surgeon, in taking the history, finds it difficult to differentiate between symptomatic hiatal hernia and duodenal ulcer, or hiatal hernia and gallbladder disease, or hiatal hernia and anxiety tension state, then he would do well to defer surgical therapy. The least satisfactory operation performed for the surgical management of hiatal hernia, disregarding technical failures, is usually related to the least satisfactory selection of the patient.

The presence of complications related to hiatal hernia offers strong indication for elective surgery. Most clinicians fail to distinguish between symptoms and complications of hiatal hernia. As stated before, symptoms usually are related to heartburn and reflux of gastric contents. The complications attributable to hiatal hernia fall into three major categories: (1) bleeding, occult or massive; (2) peptic ulceration in the gastric cardia; and (3) obstruction due to stricture or volvulus of the incarcerated stomach. Medical therapy for the patient who presents a complication attributable to esophageal hiatal hernia is for the most part useless, and should be reserved for the unfortunate patient who is disqualified as a subject for elective surgery.

Operative Procedure for Transthoracic Repair

The author's operative approach to the repair of hiatal hernia follows the Allison technique, with one major exception: the counterincision in the tendinous dome of the diaphragm has been eliminated. Emphasis is placed upon this single detail. In 1951 Allison[1] described his surgical approach to the transthoracic repair of hiatal hernia. He emphasized the importance of the phrenoesophageal ligament and fixation of the esophagogastric junction under the left leaf of the diaphragm. To accomplish this a small counterincision was made. Through the years that followed, Allison's operation has received wide application and deservedly so. However, it has come to my attention that late herniation through the counterincision occurs in a significant number of operations that utilize Allison's technique. The principles of Allison's repair can be accomplished and the desired results obtained by a simple technique that avoids direct counterincision.

The ideal operative procedure for hiatal hernia follows the basic principles of hernia repair. These principles, applicable to all hernias of the celomic cavity, are the following: (1) careful dissection of involved anatomic structures, (2) elimination of the sac element, (3) reduction of the herniated viscus, and (4) anatomic reconstruction. Alteration of gastric physiology by vagus transection and pyloroplasty does not conform to principles of hernia repair. Exotic procedures, particularly those that involve resection and anastomoses, are to be avoided except under most unusual circumstances. The basic problem with esophageal hiatal hernia is an anatomic derangement and not an underlying disturbance in physiology.

The ideal operation for hiatal hernia is one that places the stomach below the diaphragm, fixes the esophagogastric junction to the undersurface of the diaphragm, and tailors the esophageal hiatus to the size suited for the individual patient. The technique employed at the Cleveland Clinic has been previously reported.[2, 3]

Summary

Hiatal hernia is a correctable form of rupture from the celomic cavity. Many symptomatic patients and virtually all who have complicated forms of hiatal hernia are suitable subjects for elective surgical repair.

The frequency of surgical success in the management of hiatal hernia will be influenced by criteria for selection of the surgical subject and by the technique of operation. Poor selection and poor technique provide the best ammunition for those who contend that this entity is not within the surgeon's province.

The best operation for hiatal hernia is that which achieves the desired results with the least risk to the patient. Whether this is accomplished by the abdominal or transthoracic route is a matter of detail. The author's technique, which is a modification of Allison's transthoracic procedure, can be applied to almost every form of hernia involving the esophageal hiatus.

Operations that involve additional procedures such as vagus transection, pyloroplasty, or subtotal resection, should not be used for the ordinary forms of hiatal hernia. The use of these procedures is reserved for the relatively few situations in which acquired short esophagus with fibrous stricture and peptic ulceration is encountered, or when the hiatal hernia is associated with severe deformities of the pyloric antrum or duodenum.

References

1. Allison, P. R.: Reflux esophagitis, sliding hiatal hernia, and the anatomy of repair. Surg., Gynec. and Obst., 92:419, 1951.
2. Effler, D. B., and Ballinger, C. S.: Complications in surgical treatment of hiatus hernia and short esophagus. J. Thoracic Surg., 22:235, 1951.
3. Effler, D. B.: Reconstruction of the esophageal hiatus. Arch. Surg., 85:599, 1962.

Hernioplasty, Vagotomy, and Drainage Procedure in the Management of Hiatal Hernia

M. Michael Eisenberg *and* E. R. Woodward

University of Florida College of Medicine

Pathophysiology of Reflux Esophagitis

Hiatal hernia with associated peptic esophagitis is clearly a syndrome of increasing clinical importance. The cumulative literature on the subject dates back to Quincke's observation in 1879 that esophageal mucosa is especially sensitive to the corrosive action of acid gastric juice.[17] However, it is really only since Allison's classic presentation in 1951 that contemporary physicians have come to recognize the frequency with which upper gastrointestinal disorders are attended by this disease.[1] Approximately 10 per cent of all postmortem studies and 2 to 9 per cent of all gastrointestinal x-ray series for symptoms have demonstrated hiatal hernia.[20] Only duodenal ulcer has been shown to be more common under these circumstances.

The clinical and pathologic manifestations of acid peptic disease of the esophagus are remarkably similar to those of the gastroduodenal disease, and there is a growing body of evidence supporting the hypothesis that they share a basic etiologic mechanism. While esophagitis may, on rare occasions, be associated with reflux of alkaline juices, in general the dictum of *no acid—no esophagitis* appears sound. As early as 1906 Tileston observed that esophagogastric incompetence with reflux of gastric chyme is germane to the formation of esophageal ulcer.[21] Others have suggested that gastric hypersecretion, with or without duodenal or gastric ulcer, but associated with esophagitis, implies a common etiology. Of 58 patients with significant esophagitis, Neville and Bartunek found only one who had no hydrochloric acid after histamine stimulation.[14] Nine of the 58 had a past history of duodenal ulcer. Hoffman, Cruze, and Byron reported that 12 of 21 patients with esophagitis had gastric or duodenal ulcer, and they have emphasized the high correlation with acid hypersecretion.[10] Finally, Casten

Page 227

and co-workers have reported that 82 per cent of symptomatic hiatal hernias have associated gastric hypersecretion.[4]

The exquisite sensitivity of esophageal mucosa to the proteolytic action of acid pepsin is well known. Ferguson and co-workers showed experimentally that the effect of acid gastric juice on contact with esophageal mucosa is prompt and devastating.[6] Hydrochloric acid alone, in concentrations approximating that found in normal gastric juice, is far less noxious. Plzak, Fried, and Woodward demonstrated that of all mucosal surfaces in the gastrointestinal tract, esophageal mucosa is least resistant to peptic ulceration.[16] Perry and associates demonstrated the extreme vulnerability of cat esophagus to human gastric juice, particularly that obtained from patients with high concentrations of hydrochloric acid and pepsin.[15] Finally, Selye has shown that regurgitation of acid gastric juice in rats with ligated pyloric canals will regularly produce hemorrhagic esophagitis, whereas if the cardia is simultaneously ligated, no esophageal lesions are noted.[19] Many experimental studies have corroborated these findings, and it is readily apparent that these factors sharply emphasize the physiologic separation of stomach from esophagus as crucial.

Esophagitis may be divided on a clinicopathologic basis into three types, each a stage in the progression of the same process. The most mild is the pure esophagitis, manifested by a superficial mucosal erosion, and usually found in the presence of *uncomplicated* gastric reflux. The second group consists of those patients with ulceration further complicating their esophagitis, and in whom the mucosa is friable, edematous, and fissured. The third, and most difficult group from the point of view of management, is made up of those patients with cicatricial narrowing of the lumen as the end result of persistent reflux and ulceration. Mucosal destruction with fibrosis and scar formation culminating in stenosis and shortening of the lower esophagus is the outstanding feature.

The abnormal reflux of gastric secretions from the stomach into the lower esophagus is prevented by a closure mechanism of the lower esophagus, although controversy still exists over its precise anatomic construction and *modus operandi*. Surgeons have regarded the diaphragmatic hiatus as primary in importance, postulating that the thickened, sling-shaped crural fibers act as the basic valve mechanism. Others have indicated that the angle at which the esophagus joins the cardiac portion of the stomach is critical. Still others have suggested the presence of an intrinsic muscular or physiologic sphincter at the lower end of the esophagus. Meiss, Grindlay, and Ellis demonstrated that removal of the esophagogastric junction regularly culminated in esophagitis and, on the basis of this, and other experiments, postulated the existence of an intrinsic physiologic mechanism.[12] In 1950, Lerche[11] presented a physio-anatomic concept, subsequently modified by Gould and Barnhard,[8] which indicates the existence of one esophageal sacculation and ampulla, one gastric or hiatal segmental vestibule, and an inferior esophageal sphincter made up of diffuse muscle in the wall of the ampulla. This hypothesis is particularly attractive in view of the support it lends to the argument that the lower esophageal or "Schatzki" ring exists.

Whatever the relative importance of intrinsic and extrinsic factors in the integrity of the lower esophageal "sphincter," Code[5] and Fyke[7] and associates have demonstrated a final common denominator. Normally, in health, a band or zone of elevated pressure is interposed between the stomach and esophagus. With deglutition or esophageal distention this high pressure band may be temporarily abolished. The resting pressures in the stomach are always in excess of those in the esophagus and, if there were no barriers between the two organs, material would flow retrograde from the stomach into the esophagus. However, during inspiration the pressure over a band approximately 1.5 cm. wide, just below the point of respiratory pressure reversal, is always greater than the pressure in the stomach. This barrier is thought to be dependent upon contraction of circularly disposed muscle fibers. This band of increased pressure between the two organs represents the gastro-esophageal sphincter. It is the failure of this physiologic sphincter that results in the reflux of acid gastric juice into the esophagus, and the commonest cause of sphincter failure is the sliding type of hiatal hernia.

Diagnosis

Malfunction of the physiologic sphincter has been demonstrated by studies in patients with hiatal hernia in whom the pH of esophageal content is measured. Tuttle and Grossman[22] have shown that, unlike normal individuals, there is free reflux of acid material for extended distances up the esophagus. It is this abnormal regurgitation of acid chyme that generates peptic esophagitis and, in large measure, accounts for the symptoms associated with hiatus hernia. While in most reported series the incidence of reflux has been based upon its roentgenologic demonstration, this may not be a wholly accurate method. Morgan, Hill, and Selby[13] studied 115 cases of sliding hiatal hernia using the method first described by Tuttle and Grossman.[22] Reflux of acid was determined by means of a pH electrode and an open tip catheter (*vide infra*). A comparison was made with radiographic evidence of reflux of barium. Ninety-four of 115 patients (83 per cent) with symptomatic hiatal hernias were found to have reflux detected by x-ray study, and in only one patient did the fluoroscopist detect reflux not found by intraluminal pH and pressure study. The importance of these observations should not be underestimated, both as regards the validity of various techniques for demonstrating reflux, and as a clue to the underlying pathophysiology of esophagitis.

Treatment: Argument for Procedures to Alter Gastric Physiology

It is apparent that in most instances the presence of acid reflux is necessary for the development of esophagitis. It follows, then, that the successful alleviation of symptoms referable to this syndrome must depend upon one of two factors. Either reflux must be prevented by restoration of normal gastroesophageal sphincter function; or the reflux must be deprived of most or all of its acid-pepsin content. Ideally, both goals are desirable.

Simple mechanical repair of the hiatus defect does not guarantee either complete relief of distress or prevention of peptic esophagitis. Smith and Bradshaw reported that 12 of 73 patients (16.5 per cent) treated by hiatus herniorrhaphy, exclusive of those with recurrences, were not completely relieved of symptoms following operation.[20] Morgan and co-workers have reported that, of 20 patients with preoperative free or induced reflux, (again, exclusive of those with recurrences) only 14 had complete correction of the reflux after herniorrhaphy, and in at least one patient esophagogastric continence was *decreased*.[13] Other authors have reported similar examples of patients who were relieved of symptoms that recurred following "successful" herniorrhaphy by the addition of a subtotal gastrectomy or vagotomy plus a drainage procedure.[9]

In view of the growing volume of evidence that the vast majority of patients with symptomatic hiatal hernia have esophageal reflux and acid hypersecretion, and with the further evidence that simple mechanical repair of the hernial defect does not necessarily prevent reflux, an increasing number of surgeons have begun to recommend that ancillary procedures accompany the primary repair. Burford and Lischer have suggested using pyloroplasty to encourage rapid gastric emptying, thus reducing the size of the bolus available for reflux.[3] Others have suggested that subtotal gastrectomy accompany herniorrhaphy in those patients in whom gastric or duodenal ulcer or marked acid hypersecretion plays a role in the production of symptoms. Still others have recommended pyloroplasty and vagotomy as definitive for the control of acid secretion.

Herrington has reported on 22 patients with sliding esophageal hiatal hernia who have undergone herniorrhaphy combined with a procedure designed to eliminate gastric hypersecretion, either vagotomy and pyloroplasty or vagotomy and excision of the gastric antrum.[9] Patients with associated duodenal ulcer were excluded from the study. Postoperative results showed 21 of the 22 patients completely relieved of epigastric and substernal discomfort. Berman and co-workers have performed a one-stage "balanced" operation for all types of hiatal hernia in 105 consecutive cases.[2] The procedure consists of reduction of the hernia and repair of the enlarged hiatus, accompanied by esophago-gastropexy, vagotomy, and pyloroplasty. There is evidence of one recurrence in the series and only two patients with persistent complaints.

Results of Treatment Noted by Authors

The following represents our own experience with hiatal hernia and peptic esophagitis. It has been the purpose of this analysis to correlate the clinical result of surgical treatment with an objective measurement of esophageal reflux. In addition to history, a postoperative upper gastrointestinal x-ray examination was made on all patients. Esophagoscopy was utilized in patients with persistent or recurrent symptoms of esophagitis. A total of 37 patients are available for analysis. Follow-up varies from four months to four years and three months. Thirty-two of the 37 patients have been evaluated more than one year after surgery. A clinical history compatible with reflux esophagitis was present in all patients. Radiographic studies demonstrated hiatal hernia preoperatively in 34 of the 37 cases. In the remaining three, reflux was proved in the laboratory, confirming the clinical impression, and in all a sliding hiatal hernia was demonstrated at surgery. Significant reflux was found in 31 of the 37 patients preoperatively by means of intraluminal pH and pressure studies. The examination was not performed prior to sugery in the remaining six cases. There have been no cases of sliding hiatal hernia and esophagitis in whom gastroesophageal reflux has been found to be absent.

Reflux has been defined as a pH below 3.5 at a distance of 4 cm. or more above the diaphragm and was measured by the method of Tuttle and Grossman. Briefly, a tube consisting of a polyethylene catheter and a pH electrode was passed into the stomach through the nasopharynx. Pressure was recorded continuously through the polyethylene catheter using a pressure transducer and a recording polygraph. Two hundred cubic centimeters of 0.1 N hydrochloric acid were introduced into the stomach through the polyethylene catheter to insure a strongly acid gastric pH and to provide an adequate bolus for reflux. With the patient in the sitting position the tube was withdrawn in 1-cm. increments. The level of the diaphragm was determined by inversion of intraluminal pressures during the respiratory cycle. Withdrawal through the esophagus was continued with the same increments until a pH level approaching neutrality was obtained or until the pharynx was reached. The tube was then passed into the stomach again and the withdrawal procedure repeated with the patient in the reclining position. No Valsalva or other pressure changing maneuvers were used.

The operations utilized have been hiatal herniorrhaphy alone, hiatal herniorrhaphy plus pyloroplasty, and hiatal herniorrhaphy, pyloroplasty, and vagotomy. Of the 16 patients treated by hiatal herniorrhaphy alone, significant reflux persisted postoperatively in 11, although there is no evidence of recurrent hernia by x-ray. Two patients have been only partially relieved of their symptoms and two have been clinically unimproved by surgery.

This is in sharp contrast with the series of 14 patients treated by hiatal herniorrhaphy, vagotomy, and a gastric drainage procedure. Twelve of these 14 patients had active duodenal ulcer, and the remaining two had basal gastric hypersecretion. It was anticipated that peptic esophagitis would be more severe in its manifestations because of the much greater acid-pepsin potency of the gastric content available for reflux. In fact, however, the actual results have been somewhat better in this group. Eleven of the 14 patients are entirely asymptomatic and only one has had persistent mild symptoms suggestive of reflux esophagitis. The primary pathologic process, therefore, has been satisfactorily reversed in 13 of 14 patients. In addition, this group demonstrates a lower incidence of postoperative reflux, and three of these patients are asymptomatic.

Finally, the group of patients treated by hiatal herniorrhaphy and pyloroplasty shows a lower incidence of postoperative reflux (3 out of 7). Although the series is too small for extensive analysis, this suggests that a drainage procedure may indeed facilitate a more rapid gastric emptying, decreasing the opportunity for the bolus to reflux cephalad. This observation is consistent with and lends support to that made by Burford and Lischer.

Conclusion

In summary then, the following conclusions appear warranted:

1. Although the incidence of hiatus hernia in the normal population is high, many of these patients are completely asymptomatic. Within the symptomatic group only a small percentage actually require surgical intervention.

2. Peptic esophagitis secondary to gastric hypersecretion and esophageal reflux appears to account for the vast majority of those patients requiring definitive operative procedures for relief of symptoms.

3. Since simple mechanical repair of the hernia does not always correct reflux, even in the absence of a recurrence, ancillary procedures are indicated. A drainage procedure, preferably pyloroplasty, appears to be a worthwhile adjunct. Certainly, based on the limited experience available, the incidence of postoperative reflux is lower.

4. In patients *with* active duodenal ulcer disease and basal gastric hypersecretion, in whom the effects of hiatal hernia and associated peptic esophagitis are predictably more intense, the combined operation of herniorrhaphy, vagotomy, and gastric drainage procedure has produced better results than herniorrhaphy alone in a group of patients *without* duodenal ulcer. This is explained in large measure by the reduced vagally controlled basal secretory rate and, therefore, lower acidity of gastric content.

5. Finally, it is clear that peptic esophagitis is merely another manifestation of acid-peptic disease in a new location. The importance and value of preoperative gastric secretory studies is apparent.

References

1. Allison, P. R.: Reflux esophagitis, sliding hiatal hernia, and the anatomy of repair. Surg., Gynec. and Obst., 92:419, 1951.

2. Berman, J. K., and Berman, E. J.: Management of esophageal hiatus hernia syndrome and associated abnormalities with balanced operations. Dis. Chest, *39*:1, 1961.

3. Burford, T. H., and Lischer, C. E.: Treatment of short esophageal hernia with esophagitis by Finney pyloroplasty. Ann. Surg., *144*:647, 1956.

4. Casten, D. R.: Personal communication to the authors, 1963.

5. Code, C. F., Creamer, B., Schlegel, J. F., Olsen, A. M., Donaghue, F. E., and Andersen, H. A.: An Atlas of Esophageal Motility in Health and Disease. Charles C Thomas, Springfield, Ill., 1958.

6. Ferguson, D. J., Sanchez-Palomera, E., Sako, Y., Clatworthy, H. W., Jr., Toon, R. W., and Wangensteen O. H.: Studies of experimental esophagitis. Surgery, *28*:1022, 1950.

7. Fyke, F. E., Jr., Code, C. F., and Schlegel, J. F.: The gastrointestinal sphincter in healthy human beings. Gastroenterologica, *86*:135, 1956.

8. Gould, D. M., and Barnhard, H. J.: Changing concepts in the structure, function and disease of the lower esophagus. Am. J. M. Sc., *233*:581, 1957.

9. Herrington, J. L., Jr.: Hiatal hernia with esophagitis: treatment by hernia repair, vagotomy and pyloroplasty or antrectomy. Ann. Surg., *151*:812, 1960.

10. Hoffman, R. F., Cruze, K., and Byron, F. X.: Symptomatic hiatus hernia. J.A.M.A., *169*:119, 1959.

11. Lerche, W.: The Esophagus and Pharynx in Action. Charles C Thomas, Springfield, Ill., 1950.

12. Meiss, J. H., Grindlay, J. H., and Ellis, F. H., Jr.: The gastroesophageal sphincter mechanism. J. Thorac. Surg., *36*:156, 1958.

13. Morgan, E. H., Hill, L. D., and Selby, D. K.: Objective assessment of gastroesophageal reflux secondary to hiatal hernia. Dis. Chest, *43*:367, 1963.

14. Neville, W. E., and Bartunek, R. R.: A combined medical and surgical approach to the treatment of reflux esophagitis. Am. J. Gastroenterol., *35*:335, 1961.

15. Perry, J. F., Jr., Yonehiro, E. G., Ya., P. M., Root, H. D., and Wangensteen, O. H.: Digestive action of human gastric juice. Proc. Soc. Exper. Biol. and Med., *92*:237, 1956.

16. Plzak, L. F., Fried, W., and Woodward, E. R.: Relative susceptibility of the gastrointestinal tract to experimental acute peptic ulceration. S. Forum, 7:389, 1956.

17. Quincke, H.: Ulcus Oesophagus Exdigestione. Deutsche Arch. F. Klin. Med., *24*:72, 1879.

18. Schlegel, J. F., and Code, C. F.: Pressure characteristics of the esophagus and its sphincters in dogs. Am. J. Physiol., *193*:9, 1958.

19. Selye, H.: Experimental production of peptic hemorrhagic esophagitis. Canad. M. A. J., *39*:447, 1938.

20. Smith, L. C., and Bradshaw, H. H.: Esophageal hiatal hernia. Surg., Gynec. and Obst., *109*:230, 1959.

21. Tileston, W.: Peptic ulcer of the esophagus. Am. J. M. Sc., *132*:240, 1906.

22. Tuttle, S. G., and Grossman, M. I.: Detection of Gastroesophageal reflux by simultaneous measurements of intraluminal pressure and pH. Proc. Soc. Exper. Biol. and Med., *92*:225, 1958.

Prevention of Hemorrhage in Patients with Portal Hypertension

Introduction

In the present state of our knowledge, an operation that creates a shunt between the portal venous system and a large systemic vein provides the best means at our disposal of preventing death from hemorrhage from the esophageal varices of patients with severe degrees of portal hypertension. This fact was well demonstrated by the pioneer work of Whipple, and of Blakemore and Lord, who demonstrated that recurrence of massive hemorrhage from the esophageal varices could be prevented by portosystemic venous anastomosis. The techniques available include an end-to-side or side-to-side portacaval anastomosis, or a lienorenal venous anastomosis in cases where the portal vein is unavailable or where a very large spleen and hypersplenism make this procedure desirable. When neither the portal nor the splenic vein is available, the shunt between the proximal end of the divided vena cava and the side of the superior mesenteric vein is equally feasible. In a patient with bleeding esophageal varices, due consideration must be given to any concomitant ascites, ammonia intoxication, and availability of the appropriate segment of portal or splenic vein, all equally important considerations in the selection of the procedure.

Apart from the danger of progressive deterioration in hepatic function in cirrhosis of the liver, portal hypertension threatens life in two important ways: first, by causing exsanguinating variceal hemorrhage, and second, by aggravating the degree of hepatic decompensation by the accumulation of gastrointestinal blood. The only goal that the surgeon has in the treatment of portal hypertension, then, is to prevent this threat to life. It is important to appreciate that though a portal pressure above 300 mm. of water is frequently associated with bleeding varices, variceal hemorrhage may on occasion occur in patients who demonstrate a normal portal pressure, indicating that some other superimposed mechanism may precipitate the variceal hemorrhage, for example, the presence of gastric acid reflux.

It is necessary to point out that the surgical procedures mentioned above, which provide for portal decompression, are not unassociated with significant mortality and morbidity, but may be acceptable in reducing the incidence and severity of recurrent bouts of hematemesis. It must also be recognized that even after an uneventful portal decompression, subsequent thrombosis of the anastomosis may occur with redevelopment of varices and recurrence of bleeding. The development of peptic ulceration is not infrequent subsequent to a shunting procedure, this being due to the intestinal histamine-like substances, which by-pass the liver where normal degradation would occur and become responsible for gastric hypersecretion and peptic ulceration. Nevertheless, in general, it may be truly stated that the risks of recurrent massive hemorrhage from varices are greater than the risks of portal decompression; 75 per cent of patients admitted to hospital with massive variceal hemorrhage die as a result of their first hemorrhage.

Whether it is desirable to introduce prophylactic portasystemic shunting as a precaution against variceal hemorrhage in patients with portal hypertension, at present provides a source of controversy. On the one hand, acceptance of such a principle would introduce the hazards of surgery to people with portal hypertension and gastroesophageal varices who may never bleed, while subsequent thrombosis of the anastomosis may precipitate bleeding, which can no longer be remedied by appropriate surgery.

There is one situation in which few would cavil at the performance of a prophylactic shunt. This is in the patient with portal hypertension and gastroesophageal varices that have not yet bled, and with congestive splenomegaly and hypersplenism, in whom splenectomy should be complemented by a lienorenal shunt to reduce the chance of subsequent variceal hemorrhage. It may well be argued that in such cases a prophylactic portacaval shunt may reduce the congestive splenomegaly, thereby curing the hypersplenism as well as incidentally reducing the probability of variceal hemorrhage.

If one could, on the basis of clinical experience, define which patients with portal hypertension and esophagogastric varices were likely to bleed, selection of such cases for prophylactic shunting might well be acceptable; but until such criteria can be established, it would be unwise to crusade for general prophylactic portal systemic venous shunting. Such a clinical assessment would require: (1) a systematic investigation of all patients suffering from cirrhosis; (2) assessment of whether the mechanism of portal obstruction is predominantly intra- or extrahepatic; (3) the recording of splenic pulp pressure as well as splenoportography to demonstrate the architectural pattern of the portal system and the presence of esophageal varices; and (4) esophagram, esophagoscopy, and hematologic study for hypersplenism. These studies would naturally be complemented by appropriate laboratory procedures for assessment of liver function, and if repeated studies demonstrated increasing portal hypertension, increasing size or extent of varices, and increasing hypersplenism, such patients may, with some justification, be considered for prophylactic shunts. It is important to remember that spontaneous remissions and improvement may occur and contraindicate surgical intervention.

The following two chapters emphasize the alternative viewpoints in the management of portal hypertension with nonbleeding varices. It is probable that further experience in the use of prophylactic surgical portal decompression in appropriately selected cases, and controlled statistical comparison with comparable groups treated conservatively will, over a five- to ten-year period, permit a more valid rationalization of this problem, with the truth perhaps lying somewhere between the apparently antagonistic points of view.

CHARLES MARKS, M.D., F.R.C.S.
(*Guest Editor*)

Routine Prophylactic Shunting as a Precaution Against Bleeding from Cardioesophageal Varices

Eddy D. Palmer

Brooke General Hospital, Fort Sam Houston, Texas

Although nonemergent surgical portal decompression is in all cases a prophylactic move, by common usage "prophylactic shunting" has come to mean shunting that is done before the patient has had a variceal hemorrhage. Occasionally, it is true, a shunt proves to be good treatment for ascites (just as often it creates chronic ascites), but it is important to understand, when discussing the question implied in the title, that the operation does not make the patient feel better or in any way improve the underlying cause of his portal hypertension. The shunt is made simply to prevent future variceal hemorrhage. There are, of course, a great many causes of cardioesophageal varices, but because all problems are made more difficult when the underlying disease is cirrhosis, it is best to direct the discussion at management of the varices in this disease.

The question is simply this: in view of the admitted strenuousness of the operation, is it better to wait for the patient with varices to prove he can bleed from varices before eliminating the lesions, or is the danger of the first hemorrhage so great that the risk of operation is comparatively insignificant? Feelings have run high enough on the question, so that ethical considerations have prevented truly objective study by alternate patient selection. If there were some way to measure varices or the patient with varices to separate those that will bleed from those that will not, there would be no serious argument. But variceal hemorrhage is wholly unpredictable, and I must therefore urge adoption of prophylactic shunting as a routine policy. I can best explain the reason by answering certain pertinent questions from personal experience.

How Dangerous to the Cirrhotic Patient is His First Hemorrhage?

The risk of the cirrhotic patient's first hemorrhage is, of course, of paramount importance to the argument for prophylactic shunt. If the first hemorrhage proves fatal to a large proportion of the patients, the value of any effort on behalf of the group is immediately very much reduced. A good operation becomes rather useless if a large proportion of the potentially salvagable patients are lost before the surgeon gets to operate.

TABLE 1.   CAUSES OF DEATH AMONG 250 CIRRHOTIC PATIENTS WHO WERE NOT TREATED BY PORTAL DECOMPRESSION

Cause of Death	Number of Patients
Liver failure without hemorrhage	88
Liver failure due to hemorrhage	85
Exsanguination from varices	36
Hepatoma	8
Death unrelated to liver disease	33

TABLE 2.   CHRONOLOGY OF FATAL HEMORRHAGE AMONG 121 CIRRHOTIC PATIENTS WHO WERE NOT TREATED BY PORTAL DECOMPRESSION

Fatal Hemorrhage	Per Cent of Patients
First	70
Second	24
Third	5
Fourth	0
Fifth	1

In personal experience, 250 cirrhotic patients who had not been subjected to shunt have died. Among 121 (48 per cent), the direct cause of death was hemorrhage, which, in the majority of cases, proved to be from varices (Table 1). The most significant feature of the fatal bleeding was that 70 per cent of the cirrhotic patients who died of hemorrhage died of their first hemorrhage (Table 2).

How Dangerous to the Cirrhotic Patient Is Shunt Surgery?

Against these figures must be posed figures indicating the risks of shunt surgery. Statistics vary from one hospital to another, depending not on the competence of the surgeons, but rather on local indications for surgery, the level of liver function required before operation is scheduled, and other points of difference.

At any rate, nonemergent shunt surgery (either portacaval or spleno-renal) among 172 adult cirrhotic patients has resulted in 11 deaths (6.4 per cent) within the first two postoperative weeks and 7 more (total 10.5 per cent) by the end of the first month.

How Effective Is Portal Decompression in Precluding Variceal Hemorrhage?

The point of shunt surgery is preclusion of variceal hemorrhage, and this is quite easy to assess. Of the 172 patients who have been followed for a total of 5838 months since surgery, 17 have bled from the upper gastro-intestinal tract; in most instances the bleeding proved to be from varices (in the other cases the patients were not available at the moment of hemor-rhage for direct determination of the site of bleeding). Sixty-two of these 172 operations were "prophylactic" procedures, and two of these patients were among the bleeders. In most cases the cause of recurrence of varices and hemorrhage was thrombosis of the shunt.

To put the surgical results on a more quantitative basis, one may note some transfusion requirements, these being about the best measure of the severity of hemorrhage when blood is freely available for replacement. The monthly blood replacement requirement for each of the 172 patients during the year prior to surgery averaged 341 ml. Since operation each patient has required an average monthly blood replacement of 6.8 ml. It must be remembered, of course, that many of the patients initially came to medical attention because of hemorrhage, thereby accentuating the trans-fusion requirements just prior to surgery.

Evaluation of Results

The life of a cirrhotic patient is often a brief one. Elimination of varices as a bleeding source is expected to prolong life, of course, but only to a degree. Spontaneous hepatic failure becomes the big threat. To date, 80 of the 172 patients have died, but only in three instances was variceal bleeding involved. There was no exsanguination; instead, minor bleeding in these three patients merely accompanied progressive liver decompen-sation.

Some patients who are in desperate condition at the time of operation die soon after and some survive for many years. Many cirrhotics live long and productive lives. In local experience postshunt cerebral problems secondary to ammonia intoxication have been no more than a very minor problem. We can only wonder about the pessimistic reports of others in this connection. Fifty-seven patients have been followed for more than five years following shunt. Their productivity is outlined in Table 3. These figures show a remarkable record, but it should be remembered, of course,

TABLE 3. PRODUCTIVITY RECORD OF 57 CIRRHOTIC PATIENTS SURVIVING
MORE THAN 5 YEARS AFTER SHUNT

Activity	Number of Patients	
	At Time of Surgery	At End of 5 Years
Active Army duty	32	10
Other full-time employment	5	24
Housewives, active	14	11
Part-time employment	—	2
Inactive but not disabled	4	6
Invalids	2	4

that many of the potentially less productive patients did not survive the 5 years.

Conclusion

To this nonsurgeon the experience outlined here is convincing indication of the important contribution that portal decompression can make to the patient with cardioesophageal varices who has not bled, even when the underlying disease is cirrhosis:

1. The possibility that the varices will eventually bleed is very good.

2. The first variceal hemorrhage is very likely to prove fatal if the underlying disease is cirrhosis.

3. The surgical risk of nonemergency portal decompression is reasonably low.

4. The operation is very effective in precluding future hemorrhage.

5. Many shunted cirrhotics are capable of leading long and notably productive lives.

Factors Favoring Conservative Management of Patients with Asymptomatic Cardioesophageal Varices

Konrad H. Soergel

Marquette University School of Medicine

Objections to the Prophylactic Shunt

Bleeding from the upper gastrointestinal tract in patients with cirrhosis of the liver is of ominous prognostic significance: only 30 per cent of these patients are alive one year after the first bleeding episode. The occurrence of acute gastrointestinal hemorrhage during the terminal phase of the illness has been variously reported in 11 per cent,[1] 25 per cent,[2] and 32 per cent[3] of all patients with cirrhosis. These figures gain added impact when it is recalled that cirrhosis is the tenth leading cause of death in the United States, and that it ranks third among the diseases that result in loss of man's maximum productive years, between the ages of 35 and 65.[4] Since many (but not all) of these bleeding episodes arise from ruptured gastroesophageal varices, it has been suggested that this catastrophic event can be prevented by performing "prophylactic" portasystemic shunts in all cirrhotic patients with esophageal varices *before* the first hemorrhage has occurred.[5]

All available evidence indicates that the "prophylactic" shunt operation may be expected to decrease both incidence and severity of bleeding from gastroesophageal varices. This does not necessarily mean that creation of "prophylactic" shunts will actually prolong life because ". . . the natural desire is to operate upon patients earlier in their disease, before physiological function is grossly disturbed and structure irreparably altered. Such a trend undoubtedly provides lower surgical mortality and increased percentages of successful results. Unfortunately, such a trend leads to

Page 242

surgery upon the borderline patient who might never have required operation for continued freedom from difficulty."[6] Before this surgical procedure can be recommended as standard practice, a number of questions have to be answered: How many cirrhotic patients die as a direct result of their first bleeding episode from esophageal varices and might, therefore, benefit from the "prophylactic" shunt? What are the criteria for the diagnosis of cirrhosis and of asymptomatic gastroesophageal varices, and what proportion of these patients are acceptable operative risks at the time of diagnosis? Have patients with a "prophylactic" shunt fared better than non-operated control groups? And finally, are there conservative means for reducing portal hypertension?

Is Death Often Caused by the First Hemorrhage from Esophageal Varices?

A group of 115 veterans with the clinical diagnosis of cirrhosis, observed for an average of 3.3 years, was evaluated retrospectively.[7] Varices had been seen on esophagoscopy in all cases, but no episodes of gastrointestinal bleeding had occurred. Fourteen per cent of these patients died with their first upper gastrointestinal hemorrhage during the period of study. However, not all these patients could have been saved had a "prophylactic" shunt been established because:

First, "in assigning the cause of death, a distinction has to be made between those patients in whom bleeding is a final episode in the course of progressive hepatic failure and those in whom hemorrhage occurs while hepatic function is not greatly impaired."[7] Thus, in one-fourth to one-third of patients dying with the first episode of bleeding, the hemorrhage occurs as a coup de grace in the setting of terminal liver failure.

Second, the occurrence of upper gastrointestinal bleeding in patients with known cirrhosis all too often is attributed to varix rupture, despite the lack of specific evidence to this effect. In one careful study of this point, the site of acute bleeding was established in 158 cirrhotic patients admitted to the Boston City Hospital; varices were responsible for only 53 per cent of 172 bleeding episodes. In the 88 patients who died, the bleeding had originated from sites other than varices in 24 or 27 per cent.[8]

It must be remembered that reports on the natural history and clinical picture of cirrhosis apply only to the type of patient actually observed. For example, the debilitated alcoholic with Laennec's cirrhosis usually presents with deteriorating liver function, whereas problems connected with portal hypertension predominate in patients with postnecrotic cirrhosis who are seen most frequently in private hospitals.

In summary, 15 to 25 per cent of all cirrhotic patients die with their first upper gastrointestinal hemorrhage. About one-fourth of these bleed from a site other than varices, and in another one-fourth the bleeding is a terminal episode of inexorably progressing liver failure.

Criteria for Diagnosis

It seems superfluous to state that the application of the "prophylactic" shunt to the cirrhotic population would require the use of reliable and objective criteria for the recognition of hepatic cirrhosis and of gastro-esophageal varices. These criteria have not always been applied. In many published series of cases, the diagnosis of cirrhosis was based on clinical findings without the benefit of liver biopsy. This leads to the erroneous inclusion of some patients with other liver diseases, such as fatty metamorphosis, granulomatous processes, and neoplastic infiltration. A more common error is the failure to recognize the presence of any liver disease in cirrhotic patients. For example, in a Swedish University Hospital, cirrhosis was found at autopsy in 280 patients during the years 1951 to 1960. The diagnosis of cirrhosis had not even been suspected by the clinicians in 115 of these 280 cases.[1]

It is well known that esophageal varices are frequently missed on radiographic examination of the esophagus. Splenoportography also grossly underestimates the incidence of collateral circulation between the portal and the systemic venous system via the esophageal venous plexus. Therefore, the presence or absence of esophageal varices must be established by esophagoscopy. However, Palmer has pointed out the striking day-to-day variability of the extent of esophageal varices as seen through the esophagoscope.[9] In 35 of 130 patients with known esophageal varices, these dilated veins were not seen on one esophagoscopy, only to reappear on subsequent examinations. In Palmer's words, "Failure to find varices upon a single esophagoscopic examination is no assurance that varices are not potentially present."

Operability

The patient with cirrhosis and portal hypertension may for many years fail to have symptoms severe enough to cause him to seek medical attention. At the time of first hospitalization, more than half these patients have one or more signs of decompensated cirrhosis, i.e., jaundice, ascites, or encephalopathy.[10] Two out of 3 of such patients have esophageal varices,[2] and are therefore potential candidates for "prophylactic" shunt surgery. Among this group, however, many patients are already too ill to undergo this extensive surgical procedure. In a recent study,[7] 54 per cent of all cirrhotic patients in whom esophageal varices were found before the first bleeding episode were adjudged to be poor operative risks. It follows that between 30 and 50 per cent of all cirrhotic patients are known to have esophageal varices at a time when shunt surgery can be performed with acceptable operative mortality. If all these patients had a "prophylactic" shunt, about 15 per cent of the total mortality from cirrhosis could be either delayed or actually prevented.

In summary, liver biopsy and esophagoscopy are necessary to define the entire group of patients with cirrhosis and asymptomatic esophageal varices. At the time of diagnosis many are already very poor surgical risks because of advanced hepatic decompensation.

Results Following the "Prophylactic" Portasystemic Shunt

It is apparent that only a small fraction of all cirrhotic patients will be eligible for a "prophylactic" shunt. It remains to be seen how the performance of this procedure in selected patients affects their further course when compared with that of a carefully matched control group. In this evaluation, the benefits derived from lowering the portal venous pressure must outweigh not only the operative mortality, but also the morbidity following the successful establishment of a portasystemic shunt, that is, the increased incidence of peptic ulcer and chronic hepatic encephalopathy.

The problem of finding adequate control groups is formidable. However, comparison of patients with a "prophylactic" shunt with patients in whom a "therapeutic" shunt has been constructed after survival from an upper gastrointestinal hemorrhage,[5] will not give the desired information, since the two groups a priori represent different stages of the cirrhotic disease process. Ninety-two prophylactic shunts were performed by four different groups, [5, 11-13] and the operative mortality was only 6.5 per cent. This low mortality rate was achieved by the careful selection of patients and by the skill of experienced surgical-medical teams operating in large medical centers.

In two studies, one from West Haven Veterans Administration Hospital[12] and the other by the Boston Inter-Hospital Liver Group,[13] a total of 79 patients with cirrhosis and established varices were randomly assigned to a nonoperated control group or to a "prophylactic" shunt group. The results after rather short follow-up periods, ranging from 4 to 60 months, speak for themselves and are shown on Table 1.

TABLE 1. RESULTS OF TREATMENT OF PORTAL CIRRHOSIS

	Control	Prophylactic Shunt
Total number of cases	38	41
Total mortality	10	12
Hemorrhage from varices	8	1
Hemorrhage from peptic ulcer	0	2
Continued hepatic encephalopathy	1	5
In good health	22	16
Mean duration of hospitalization[7]	90 days	150 days

In summary, available evidence does not support the contention that the "prophylactic" shunt prolongs life or that it improves the general state of health. The effect of the operation on survival, on freedom from hepatic encephalopathy, and on the ability to return to work will be known only when a longer follow-up of a larger number of patients is completed.

Results of Conservative Treatment

Unfortunately, the problem of preventing varix bleeding in patients with cirrhosis is far from being solved by conservative efforts. There are, however, two situations in which medical therapy can indirectly lower the degree of portal hypertension: (1) in patients with Laennec's cirrhosis of mild to moderate degree, in whom prolonged rest and diet therapy effects a decrease in fatty infiltration, inflammatory reaction, and liver cell necrosis,[14] and (2) in some cirrhotics in whom a good dietary and diuretic regimen causes the disappearance of ascites.[15] In the presence of varices, antacid treatment of patients with hiatal hernia or peptic ulcer and heartburn seems to be a reasonable measure, but its effectiveness in preventing varix bleeding by decreasing esophageal irritation due to acid gastroesophageal reflux remains conjectural.

In summary, medical therapy may temporarily decrease the risk of varix hemorrhage in certain patients. A permanent protective effect of conservative management is unproved and unlikely.

Conclusion

The poor prognosis of the cirrhotic patient with gastroesophageal varices is more often related to progressive deterioration of liver function than to the risk of varix bleeding. Frequently these patients no longer represent an acceptable operative risk at the time of diagnosis. In a small number of selected, good-risk patients, "prophylactic" portasystemic shunt has not decreased the mortality or morbidity rate. The "prophylactic" portasystemic shunt needs to be evaluated further in carefully controlled studies before its ultimate usefulness can be assessed. In the meantime, efforts at the prevention of varix rupture remain restricted to the well established modalities of diet, rest, and diuretics.

References

1. Hällén, J. and Krook, H.: Follow-up studies on an unselected ten-year material of 360 patients with liver cirrhosis in one community. Acta med. scandinav., *173*:479, 1963.
2. Nachlas, M. M.: A critical evaluation of venous shunts for the treatment of cirrhotic patients with esophageal varices. Ann. Surg., *148*:169, 1958.
3. Cohn, R., and Blaisdell, F. W.: The natural history of the patient with cirrhosis of the liver with esophageal varices following the first massive hemorrhage. Surg., Gynec. and Obst., *106*:699, 1958.
4. Schwartz, J. L., and Lipscomb, W. R.: Loss of life due to cirrhosis of the liver: California. J. Chron. Dis., *14*:386, 1961.
5. Sullivan, B. H., Jr., Cohen, A., and Palmer, E. D.: Prophylactic portacaval shunts Gastroenterology, *39*:414, 1960.

6. Bennett, H. D., Lorentzen, C., and Baker, L. A.: Transient esophageal varices in hepatic cirrhosis. Arch. Int. Med., *92*:507, 1953.

7. Baker, L. A., Smith, C., and Lieberman, G.: The natural history of esophageal varices. A study of 115 cirrhotic patients in whom varices were diagnosed prior to bleeding. Am. J. Med., *26*:228, 1959.

8. Merrigan, T. C., Jr., Hollister, R. M., Gryska, P. F., Starkey, G. W., and Davidson, C. S.: Gastrointestinal bleeding with cirrhosis. A study of 172 episodes in 158 patients. New England J. Med., *263*:579, 1960.

9. Palmer, E. D.: On the natural history of esophageal varices which are secondary to portal cirrhosis. Ann. Int. Med., *47*:18, 1957.

10. Garceau, A. J., Chalmers, T. C., and the Boston Inter-Hospital Liver Group: The natural history of cirrhosis. I. Survival with esophageal varices. New England J. Med., *268*:469, 1963.

11. Mikkelsen, J. P., Turrill, F. L., and Pattison, A. C.: Portacaval shunt in cirrhosis of the liver. Clinical and hemodynamic aspects. Am. J. Surg., *104*:204, 1962.

12. Conn, H. O., and Lindenmuth, W. W.: Prophylactic portacaval anastomosis in cirrhotic patients with esophageal varices. A preliminary report of a controlled study. New England J. Med., *266*:743, 1962.

13. Garceau, A. J., Donaldson, R. M., Jr., O'Hara, E. T., Callow, A. D., Muench, H., Chalmers, T. C., and the Boston Inter-Hospital Liver Group: A controlled trial of prophylactic portacaval-shunt surgery. New England J. Med., *270*:496, 1964.

14. Leevy, C. M., Zinke, M., Baber, J., and Chey, W. Y.: Observations on the influence of medical therapy on portal hypertension in hepatic cirrhosis. Ann. Int. Med., *49*:837, 1958.

15. Reynolds, T. B., Geller, H. M., Kuzma, O. T., and Redeker, A. G.: Spontaneous decrease in portal pressure with clinical improvement in cirrhosis. New England J. Med., *263*:734, 1960.

Treatment of Acute Hemorrhage from Esophagogastric Varices

Introduction

Acute bleeding from esophagogastric varices is now the most common cause of gastrointestinal hemorrhage. Too many physicians believe that gross hemorrhage from varices associated with portal hypertension is either invariably fatal or heralds the onset of a worsening hepatic failure with subsequent irreversible coma. This need not necessarily be the case, and as pointed out by one of our contributors (Wantz), adequate decompression of the portal system by an emergency or early portacaval shunt will control hemorrhage from esophagogastric varices with an overall mortality of less than 40 per cent. On the other hand, the mortality of emergency operations in poor-risk patients approximated 60 per cent, which is nearly twice that seen in poor-risk patients with portal hypertension who were subjected to the prophylactic procedure. The importance of temporary nonoperative control of bleeding is therefore recognized, and certainly justifies Wangensteen's continued search for a method other than balloon tamponade for control of esophageal bleeding. Preliminary studies of esophagogastric cooling indicate that it may have some advantages over other nonoperative methods.

The other contributors to this section propose new and novel approaches to this serious problem, based on recent and additional observations on the pathophysiology of portal hypertension. Information indicating that increased formation of lymph in the liver, with further distention of the organ, can result from an increased resistance of flow of blood in the hepatic vein, has led Dumont and Witte to advocate thoracic duct cannulation. They suggest that this can be a simple surgical procedure, performed under local anesthesia at the bedside when bleeding from esophagogastric varices is refractory to the usual nonoperative methods. The resultant decrease in hepatic interstitial fluid is thought to facilitate transhepatic portal flow, with a lowering of pressure within the portal system.

The presentation by Womack and Peters includes an excellent review of the data supporting a concept that arterial flow into the portal venous system plays a major role in portal hypertension. The authors, in turn, propose splenectomy and ligation of a portion of the arterial blood supply to the stomach as an adjunct to transgastroesophageal plication of bleeding varices.

E. H. E.

Emergency Portal Decompression in the Treatment of Acute Hemorrhage from Esophagogastric Varices

George E. Wantz, Jr.

The New York Hospital-Cornell Medical Center

Abundant evidence indicates that in patients with portal hypertension, adequate portal decompression is followed by the disappearance of esophagogastric varices and, therefore, the elimination of massive and possibly catastrophic variceal hemorrhage. However, since portal decompression is associated with significant, although acceptable, mortality and morbidity, and since not all patients with esophagogastric varices necessarily bleed, the procedure has been generally reserved for those patients who have already recovered from variceal hemorrhage and who, after prolonged diet therapy, are in top condition. Yet, this approach to portal hypertension excludes altogether the patient with bleeding esophagogastric varices. Therefore, the management of the patient who is bleeding from esophagogastric varices is the crucial problem. Variceal hemorrhage is always serious, invariably recurrent, and all too frequently results in death, if not by exsanguination, by the induction of irreversible hepatic decompensation. Although hemorrhage may cease spontaneously in some patients, in many other patients it does not. In the latter instances, the esophageal tamponade has proved of great value in controlling the bleeding and minimizing the immediate danger of exsanguination. Unfortunately, esophageal tamponade does not control the hemorrhage in all patients bleeding from esophagogastric varices, nor does it assure that hemorrhage will not recur upon deflation of the balloon. Too frequently the bleeding recurs immediately or while the patient is undergoing evaluation and preparation for operation, thus further reducing the patient's chance of recovery. Furthermore, the esophageal balloon is in itself hazardous, since it may lead to pressure necrosis of the nose, pharynx, esophagus, or stomach; perforation of the esophagus or stomach; or aspiration pneumonia.

To overcome these disadvantages, a variety of measures and procedures have been advocated as a substitute for, or as an adjunct to, esophageal tamponade. Whether these measures be local gastric hypothermia, intravenous vasopression, or operations directed at controlling the bleeding varix per se, e.g., esophagogastrectomy, gastric transection, or variceal ligation, they all have the same disadvantages as esophageal tamponade in that they neither ensure cessation of hemorrhage nor prevent its recurrence. Furthermore, in the case of operation, the substitute is not necessarily less formidable or stressful than portacaval shunt.

A logical solution to the problem would be to treat the initial acute hemorrhage definitively by emergency portal decompression. There is ample evidence that this procedure abruptly and permanently checks hemorrhage from esophagogastric varices, thus averting the chance of exsanguination, the perils of recurrent variceal bleeding, and the risks of other operative procedures which, at best, only temporarily control the hemorrhage.

Nevertheless, portal decompression is obviously a major undertaking and, even under elective conditions, not all patients are candidates for it. Moreover, for a successful outcome there are additional problems to be carefully considered: the preparation of the patient, the timing of the procedure, and the choice of procedure. Finally, certain vital questions must be answered: Do the results of emergency portal decompression justify its performance? Is the salvage rate of these desperately ill patients increased? Does portacaval decompression actually prolong life?

Definition of Emergency Portacaval Shunt

The term "emergency portacaval shunt" should not imply that the patient is subjected to operation immediately after the diagnosis is made. Rather, the operation is performed at an optimal time after the patient has been prepared, the bleeding controlled by esophageal balloon, and the vital signs stabilized. There is nothing to be gained by rushing the patient to the operating room, unless the patient is a good-risk candidate who is bleeding uncontrollably and exsanguination is imminent. The time taken to decide to operate or to prepare the patient may make the difference between a successful or an unsuccessful outcome. "Early portacaval shunt" perhaps would be a more accurate and descriptive term since, in most instances, the esophageal tamponade eliminates the immediate necessity to decompress the portal system for the control of acute hemorrhage from esophagogastric varices.

Selection of Candidates

The best results are generally obtained in patients with the greatest amount of hepatic reserve because operative mortality and morbidity parallel the degree of hepatic disease. Consequently, the criteria for selecting patients for elective portacaval shunt apply equally to the candidates for emergency operation. Under no circumstances should the procedure be performed on patients who are in hepatic coma or shock, exhibit frank hepatic decompensation, or are obviously moribund. For patients in these states, operative mortality is simply too high to justify an aggressive approach.

Likewise, patients whose general health has progressively deteriorated before hemorrhage and in whom the bleeding represents an additional manifestation of hepatic decompensation should be given a trial of balloon tamponade. In general, all patients with little hepatic reserve should be treated conservatively, since hepatic function may be so improved by a period of diet therapy that they become good-risk candidates rather than poor ones. Moreover, the advisability of emergency portal decompression in patients with advanced cirrhosis, even though stabilized, is questionable. Under the most ideal elective conditions, the results of portacaval shunt in such patients are far from satisfactory, since they have so little hepatic reserve that operative mortality is excessive, morbidity from hepatic coma distressingly common, and the chance for survival as integrated human beings for as much as two years extremely low. However, if hemorrhage continues or recurs despite the proper nonoperative treatment, in a patient with advanced portal cirrhosis who is able to maintain a relatively stable state of hepatic function and who is not intensely icteric or moribund, operative intervention sometimes may be justified as the only means of controlling the hemorrhage and preventing exsanguination.

Recognition of good-risk candidates when they are bleeding intensely is not too difficult. A complete battery of hepatic function tests, although admittedly valuable, is not necessary, nor is it readily available at most hospitals at all times during the week. An accurate clinical history and careful physical examination, plus only the hepatic function determinations of serum albumin and serum bilirubin, make it possible to accurately and quickly assay the patient's hepatic reserve. Typically, good-risk patients exhibit, at most, only moderate muscle wasting; have rarely, if ever, been in hepatic coma or exhibited frank icterus; usually do not have ascites, but if they do, the ascites either is easily manageable or is refractory without concomitant severe hypoalbuminemia and malnutrition; usually have serum albumin levels exceeding 3.0 Gm./100 ml. and serum bilirubin levels less than 3.0 mg./100 ml.; and have been able to carry on their normal daily activities.

The results of hepatic function tests require careful evaluation. Blood for hepatic function tests should be drawn shortly after admission, since the effects of both the hemorrhage and multiple transfusions may adversely affect their results and inaccurately reflect the patient's hepatic reserve at the onset of the hemorrhage. For example, hemorrhage of any degree can quickly impair hepatic function, resulting in icterus, hypoproteineuria, and other manifestations of hepatic decompensation. But the hemolysis of the transfused blood also may produce a significant misleading elevation of the serum bilirubin. Generally, it is ill advised to operate on a patient with portal cirrhosis who has a serum bilirubin exceeding 4.0 mg./100 ml. because, although serum bilirubin levels of 1.0 to 2.0 mg./100 ml. are common, frank and obvious icterus is usually encountered in patients with portal cirrhosis only when hepatic decompensation is present. Indeed, jaundice sometimes may precede all other clinical evidence of approaching hepatic collapse. Biliary cirrhosis is the exception to this generalization, since in this condition marked jaundice may occur in the presence of otherwise good hepatic function.

Likewise, hemorrhage is frequently followed by the sudden development of ascites which, combined with the blood loss, may produce a sudden severe hypoalbuminemia. In these circumstances a marked hypoalbuminemia is not necessarily a manifestation of far advanced cirrhosis or a contraindication to operation, because it is not a true reflection of the ability of the liver to manufacture albumin.

The amount of muscle wasting is one of the best indications of the degree of hepatic disease. Marked muscle wasting, as manifested by spindly arms and legs and atrophy of the muscles of the shoulder girdle, is a typical feature of advanced liver disease and is associated with a marked increase in operative mortality. On the other hand, the absence of muscle wasting, unless there is acute hepatic decompensation, indicates good hepatic functional reserve.

The hemorrhage itself will aid in the evaluation of hepatic reserve, since those patients who do not develop manifestations of hepatic coma after a massive hemorrhage will probably have good hepatic function. The converse, however, is not necessarily true, and massive hemorrhage in a good-risk candidate may result in frank hepatic coma if sufficient nitrogenous products from the blood in the intestine are absorbed and shunted around the liver into the systemic circulation by collateral circulation.

Finally, adequate renal function is necessary for safe operative intervention. The state of the kidneys is indicated by the quantity and quality of urine being excreted and by the blood urea nitrogen level. However, since elevation of the blood urea nitrogen may be caused merely by the absorption of blood in the intestinal tract, it sometimes may be necessary to do a urea clearance test to rule out primary and secondary renal disease as well as the hepatorenal syndrome, all of which are contraindications for operation.

Preparation of the Patient

The preparation of the patient for operation actually encompasses all aspects of management of an individual with acute bleeding from esophagogastric varices. Within the scope of this paper, however, only the salient points for ensuring a successful emergency portal decompression will be discussed.

It is particularly important to control the hemorrhage, not merely because of the possibility of exsanguination, but especially because of the serious consequences it has on the liver. Therefore, unless the hemorrhage has already ceased or is extremely mild, an active effort should be made to stop it to permit the patient's vital signs to become stable without the undesirable necessity of administering huge quantities of whole blood. The immediate control of variceal hemorrhage is most assuredly accomplished by the esophageal balloon. Moreover, the esophageal balloon, by checking the hemorrhage, will also confirm the diagnosis of esophagogastric varices. Too frequently, the performance of various other diagnostic procedures, e.g., string test and esophagoscopy, results in undue delay in controlling the hemorrhage. Furthermore, the fact that the esophageal balloon is also potentially dangerous often produces procrastination in the hope that the bleeding either will cease spontaneously or is not variceal in origin.

Although it is not always available, whole fresh blood is preferable to old bank blood for the replacement of blood lost by patients with cirrhosis. Enormous quantities of blood frequently are needed, and the use of freshly drawn blood will minimize the danger of clotting disorders. The possibility of overtransfusion is always present when large quantities of blood are hurriedly administered. Even slight overtransfusion, however, is hazardous in patients with portal hypertension, since it may reinstitute the hemorrhage by elevating portal pressures. Therefore, it is best to maintain the hematocrit in the range of 30 to 33 per cent. Patients with cirrhosis and portal hypertension usually have long been anemic and tolerate low hematocrit levels without clinical manifestation. Hydration should, of course, be maintained by 10 per cent glucose in water. Saline should be strictly avoided, since it will only aggravate the retention of fluid.

It is important to evacuate and sterilize the bowel. While these objectives are always important in treating hepatic coma, they are especially important in candidates for an emergency portacaval shunt, even though they may not show manifestations of hepatic encephalopathy. If the bowel is not evacuated, an enormous quantity of protein, the result of hemorrhage, will lie stagnant and irremovable in the postoperative bowel because of paralytic ileus, and may cause severe and untreatable ammonia intoxication. A good way to evacuate the bowel is to administer magnesium citrate into the stomach via the aspirating lumen of the esophageal balloon. Magnesium citrate is a powerful cathartic, is easily injected down the lumen, and unlike castor oil, does not rot rubber tubing. Tap water enemas also will evacuate the colon, but when combined with cathartics may exhaust the patient if given too frequently.

Oral neomycin is an excellent agent to sterilize the bowel. An initial dose of 4 Gm., followed by 1 Gm. every four hours, is adequate. However, complete sterilization of the bowel is unlikely, since the time available for preparation is insufficient and since the antimicrobial agent will be quickly evacuated from the bowel along with the blood and stool. Nevertheless, the number of coliform bacteria will be diminished and the metabolic activity of those remaining reduced; this will result in a significant and beneficial reduction in the formation of ammonia.

Finally, preparation of the patient for operation should include spleno-manometry and splenoportography. Not only will these studies permit straightforward establishment of the diagnosis, but they will aid the surgeon in planning the course of the operative procedure. These studies have low morbidity and can be easily done, with the aid of local anesthesia, just prior to the contemplated surgery.

Choice of Operative Procedure

For a successful result, portal decompression obviously must be ade-quate. Portal decompression is adequate when the final portal pressure is less than 25 cm. of water or, better, when it is identical to or within several centimeters of, that of the inferior vena cava. The best way to achieve adequate portal decompression is by a portacaval shunt. The expe-rience of those interested in the problem of portal hypertension indicates that portacaval shunts are not only large enough to be regularly adequate, but also remain permanently patent. Both end-to-side and side-to-side porta-caval shunts are equally effective in the elimination of esophagogastric varices, but the latter is more efficient in dealing with ascites, since it decompresses both the splanchnic side and the hepatic side of the portal system. Furthermore, the absence of ascites does not necessarily preclude the need of a side-to-side portacaval shunt. The procedure is also manda-tory when the hepatic production of lymph is excessive, as indicated by unusually large hepatic lymphatic channels, and when, upon occlusion of the portal vein, the pressure on the hepatic side of the occlusion approxi-mates or is greater than the unoccluded portal pressure, suggesting thereby that the portal vein is acting as an outflow tract of the liver. If an end-to-side portacaval shunt is performed in these circumstances, the post-operative course may be seriously jeopardized by the development of intense ascites, albeit the ascites is only transitory.

If for any reason the portal vein is occluded and it is impossible to perform a portacaval shunt, one of the alternative shunts, either splenorenal or end-to-side inferior vena cava–superior mesenteric, may be done. Inferior vena cava–superior mesenteric shunts are large and usually result in adequate portal decompression. The record achieved by splenorenal anastomoses in accomplishing an adequate portal decompression is far from satisfactory, and the procedure is, therefore, not advisable as a first choice for emer-gency portal decompression. In the rare event that adequate portal decom-pression is not obtained, an operative procedure that deals directly with the varices, such as interruption of the coronary vein and short gastric veins, gastric transection, or variceal ligation, should be attempted in an effort to ensure the cessation of hemorrhage.

The anesthetic agent should be one that least affects the liver. Also the level of anesthesia should be as light as is feasible for performance of the shunt. Mild hypothermia is a useful adjunct, since it diminishes metabolic activity of the liver and reduces the stresses of anesthesia and operation. Its use need not be routine for successful portacaval shunt, but it is probably indicated in the more critically ill and is especially valuable in all the patients who are febrile.

Finally, it should be emphasized that the entire procedure should be performed neatly, expeditiously, and with minimal trauma and blood loss. Portacaval shunts are difficult under elective conditions, but under emergency conditions they become even more taxing. Consequently, even surgeons experienced in the technique of portal decompression should approach the procedure carefully and cautiously.

Results of Portacaval Shunts

As stated earlier, adequate portal decompression will abruptly halt hemorrhage from esophagogastric varices. Furthermore, it will accomplish this objective without the aid of the esophageal balloon or any other adjunctive procedure, and when the patients are bleeding massively and uncontrollably. In selected good-risk patients, the risk of emergency portal decompression is very acceptable and is roughly equal to that for an elective portacaval shunt. At the New York Hospital–Cornell Medical Center the current mortality for elective portacaval shunt in good-risk candidates is 8.1 (eight deaths in 99 patients) and is 6.2 per cent (one death in 16 patients) for emergency portacaval shunt. Thus, it would appear that portacaval shunt need not be delayed in good-risk patients and that it is a justified procedure, since it will result in an increased salvage rate of the patients by eliminating the double stress of the hemorrhage and of subsequent operation.

The mortality of emergency portacaval shunt in the patients with advanced liver disease, however, is discouragingly high, and is 60.9 per cent (14 deaths in 23 patients), whereas for the elective procedure it is 35.2 per cent (6 deaths in 18 patients). However, considering the fact that nearly 40 per cent of these poor-risk patients did survive and that all, with two exceptions, were bleeding either uncontrollably or recurrently, and therefore unrelentingly, indicates that the procedure is not completely without merit. Nevertheless, patients with little hepatic reserve have the most to gain by a period of prolonged diet therapy; therefore, although they tolerate the hemorrhage very poorly, and frequently the bleeding tends to be more severe, a trial period of balloon tamponade is justified, since mortality from immediate operation is not significantly different from the rate for operation that is delayed a day or so.

Furthermore, this approach is justified by the fact that there is considerable doubt whether portal hypertension in the patient with advanced liver disease should be treated at all, because of the almost uniformly unsatisfactory results from portacaval shunt and because of the very short life expectancy of the patient in this stage of the disease. In general, we have in recent years increasingly declined to recommend operative intervention in such patients. Nevertheless, occasionally such individuals deserve consideration for portacaval shunt, especially when death seems to be the only certain alternative to operation.

There remains the final question: Is the life of a patient surviving portal decompression actually prolonged? Adequate control series do not exist, making definitive answer unobtainable. Further, although this question is not actually appropriate to this discussion of emergency portal decompression, it is, nevertheless, a legitimate one, since nearly all patients with portal hypertension have an underlying liver disease which, irrespective of treatment, progresses inexorably, terminating only in death. Moreover, some patients undergoing portal decompression may unpredictably develop hepatic encephalopathy. This condition, readily treated in many patients, may be totally incapacitating in occasional patients long before the end stages of the cirrhosis are approached.

Nevertheless, there is some evidence to warrant a continued aggressive approach to the problem. For example, adequate portal decompression is usually impossible in children who have extrahepatic portal obstruction. Although these patients generally have relatively normal liver function, few survive the ravages of repeated hemorrhage from esophagogastric varices for even a few years. On the other hand, our experience, and that of others, indicate that more than 85 per cent of the good-risk adults who have established cirrhosis will survive after portal decompression for at least three years, and many for as long as 10 or more years (if they abstain from liquor), without the serious hazards of vericeal hemorrhage.

References

1. Child, C. G., III: The Shatluck lecture: The portal circulation. New England J. Med., 252:837, 1955.
2. Linton, R. R., and Ellis, D. S.: Emergency and definitive treatment of bleeding esophageal varices. J.A.M.A., 160:1017, 1956.
3. Mikkelsen, W. P., and Pattison, A. C.: Emergency portacaval shunt. Am. J. Surg., 96:183, 1958.
4. O'Sullivan, W. D., and Payne, M. A.: Emergency portacaval shunt. Surg., Gynec. and Obst., 102:668, 1956.
5. Rousselot, L. M., Gilbertson, F. E., and Panke, W. F.: Severe hemorrhage from esophagogastric varices, its emergency management with particular reference to portacaval anastomosis. New England J. Med., 262:269, 1960.
6. Wantz, G. E., and Payne, M. A.: Experience with portacaval shunt for portal hypertension. New England J. Med., 265:721, 1961.
7. Wantz, G. E., and Payne, M. A.: Emergency portacaval shunt. Surg., Gynec. and Obst., 109:549, 1959.

Esophagogastric Cooling in the Management of Bleeding Esophageal Varices*

Stephen L. Wangensteen *and* Robert B. Smith, III

Columbia University College of Physicians and Surgeons

Bleeding esophageal varices is a common cause of death in patients with portal hypertension and cirrhosis of the liver. The fact that approximately one-half of these patients have succumbed during their initial bleeding episode serves to indicate the seriousness of the problem. Esophagogastric cooling, a modification of gastric cooling, has emerged as a new modality for the temporary control of massive hemorrhage from bleeding esophageal varices. Our reasons for selecting esophagogastric cooling as the initial therapeutic method for major hemorrhage from esophageal varices are based principally on our preference for an early nonoperative means of control of hemorrhage and shock, and on the effectiveness of this form of cooling in the control of such bleeding.

Advantages of Early Conservative Approach

Linton,[2] Blakemore,[1] and others have aptly stressed the importance of liver function as a prime factor in the prognosis of patients with cirrhosis of the liver and bleeding from esophageal varices. The liver function in cirrhotic patients with portal hypertension may vary from good compensation to severe impairment of function when bleeding seems to occur as a terminal event. Somewhere in the mid-range of this spectrum of liver function is a significant group of patients with moderate hepatic dysfunction, upon whom the effects of hemorrhage may cause temporary reversible liver decompensation. It is our opinion that if the stress of an emergency major surgical procedure is added to the stress of shock-producing hemor-

* Supported by Research Grant H–5372CS1 from the National Institutes of Health, United States Public Health Service.

rhage, the damaging process within the liver may become irreversible with ensuing death. Unfortunately there are no completely reliable indices available to assess the ultimate effects of hemorrhage on the liver from the outset, although jaundice, ascites, and stupor are grave signs. Furthermore, if hemorrhage can be controlled conservatively and if liver function improves after a four- to six-week period of bed rest, the operative mortality from a portacaval shunt is lessened. Voorhees[4] recently emphasized the importance of the time interval between hemorrhage and operation, citing its effect on operative mortality. The passage of time allows: (1) a natural selection of patients, in that the patients with irreversible liver damage do not survive, (2) clearance of residual blood from the gastrointestinal tract, which might otherwise lead to a fatal coma, and (3) an accurate diagnosis, which is of considerable importance in view of the known coincidence of peptic ulcer in patients with cirrhosis.

Cooling in Preparation for Shunt

It is now generally recognized that portal bed decompression in the form of a portal-systemic shunting procedure represents the best surgical approach currently available to prevent further bleeding from esophageal varices. We regard the control of hemorrhage achieved by esophagogastric cooling as temporary, and after control is established the patient is prepared for a definitive portal-systemic shunting procedure. If conditions permit, the time interval between hemorrhage control by cooling and portal decompression is three to six weeks. During this period liver function is assessed repeatedly, and vigorous attempts are made to improve the overall condition of the patient.

Control Achieved by Cooling

In our hands esophagogastric cooling has controlled hemorrhage from esophageal varices far more consistently than other nonoperative measures. A 90 per cent control rate, believed possible by Blakemore[1] with the use of the Sengstaken-Blakemore tamponade device, unfortunately has not been realized. A review of the experience at the Presbyterian Hospital[3] with the balloon tamponade revealed that it controlled hemorrhage in approximately half the cases. Employment of esophagogastric cooling in 31 patients bleeding from esophageal varices has led to control of hemorrhage in all but one. The single failure occurred in a patient in whom a gastric varix had eroded into the left gastric artery, causing immediate exsanguination. Rebleeding following the termination of cooling occasionally has been a problem, but with re-institution of local cooling, bleeding again has been uniformly controlled. The hospital mortality of patients treated by cooling has been high, but included in our overall experience is a substantial number of patients who were in a terminal phase of their cirrhosis. In addition, nearly a third of the patients underwent esophago-gastric cooling after balloon tamponade had failed. Previously we reported our experience with esophagogastric cooling in patients bleeding from esophageal varices,[5] and the overall hospital mortality rate was 68 per cent. More recently we treated an additional 10 patients, of whom three suc-cumbed and seven survived. The number of patients treated in this fashion is as yet too small to draw any definite conclusions; however, it appears that as we gain more experience with local cooling and as we treat patients that are less carefully selected, we are becoming more successful. Never-theless, it remains true that the ultimate survival of a patient with cirrhosis of the liver bleeding from esophageal varices is dependent on the capacity of the liver to survive.

Technique of Esophagogastric Cooling

To achieve effective esophagogastric cooling capable of controlling serious hemorrhage, an efficient mechanical apparatus is necessary. There are several machines that have a wide range in cost and complexity. A cooling apparatus selected for clinical use should be simple to operate and safe for the patient. Although the technique of esophagogastric cooling is not particularly complex, those who plan to use the technique should gain experience with the apparatus, preferably in the animal laboratory, prior to undertaking management of the human patient. Avoidable disasters have resulted from gastric cooling primarily through lack of understanding of the apparatus and technique. In our hands a skilled "team approach" has been most useful.

The patient is suitably sedated, and the head of the bed is raised moderately. The nasopharynx is topically anesthetized, and a large-bore nasogastric tube is passed into the stomach to remove all blood clots which, if allowed to remain in the stomach, may act as insulators and impair the cooling effect or may cause the stomach to rupture upon inflation of the balloon. The nasogastric tube is left in place during the cooling process and attached to suction, for it serves as the best guide to further bleeding.

There are two types of latex balloons available for esophagogastric or gastric cooling. One of these cools a major portion of the esophagus and upper stomach; the other applies cooling to the stomach only. The balloon selected depends on the clinical certainty of the bleeding site. If there is some question whether bleeding is from esophageal varices, the gastric balloon is selected, for it generally controls bleeding from esophageal varices, and it is also effective in controlling hemorrhage from gastric or duodenal ulceration.

Following thorough irrigation of the nasogastric tube to remove blood from the stomach, the esophagogastric or gastric balloon is passed into the stomach through the nasopharynx. Chilled fluid is then introduced into the balloon by increments until the desired circulating volume is attained. Initially 600 to 800 cc. of fluid is placed into the balloon.

When the esophagogastric balloon is employed, tension is exerted on the plastic tubing at the point where it emerges from the nose. This maneuver directs the elongated esophageal portion of the balloon into the esophagus, while the globular gastric portion of balloon remains within the stomach. Resistance is noted as the gastric portion is drawn up against the diaphragm. When resistance is detected, tension is relaxed, and the tubing is allowed to slip back slightly so that no pressure or tamponade effect is produced. After the esophagogastric balloon has been placed, we frequently check its position by introducing a water-soluble radiopaque contrast agent into the circulating fluid and by portable x-ray examination.

Control of hemorrhage generally is achieved in one to two hours. Despite early control of hemorrhage, we usually continue local cooling for 48 to 72 hours in the patient bleeding from esophageal varices. During this period the patient is gradually "weaned" from the cooling process. Circulating fluid temperatures in the range of 2° to 4° C. are used during the initial hours of treatment. After hemorrhage has been controlled for several hours, the fluid temperature is gradually raised until the temperature reaches 18 to 20°C. at the completion of treatment. We theorize that use of lower fluid temperatures initially leads to lower local blood flow and greater ease in hemorrhage control. Raising the temperature later insures against local tissue damage. Similarly, the balloon volume is slowly decreased during the interval of treatment until about 300 cc. remains in the balloon at the termination of the procedure.

During intragastric cooling, body temperature is maintained by external heating with thermal blankets, and body temperature is monitored by a thermistor probe inserted in the rectum. Maintenance of body temperature is infrequently a problem, but precipitous drops in body temperature may occur if esophagogastric cooling is combined with the rapid transfusion of chilled bank blood.

Complications of Cooling

The complications resulting from local cooling have not been numerous. The principal problems we have encountered are pneumonia and gastric rupture. It is our opinion that if the technique is properly performed and the patient carefully observed, serious complications should be rare. We believe that the most catastrophic of all its complications, namely, stomach rupture, should no longer occur. Gastric rupture was caused by air leakage into the circulating fluid system of the cooling apparatus, which resulted in massive overdisplacement of fluid into the gastric balloon. Advances in design by commercial manufacturers have obviated this possibility. To date we have not recognized a single instance of nasal septal necrosis, esophageal ulceration, or aspiration. Since tamponade is not performed, the patient may swallow his own secretions around the balloon within the esophagus. In our experience with esophagogastric or gastric cooling, we have not detected any direct evidence to indicate that local cooling itself impairs hepatic function in the human patient.

Conclusions

1. Survival of the cirrhotic patient bleeding from esophageal varices is dependent on maintenance of adequate liver function.

2. Our experience indicates that esophagogastric cooling controls massive hemorrhage from esophageal varices more uniformly than other nonoperative measures.

3. Control of hemorrhage by cooling is considered temporary, and the patient is prepared for elective portal decompression.

4. If the technique of esophagogastric cooling is performed carefully by experienced personnel, complications should be rare.

References

1. Blakemore, A. H.: Differential Balloon Tamponade in Diagnosis and Treatment of Ruptured Varices. *In* Mulholland, J. H., et al. (Ed.): Current Surgical Management. Vol. I, Philadelphia, W. B. Saunders Company, 1957, pp. 88–97.
2. Linton, R. R.: Surgery of portal cirrhosis. Am. J. Med., *24*:941, 1958.
3. Voorhees, A. B.: Management of portal hypertension. Bull. New York Acad. Med., *35*:223, 1959.
4. Voorhees, A. B.: Surgical aspect of portal hypertension associated with cirrhosis of the liver. M. Clin. North America, *47*:579, 1963.
5. Wangensteen, S. L., Orahood, R. C., Voorhees, A. B., Smith, R. B., and Healey, W. V.: Intragastric cooling in the management of hemorrhage from the upper gastrointestinal tract. Am. J. Surg., *105*:401, 1963.

Thoracic Duct Cannulation:

A New Approach to

the Emergency Treatment

of Bleeding Esophageal Varices

Allan E. Dumont *and* Marlys H. Witte

New York University School of Medicine

At Bellevue Hospital the typical patient bleeding from esophageal varices presents with cachexia, jaundice, ascites, and impending hepatic coma, in addition to shock from blood loss. Successful management of such desperately ill patients is rarely achieved by current methods. Recent studies of thoracic duct lymph in patients with Laennec's cirrhosis have disclosed some previously unrecognized aspects of the disease.[3, 4] Data obtained implicate the lymphatic system as a key factor in portal hypertension, and provide the rationale for thoracic duct cannulation in the treatment of acute bleeding from esophageal varices.

Sustained portal hypertension is not produced by ligation of the portal vein in either man or monkey,[1, 8] nor by ligation of the supradiaphragmatic vena cava in dogs.[2] Any pressure created by these maneuvers is shortly dissipated by edema, increased lymph formation, and collateral flow. On the other hand, increase in portal pressure does follow simultaneous ligation of the thoracic duct and supradiaphragmatic vena cava in dogs.[5]

Determinations of thoracic duct lymph flow, pressure, and composition in 53 patients with cirrhosis demonstrated striking alterations. The thoracic duct was cannulated in the neck under local anesthesia. At operation the duct was found to be 2 to 4 times the normal diameter, and hemorrhagic lymph flowed under pressures of 15 to 70 cm. of water at 3 to 15 times the normal rate of 1 cc. per minute. Thoracic duct end-pressure was almost identical with portal pressure, and in patients actually bleeding from esophageal varices, lymph flow rates regularly exceeded 10 cc. per minute. The hemorrhagic component of the lymph, measured as hematocrit, varied from 1 to 6 per cent and was due to intact red blood cells.

Within 24 to 48 hours, important changes occurred in the clinical status of many of these patients. Liver size decreased markedly, ascites became much less prominent or disappeared, and bleeding from esophageal varices ceased. The total number of patients actively bleeding from varices who underwent cannulation and provided data is still too small for statistical validity. Cannulation was followed by prompt cessation of bleeding in 8 of 13 patients. Portal pressure (umbilical vein or splenic pulp) fell significantly in the 4 patients in whom measurements were made. Rebleeding occurred in 5 patients within 72 hours of removal or obstruction of the cannula, and in the remaining 3 patients several days later with the cannula in place and flowing.

The curious effects of this procedure on liver size, ascites, and bleeding from varices must be related to the outlet that is provided for excess lymph under pressure. Normally about one-half of thoracic duct lymph originates in the liver, and about 80 per cent of the total liver lymph flows from hilar lymphatics to the cisterna chyli and thoracic duct. Clusters of dilated lymphatics around the porta hepatis, frequently seen at laparotomy* and at autopsy in patients with cirrhosis, are evidence that the liver is the major source of the increased thoracic duct lymph.

Forces responsible for the increased formation of liver lymph are more obscure. Protein concentration in liver lymph is almost identical with that in plasma, and there is thus no effective oncotic gradient between the sinusoid and hepatic interstitial space. Accordingly, very small increments in hepatic vein resistance to flow result in significant increases in liver lymph formation, not only by increasing hydrostatic pressure in capillaries, but also by decreasing venous reabsorption. Starling[7] recognized that the unique permeability of normal hepatic capillaries enables the liver to drain a fluid portion of the blood when hepatic venous outflow becomes impaired. The presence of intact blood cells in lymph in cirrhosis suggests that the sinusoids become permeable even to formed elements in this disease. Greater permeability also enhances hepatic capillary filtration, and hence liver lymph formation.

The thoracic duct drainage system is, however, a phylogenetic late-comer.[6] It does not seem to adapt, except in limited fashion, to transport of excess volumes of lymph. With excess lymph formation, marked distensibility of the thin-walled duct, and resistance to flow at the veno-lymphatic junction in the neck combine to bring about early overloading of the system. The liver distends because of increased volume of undrained interstitial fluid or lymph, rather than because of regenerating nodules, excess lipid deposition, or scar formation. Evidence for this belief is the finding that the cirrhotic liver has a very low specific gravity,[5] and that the liver decreases in size promptly after thoracic duct cannulation.

Overloading of the lymph channels draining the liver and extrahepatic

---

* In a recent instance at Bellevue Hospital a markedly distended lymphatic containing grossly hemorrhagic lymph was mistakenly identified as the portal vein and mobilized for a portacaval anastamosis.

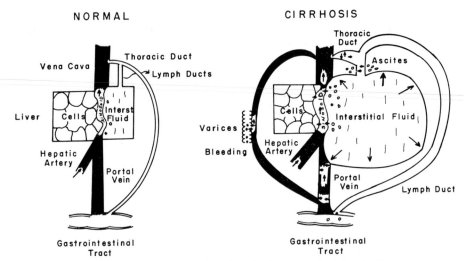

Fig. 1. In cirrhosis, overloading of the lymphatic system draining the liver and extra-hepatic portal bed in association with hepatic venous outflow obstruction leads to: (1) distention of the lymphatics, (2) expanded liver interstitial fluid volume, (3) hepato-megaly, (4) increased hepatic interstitial pressure, (5) ascites formation, (6) progressive resistance to transhepatic portal blood flow, and (7) varix formation and bleeding.

portal capillary bed, in combination with hepatic venous outflow obstruc-tion, are probably sufficient to raise portal pressure in Laennec's cirrhosis (Fig. 1). It seems paradoxical that closure of an end-to-side portacaval shunt, a complication simulating experimental portal vein ligation, is fol-lowed by elevation of portal pressure and recurrent bleeding from varices. Increased formation of extrahepatic lymph following portal vein obstruc-tion in this situation is, however, superimposed on pre-existing hepatic venous outflow obstruction and excess hepatic lymph. It is reasonable to speculate that thoracic duct cannulation in the patient bleeding from varices is effective on the one hand in decreasing hepatic interstitial fluid volume and pressure, thereby facilitating transhepatic portal flow, and on the other in providing free lymph exit for the extrahepatic portal capillary bed.

In frogs and other amphibia, capillaries are highly permeable to protein, and in order to maintain homeostasis, the lymphatic system must transport a volume of fluid in 24 hours that may be 50 times the blood volume. Lymph hearts are required to return this quantity of lymph to the blood. Patients with Laennec's cirrhosis are similarly in need of a pump to trans-port excess lymph back to blood. In an attempt to meet this need and to prevent deficits in fluids, electrolytes, proteins, and clotting factors, lymph of several patients was allowed to flow freely into a large chest drainage bottle, and a constant infusion pump recirculated lymph from the reservoir into an inlying venous cannula. Further experience may disclose a method for draining or pumping excess lymph into the venous system in situ with-out external collections.

The therapeutic value of thoracic duct cannulation in patients with cirrhosis of the liver is uncertain at this time. More data are required. When bleeding from esophageal varices is refractory to available nonoperative methods of treatment, cannulation can, if necessary, be performed at the bedside under local anesthesia. This simple surgical maneuver may stop the hemorrhage and enable the surgeon to prepare the patient for a semi-elective definitive procedure.

References

1. Child, C. G., III: The Hepatic Circulation and Portal Hypertension. Philadelphia, W. B. Saunders Co., 1954.
2. Drapanas, T., Schenk, W. G., Pollack, E. L., and Stewart, J. D.: Hepatic hemodynamics in experimental ascites. Ann. Surg., 152:705, 1960.
3. Dumont, A. E., and Mulholland, J. H.: Flow rate and composition of thoracic duct lymph in patients with cirrhosis. New England. J. Med., 263:471, 1960.
4. Dumont, A. E., and Mulholland, J. H.: Alterations in thoracic duct lymph flow in hepatic cirrhosis: significance in portal hypertension. Ann. Surg., 156:668, 1962.
5. Dumont, A. E.: Unpublished observations.
6. Mayerson, H. S.: Lympathic system with particular reference to the kidney. Surg., Gynec. and Obst., 116:259, 1963.
7. Starling, E. H.: The Fluids of the Body. Chicago, W. T. Keener, 1909.
8. Taylor, F. W.: Experimental portal hypertension. Ann. Surg., 146:683, 1957.

Ligation of Gastric Arterial

Supply and Splenectomy

in the Treatment

of Acute Hemorrhage

from Gastroesophageal Varices

Nathan A. Womack *and* Richard M. Peters

University of North Carolina School of Medicine

Vascular Aspects of Cirrhosis

In the treatment of patients with severe hemorrhage from vascular distortions in the lower esophagus and upper stomach, the basic underlying problem has been considered to be portal hypertension, resulting from either extrahepatic or intrahepatic obstruction of the portal venous bed. This obstruction is thought to be passive in type, and one that produces an increase in resistance to portal flow. In the extrahepatic areas this is usually considered to be due to intravascular clotting, although the demonstration of such thrombus formation has at times been difficult. For a long time the obstruction within the liver was thought to be due solely to a contraction of fibrous tissue, in spite of the fact that fibrosis of the liver from causes other than cirrhosis seldom gave such a vascular picture, and in spite of the fact that often in cirrhosis the liver was increased in size, not decreased. More recently distortion of the hepatic vasculature, particularly the hepatic venous system, by expanding regenerating nodules of liver parenchyma has been considered the agent causing obstruction.

With an increase in resistance to portal blood flow, it has been postulated that there follows chronic passive congestion of the tissues drained by the portal circulation. Often, however, this sequela is difficult to demonstrate. Indeed apparent edema of the wall of the stomach and intestines is notably lacking, even when surrounded by ascitic fluid. Nevertheless it is

Page 268

assumed that as a result of the increase in pressure and congestion, collateral channels of portal venous return are opened, soon become distended, and often are the source of the bleeding. Other stigmata of cirrhosis, such as splenomegaly and ascites, develop.

To correct this undesirable sequence of events, surgical procedures have been devised to divert the high pressure portal venous blood into the low pressure vena caval system. So well established have these dramatic shunting operations become in our surgical armamentarium that any recommendation of deviation from them must have justification from sound physiologic considerations. It is from such a point of view that we shall approach the subject, although at times clinical representation will be used.

Our attention was called to the ineffectiveness of this classic concept of passive intrahepatic obstruction as a cause of some of the vascular findings in cirrhosis when we had an opportunity to observe the results from excision of many of these collateral pathways. One would anticipate that such a procedure, by blocking much of the portal venous return, should worsen the condition of the patient. On the other hand, Phemister and Humphreys reported in 1947,[6] that two patients with Banti's syndrome, who had been operated on by them for massive bleeding, had been improved when the lower esophagus and upper stomach had been excised in one patient and a total gastrectomy performed in another. Shortly afterward we verified such observations by removing the lower esophagus, the upper stomach, and the spleen from seven patients entering the hospital because of severe bleeding from varices due to cirrhosis. One of these patients died shortly after operation, from pulmonary emboli. One, a child, died from progressive cirrhosis a year and a half later. One patient lived 10 years, and three have lived over 12 years and were without clinical evidence of cirrhosis when last seen.

These patients illustrate the fact that the excision of the collateral circulation did not worsen the circulatory status of the patient and, certainly in most instances, prevented a return of bleeding. Furthermore, if this could be done, even far advanced cirrhosis could become a reversible disease. This operation, however, was associated at times with esophagitis. A better procedure was needed, but would be difficult to devise until we knew more about the underlying nature of our lesion.

Shortly afterward we had the good fortune to have a patient referred to us who presented a physiologic model of our problem, and without having cirrhosis of the liver. There was a history of numerous episodes of massive hematemesis during the preceding 10 years. She had received approximately 300 blood transfusions during this period. A partial gastrectomy had been performed, but her episodes of hemorrhage had persisted. Physical examination was within normal limits except for small telangiectases of the skin and buccal mucosa. At operation the vascular findings within the abdomen were similar to those seen in cirrhosis, but the liver itself appeared normal. The spleen was enlarged, the splenic artery was approximately 1 cm. in diameter, and the splenic vein 2 cm. in diameter. Several large arteries, 0.25 cm. in diameter, extended from the splenic artery to the fundus of the stomach, and there was pulsation in the tail of the pancreas. Abnormal arteriovenous anastomoses were considered to be present, and the spleen and tail of the pancreas were removed and the arteries to the fundus of the stomach ligated. At first the patient did well, but at a later date there was additional bleeding and a large angioma of the stomach was removed; there has been no further hemorrhage. At this last operation portovenogram and portal venous pressures were normal, and there were no enlarged veins noted. This patient had many of the vascular stigmata of cirrhosis, but without cirrhosis.

The problem was further delineated shortly afterward by observations made on a patient with so-called Banti's syndrome. There had been several episodes of massive hematemesis, and esophageal varices were huge, extending to the level of the carina. The spleen was unusually large, and there was leukopenia with a low platelet count. All of the so-called liver function studies were within normal limits. A splenoportogram showed the splenic and portal veins to be 2 cm. in diameter, approximately the size of the vena cava. Although there were large gastric and gastroepiploic tributaries, most of the blood seemed to return through the liver, and the intrahepatic radicles of the portal vein were clearly defined without evidence of obstruction. Surgical approach was through a left transthoracic incision. The spleen was huge. The splenic artery was 0.6 cm. in diameter, and there was a readily palpable thrill. The splenic vein had a thrill, but one that was less apparent. It was noted that in the splenic vein and in the hemiazygous there was swirling and eddying of streams of bright red blood. Samples of arterial and venous blood were taken for estimation of the degree of oxygen saturation. In the aorta it was found to be 96 per cent, in the splenic artery 98 per cent, in the splenic vein 95 per cent, and in the hemiazygous vein 90 per cent. Here then was arterial blood within the venous system. Venous pressure was 30 cm. of saline in the hemiazygous and 27.6 cm. of saline in the splenic vein. When a bulldog clamp was applied to the splenic artery, the thrill and the swirling of blood disappeared from the splenic vein, and the pressures fell to 15 cm. of saline in the splenic vein and 5.5 in the hemiazygous, a considerable reduction. Studies now showed the oxygen saturation of the splenic venous blood to be 60 per cent. Unfortunately the blood removed from the hemiazygous clotted before the determination could be made. Since then, however, such determinations have been repeated on similar patients, and the hemiazygous saturation noted also to be in the region of 75 per cent following such a procedure.

These findings of an increase in the oxygen saturation of the portal venous blood concomitant with a rise in portal venous pressure, and a fall in the oxygen saturation with a drop in venous pressure following splenic artery ligation, obviously necessitated a review of the hemodynamics of the portal system. Obstruction of the portal vein, either before or after it reached the liver, would not explain these phenomena.

Effects of Obstruction of Portal Vein

Nevertheless an experiment was designed to test the effect of obstruction.[9] Using adequate controls it was found that when the portal vein of a dog was partially occluded or completely occluded, there was an immediate rise in portal venous pressure from 5 to 10 mm. of mercury to 28 to 40 mm. of mercury, while the oxygen saturation of the portal venous blood fell to approximately 70 per cent of normal. The cardiac output was decreased and the arterial blood pressure fell to shock-like levels. This is the reverse of what was noted in our patients with varices. We were impressed by the fact that when the portal obstruction was released, the return to normal arterial pressure was delayed when compared to that following similar obstruction of the vena cava above or below the renal veins. This suggested some injury to the liver, perhaps to a system sensitive to anoxia.

Unfortunately such experiments must be performed rapidly on the dog, since this animal, as a rule, will not survive portal obstruction for more than a few hours. The monkey, however, will survive such obstruction, and pertinent observations following obstruction to the portal vein in the Macaca monkey have been made by Child.[2] He reports that immediately after portal vein occlusion, the spleen becomes tense and the veins of the stomach, the small bowel, and the right colon congested. There is a uniform fall in systolic blood pressure, which returns to pre-occlusive levels within 30 minutes to an hour. There is an immediate rise in portal venous pressure from 8 to 10 centimeters of saline to 30 to 60 centimeters of saline, where it remains for several hours. It then begins to fall and, after six to ten days, returns to pre-occlusive levels. There is a development of many collaterals, which eventually give way to several large ones that by-pass the site of the obstruction, and the portal blood again enters the liver. There are no submucosal varices described in the esophagus and the stomach, nor is there ascites or splenomegaly. We have encountered complete obstruction of the portal vein of long standing in the human, and noted the portal pressure at such times to be 18 cm. of saline and the spleen to be small. The absence of splenomegaly under such circumstances interested us. Just what is the effect of obstruction of the splenic vein on the spleen?

Effects of Obstruction of Splenic Vein

The spleen is a viscus that lends itself nicely to the study of obstruction, and we have carried out such studies with the dog's spleen.[10] Immediately after obstruction of the splenic vein, pressure distal to it rises abruptly, and the spleen becomes large and tense. Equilibrium is soon established, and decrease in flow through the splenic artery is noted. Within a few weeks the spleen decreases to about a third of its preligation size, and the pressure in the splenic vein returns to preligation level. When the arterial inflow to the spleen was measured by means of an electromagnetic flowmeter it was noted that within a few minutes after occlusion of the splenic vein the flow rate in the artery would fall as much as one-half of its pre-occlusion value, the fall being in proportion to the complete-ness of the venous occlusion.

These results from occlusion of the splenic vein could have been anticipated, for it is obvious that appreciable decrease in venous outflow from a viscus must reflect itself in decrease in the arterial inflow or catas-trophe soon supervenes. Obstruction of the portal vein thus falls short in explaining the many phenomena relating to the vascular bed in cirrhosis of the liver.

Oxygen Saturation in Blood of Portal Vein

Early in our observations we were intrigued by the fact that under normal circumstances the oxygen saturation of the blood in the portal vein is elevated. The level is usually from 25 to 30 per cent higher than that in the vena cava below the renal veins, and also higher than the mixed venous blood in the right atrium. Blalock had noted this increase in saturation in dogs as early as 1937, and Blakemore in the human in 1951. We were able to verify their findings. This rise in oxygen saturation could be caused by (1) a failure of cells to extract oxygen from the blood as it passed through the capillary bed, due to lack of tissue need for oxygen, or (2) an unusually rapid capillary flow, or (3) a shunting mechanism between the arterial and venous beds. An experiment was devised to explain this phenomenon, and it was soon found that such could not be explained by a failure of cells to extract oxygen from the blood owing to either a lack of tissue need for oxygen or an unusually rapid capillary flow. By inference, arterial blood must be entering the venous channels proximal to the capillary bed. A shunting mechanism between the arterial and venous beds must therefore exist.[9]

Studies in Arteriovenous Anastomoses

We selected the stomach as the first organ in the splanchnic bed to study for the presence of such arteriovenous anastomoses. Indeed we found that these structures had already been described in the stomach by several investigators in recent years. Watska[8] in 1936, and de Busscher,[3] in 1948, had demonstrated such structures by reconstruction techniques. Barlow,[1] in 1951, using a double colored injection technique, demonstrated clearly anastomotic channels between the arteries and veins in the submucosa of the human stomach, and Walder[7] was able to perfuse beads as large as 140 μ across these connections in the human stomach. We repeated these findings,[4] and in the experimental animal demonstrated that these A-V anastomoses had a sphincteric mechanism highly sensitive to certain vaso-active substances. Following the injection of histamine, for instance, and to a lesser extent when the vagus nerves were stimulated, there was rich perfusion of the gastric mucosal capillaries, an increase in gastric acid output, and slight increase in portal venous pressure with little change in oxygen saturation. When such a stomach was perfused with a solution containing glass beads, very few could be recovered in the vein and none of these were over 25 μ in diameter. This suggested that during the phase of active gastric acid secretion, there was little if any flow through the shunts. When epinephrine was given the reverse took place. Following the injection of epinephrine there was little perfusion of the gastric mucosal capillaries, and gastric secretion ceased or was very slight. Portal venous pressure was doubled in amount and oxygen saturation of the venous blood was almost that of the artery. Glass beads as large as 125 μ could be recovered in the veins following arterial injection.

Here then is both anatomic and physiologic demonstration of the shunting mechanism in the stomach. Of importance is the realization that it regulates capillary perfusion to a region, phasic with the function of this region. This ability to shift the relatively small amount of available blood from one capillary bed to another is obviously a physiologic necessity for the organism. Furthermore, it can be mediated by humoral factors. When this mechanism is incompetent, there will be, among other things, an increase in the size of particular venous channels, an increase in blood volume and an increase in cardiac output. The size of the veins is increased in cirrhosis, and a number of studies have demonstrated elevated blood volume and cardiac output.

Studies of arteriovenous anastomoses were next carried out on the spleen, and a similar pattern was found.[10] Communications between arteries and veins that by-passed the splenic pulp could be identified by an injection-corrosion technique with a plastic too viscid to penetrate the penicilli of the splenic arteries. Arteriovenous differences in the oxygen saturation of the blood were determined in the normal spleen and the spleen in contraction following a single injection of .02 mg./kg. of norepinephrine. This was correlated with splenic venous pressure. It was noted that the mean arterial saturation in the control animals was 98 per cent, and the splenic venous saturation 88 per cent, with a splenic venous pressure of 9.2 mm. of mercury. Following the administration of norepinephrine, the mean arterial saturation remained at 98.5 per cent, while the splenic venous pressure rose to 20.7 mm. of mercury and the oxygen saturation approached arterial levels. These changes are significant below the 1 per cent level and mimic those at times seen in cirrhosis.

In the liver, shunts between the hepatic arterial and portal venous blood have been previously demonstrated by others. These are in the perilobular as well as in the presinusoidal areas. There are also presinusoidal sphincters afferent to the sinusoid regulating portal inflow, as well as efferent sphincters between the sinusoid and hepatic venous system. That this sphincteric mechanism in the liver responds to humoral stimulation has also been well demonstrated by others.

As is readily apparent, the shunting mechanism in the viscera that we have described, as well as that elsewhere in the body, is important both from the standpoint of structure and of function. Much of the control of this mechanism seems to be humoral. Since these shunts are controlled by smooth muscle sphincters, this regulation is always a mechanically hazardous venture as has been pointed out by Burton.[1a] Burton and his colleagues have called attention to a formula of Laplace. As applied to blood vessels this can be expressed by the equation $T = r(P_i - P_e)$, where "T" equals tension in dynes per square centimeter on the vessel wall, "r" the radius in centimeters, "P_i" the intraluminal blood pressure and "P_e" the tissue pressure. This means that the larger the radius of the vessel (r), the greater the tension or strain on the vascular wall for the same pressure. Likewise the lower the tissue pressure (P_e) or tissue tension, the greater the strain on the vessel wall.

As will be noticed the smaller the radius of the tube, the greater the pressure that can be accommodated without appreciably altering the tension in the wall. When this principle is applied to the vascular bed it can be seen that the walls of the larger vessels are more vulnerable to increases in intraluminal pressure than are those of vessels of smaller diameters. If in cirrhosis the vascular problem were simply one of portal hypertension, the vein most vulnerable would be the portal vein itself. This vein, of course, is rarely the site of varicosity and never the site of spontaneous hemorrhage. This is also true of the superior mesenteric vein. Most consistently the vessels that are varicose and that bleed are in the submucosa of the lower esophagus and upper stomach. The diameter of these vessels is regulated by smooth muscle sphincters, which are in turn controlled by vaso-active substances. There is evidence that in cirrhosis the liver does not adequately metabolize these substances, and it is at this point that the chain of events leading to vascular decompensation begins.

Morphology of Esophagogastric Varices

An examination of the morphology of these varicosities in the esophagus and stomach of patients with cirrhosis is of interest.[5] The vessels are usually many times larger in the submucosa than in the subserosa. Often eccentric areas of smooth muscle may be seen in these structures, both in the esophagus and in the stomach, suggesting the region of a sphincter. At other times there is mucosal atrophy of the stomach, presumably from sphincteric decompensation, with the erosion of fairly large vessels that do not appear varicose on surface examination, a condition sometimes called chronic gastritis.

We have called attention to the frequency in which a thrill is felt in the splenic vein as well as in the splenic artery in patients with cirrhosis. The infrequency with which there is splenic pulsation or even a bruit over the spleen suggests that anastomoses here may be near the hilum involving larger vessels, and this proves to be true. Again injection-corrosion specimens reveal streaming of the arterially injected mass in large branches of the splenic vein suggesting communications of considerable size. Where such communications exist in the patient with cirrhosis, the back flow down the smaller radicles of the splenic vein results in an increase in venous pressure within the spleen, producing splenomegaly without decreasing but even increasing flow through the splenic artery.

For over half a century it has been known that there is increased arterial flow into the cirrhotic liver. The increase in radius of even the smaller arteries to the extent that they become larger than the portal radicles has recently been demonstrated by Hales and his colleagues.[3a] We have made similar observations. That such increase in arterial size and flow may be due to a decrease in resistance can be seen by the large diameter of the numerous anastomoses between the hepatic arteries and portal vein branches encountered in the chaotic vascular bed within the cirrhotic liver.

Summary

These then briefly are some of the features of the vascular aspect of cirrhosis—a much more complex story than the concept of portal hypertension produced by hepatic scarring and regeneration. Here one sees the basis for many of the other phenomena noted in cirrhosis: the pulmonary shunts with cyanosis in childhood cirrhosis, shunts in the skin as spiders, liver palms, the eccentric location of varices in the lower esophagus and upper stomach rather than diffusely through the gastrointestinal tract, arterial blood in the varices, the portal hypertension, the increase in systemic venous pressure, the rise in peripheral venous oxygen saturation, the decrease in systemic arterial oxygen saturation, the decrease in peripheral vascular resistance, the increase in hepatic lymph formation with its resemblance to blood plasma, the increase in blood volume, the increase in cardiac output, and many other similar phenomena.

Static obstruction of the portal bed, either outside or within the liver, will not explain adequately many of these phenomena. A concept of cirrhosis as a vasoactive disease emerges instead.

Rationale of Treatment

The bleeding in cirrhosis of the liver that concerns the surgeon has its origin in large distorted vessels that contain a mixture of venous and arterial blood. In the production of the bleeding, pressure probably plays a part, for when the pressure is lowered, as by a shunt operation, the tendency to bleed is lessened. That this is not the sole cause, however, may be seen when varicosities are noted, and when bleeding occurs with portal pressure within normal limits. As we have demonstrated, mucosal ischemia certainly plays a part, as does peptic ulceration, gastritis, esophagitis, and local trauma.

Our very earliest experience demonstrated that the surgical eradication of the abnormal vasculature produces beneficial results. Unfortunately, however, resection of the terminal esophagus and upper stomach resulted in stomal complications often enough for us to try other, even less effective, procedures. Transmucosal plication or excision of the esophageal varices was not always satisfactory, as this often was not the site of the bleeding. Splenectomy alone has frequently given satisfactory immediate results, but in many instances, there has been a tendency for recurrence of bleeding.

Technique for Ligation of Gastric Arterial Supply and Splenectomy

Often we have observed that many times when the site of hemorrhage could be exposed surgically, the bleeding was in rhythmical spurts. At such times when the artery feeding such a bleeding site was occluded, the bleeding ceased. This observation led us to the surgical procedure that has been most effective and the safest to date in our hands.

Exposure is preferable through the left chest. The diaphragm is incised at the hiatus, and the terminal esophagus and upper stomach exposed. As a rule the bleeding point cannot be located by external observation, although the most common site is at the junction of the squamous epithelium of the esophagus and the glandular epithelium of the stomach. An occlusive tape is placed around the esophagus about 10 cm. from its termination, and another around the upper stomach to control bleeding. A longitudinal incision is made through the wall of the esophagus for about 7 cm. and another through the anterior wall of the upper stomach. Occasionally it is necessary that this be a single incision, although when possible that portion of the esophageal musculature at the esophagogastric junction is preserved. All bleeding points along the margin of the incision are ligated. When a single source of the hemorrhage is noted in the esophagus or stomach, the blood supply to this is ligated and the area excised. Apparent varices in the submucosa of the esophagus and stomach are either plicated or excised and the mucosa approximated. The incisions are then closed and the spleen removed. In the patient who is not bleeding at the time of surgery, it is usually easier to remove the spleen first.

The spleen is removed by first ligating the splenic artery shortly after it crosses the aorta. This usually will not disturb too greatly the blood supply to the pancreas. The blood supply to the stomach from the splenic artery must be secured, and this at times will require excision of a small margin of the proximal part of the greater curvature of the stomach. An occasional vessel from the aorta to the lower esophagus should be sought as well as large branches from the phrenic arteries.

Care must be taken not to destroy so much of the arterial supply as to lead to necrosis. Unless the left gastric artery is considerably enlarged, it may be left undisturbed or only the ascending branch ligated. Because of the considerable variation in the blood supply to this area it is well to consider each patient individually. While we have never noted necrosis of a suture line to develop, we have on two occasions seen what was apparently ischemic ulceration of the stomach mucosa. In both instances spontaneous healing occurred.

Results of Treatment

The operation of splenectomy along with control of the blood supply to the area of the varicosities has in our experience been a satisfactory procedure. It is not without its troubles for it is not aimed at the cure of a fundamental lesion, but at certain manifestations of this lesion. It is an operation that should be done with dispatch and with the patient's blood well oxygenated. It is obvious that patients in severe hepatic failure will not tolerate such surgery as favorably as will others in better condition.

On several occasions hemorrhage has recurred, and while at times a second operation has been advisable in order to ligate additional arterial supply, this recurrent hemorrhage has never been massive. It is also worthy of note that recurrence of the bleeding is generally seen at the time of reappearance of hepatic failure. Conversely, we have been pleased to note that on many occasions, when there has been no repetition of the bleeding, there has been clinical evidence of subsidence of the hepatic damage, affording the optimistic impression that on occasion cirrhosis of the liver may be a reversible disease.

References

1. Barlow, T. E.: Arteriovenous anastomoses in the human stomach. J. Anat., 85:1, 1951.
1a. Burton, A. C.: Laws of Physics and Flow in Blood Vessels. Ciba Foundation Symposium on Visceral Circulation. Boston, Little, Brown, and Co., 1953.
2. Child, G., III, Milnes, R. F., Holswade, G. R., and Gore, A. L.: Sudden and complete occlusion of the portal vein in the *Macaca mulatta* monkey. Ann. Surg., 132:475, 1950.
3. De Busscher, G.: Les anastomoses arterio-veneuses de l'estomac. Acta Neer. Morphologiae Norm et Path., 6:87, 1948.
3a. Hales, M. R., Allan, J. S., and Hill, E. M.: Injection-corrosion studies of normal and cirrhotic livers. Am. J. Path., 35:909, 1959.
4. Peters, R. M., and Womack, N. A.: Hemodynamics of gastric secretion. Ann. Surg., 148:537, 1958.
5. Peters, R. M., and Womack, N. A.: Surgery of vascular distortions in cirrhosis of the liver. Ann. Surg., 154:532, 1961.
6. Phemister, D. B., and Humphreys, E. M.: Gastro-esophageal resection and total gastrectomy in the treatment of bleeding varicose veins in Banti's syndrome. Ann. Surg., 126:17, 1947.
7. Walder, D. N.: Some Observations on the Blood Flow of the Human Stomach. Visceral Circulation. (Ciba Foundation Symposium) Boston, Little, Brown and Company, 1953, p. 210.
8. Watzka, M.: Über Gefässperren und arteriovenöse Anastomosen. Ztschr. mikr.-anat. Forsch., 39:521, 1936.

9. Womack, N. A. and Peters, R. M.: An investigation of the relationship between portal venous pressure and inferior vena caval and portal venous oxygen saturation. Ann. Surg., *146*:691, 1957.
10. Womack, N. A., and Peters, R. M.: The significance of splenomegaly in cirrhosis of the liver. Ann. Surg., *153*:1006, 1961.

Control of
Ascites from
Portal Hypertension

Introduction

It is apparent to all that ascites, for the most part, is a serious and late complication of far advanced cirrhosis, and that any attempt to control it must include measures designed to protect against further liver damage by elimination of alcoholism or removal of toxic substances from the patient's environment. The contributors to this section have summarized the indications, methods, and anticipated results for both medical and surgical control of ascites in patients with portal hypertension, and in this instance both Levitan and Welch agree that medical treatment deserves first priority, and that surgery had best be confined to those patients in whom conservative management has failed. A discussion of the pathophysiology of cirrhotic ascites is included by both authors, and it was of interest to the editors that some disagreement was noted.

The controversy lies in the choice of patient for a side-to-side shunt from portal vein to vena cava, and in the risk involved in operating on patients who fail to respond to medical treatment. The final decision as to treatment of any particular patient rests in the hands of the reader. It is he who must weigh the evidence for and against operation in these extreme situations.

E. H. E.

Use of Supportive Measures without Operation to Control Ascites in Portal Hypertension

Ruven Levitan
Tufts University School of Medicine

and Philip Kramer
Boston University School of Medicine

Introduction

Ascites is not a disease. It occurs as a consequence of abnormal fluid retention in a large variety of pathologic conditions,[12] which may be classified into groups as follows:

1. Local peritoneal (e.g., tuberculosis, carcinomatosis)
2. Severe hypoproteinemias (e.g., nephrosis, starvation)
3. Posthepatic "outflow block" (e.g., constrictive pericarditis, tricuspid insufficiency, right sided heart failure, hepatic vein thrombosis)
4. Prehepatic "inflow block" (e.g., portal vein thrombosis)
5. "Intrahepatic block" (e.g., cirrhosis—Laennec's, postnecrotic, biliary; hemochromatosis; Wilson's disease; acute hepatitis)

Ascites, therefore, is a symptom or a physical sign; its management is symptomatic, especially in conditions caused by intrahepatic block, since the underlying disease that causes ascites, in most instances, cannot be treated effectively.

The present discussion is limited to the management of ascites in cirrhotic patients. We believe that medical management is by far the treatment of choice, since it can control ascites in most cirrhotic patients without subjecting them to a surgical procedure that cannot alter the natural course of cirrhosis, is often ineffective in relieving ascites, and is associated with a relatively high mortality and morbidity.

In order to understand the rationale of medical management of ascites due to cirrhosis, it is necessary first to consider the mechanisms leading to its formation.

Page 281

Mechanisms of Ascites Formation

Despite extensive studies, the source of the fluid and the mechanisms involved in ascites formation in cirrhosis are still not entirely understood.[8] Some believe that the fluid originates from the liver (weeping liver), and others claim that it originates from the splanchnic area.[7] The main factors presumably leading to ascites formation are summarized in Table 1.

TABLE 1.   FACTORS PROMOTING ASCITES FORMATION IN CIRRHOSIS
OF THE LIVER

A. Local factors acting on the peritoneum
   1. Portal hypertension
   2. Decreased plasma colloid osmotic pressure
   3. Increased hepatic lymph flow
   4. ? increased peritoneal permeability
B. Factors acting on the kidney
   1. Increase in circulating aldosterone level
   2. Increase in circulating antidiuretic hormone
   3. Increase in circulating estrogenic hormones
   4. Alterations in renal hemodynamics

Local Factors Acting on the Peritoneum

PORTAL HYPERTENSION.   The role played by portal hypertension in the genesis of ascites remains controversial.[3] All investigators agree that this factor is important; however, there is a considerable overlap in the portal venous pressure levels found in patients with and without ascites. Furthermore, severe portal hypertension is not always associated with ascites and the operative decompression of the portal bed in man does not always lead to disappearance of ascites. It is also well established that sodium restriction will cause the ascites to disappear without altering the pressure in the portal system. Portal hypertension therefore is not the sole factor responsible for ascites formation.

PLASMA COLLOID OSMOTIC PRESSURE.   The plasma albumin concentration largely determines the plasma colloid osmotic pressure. Hypoalbuminemia is common in severe cirrhosis and is an important factor leading to ascites formation. However, there is no agreement as to the critical level of plasma albumin at which ascites will form. It has been suggested that the presence or absence of ascites can be best correlated with the reciprocal relationship of the portal venous pressure and the plasma colloid osmotic pressure rather than to either factor alone.[1] Thus a high portal pressure and a low colloid osmotic pressure results in ascites accumulation, according to this concept.

INCREASED HEPATIC LYMPH FLOW.   This condition has been found in patients with ascites. As a rule the thoracic duct is dilated and contains hemorrhagic lymph in such patients. The increased lymph flow results in an elevated lymph hydrostatic pressure in the thoracic duct.[2, 6] In 7 cirrhotic patients the pressure was 15 to 70 cm. of saline as compared to the pressure of 6 to 15 cm. in the controls.[2] In acute experiments drainage of the thoracic duct lymph has resulted in a decrease or disappearance of ascites in all of 7 patients,[2] suggesting that this increased hepatic lymph flow may have contributed to ascites formation. Whether this factor is cause or effect is unsettled; further studies are required to settle this point.

INCREASED PERITONEAL PERMEABILITY had been implicated as a source of ascites. At present there is no good method available to evaluate such a theory in the living human.

Factors Acting on the Kidney

INCREASED PLASMA ALDOSTERONE LEVELS are found in patients with ascites.[5] Aldosterone plays a crucial role in the formation and maintenance of ascites because it causes sodium retention by the kidney. More specifically, aldosterone acts on the distal tubules by increasing sodium reabsorption. In cirrhosis, aldosterone secretion is increased and its inactivation by the liver is impaired. The rate of fluid accumulation by the cirrhotic patient correlates with the rate of aldosterone secretion. Further evidence to support the role of aldosterone in ascites formation is suggested by the following facts: (1) adrenalectomy results in the disappearance of ascites, (2) inhibition of aldosterone production (by Metopirone, for example) will often cause ascites to disappear, and (3) blockage of aldosterone at the distal renal tubular level by aldosterone antagonists (e.g., Aldactone, Aldactone-A) will cause diuresis. It should be emphasized, however, that aldosterone by itself seems to be incapable of producing ascites in the absence of portal hypertension or decreased plasma colloid osmotic pressure. The mechanism that initiates the increased aldosterone secretion in the cirrhotic patient is unknown.[5]

INCREASE IN PLASMA ANTIDIURETIC HORMONE (ADH). This situation is suggested as a factor in ascites formation.[12] It should be pointed out that the methodology for ADH determination leaves much to be desired. With this reservation, it appears that ADH blood levels in cirrhotic patients with ascites is no higher than those found in other diseases not associated with fluid retention. Urinary levels of ADH are normal in cirrhotic patients, and the cirrhotic liver likewise inactivates this hormone normally. In conclusion, it appears that ADH does not have a primary essential role in the pathogenesis of ascites formation, although it is possible that it may be a contributing factor leading to hyponatremia and further water retention once ascites has started to accumulate.[12]

INCREASE IN CIRCULATING ESTROGENIC HORMONES. This situation is found in cirrhosis because the cirrhotic liver is unable to inactivate these hormones.[12] Estrogens may cause sodium retention by the kidney, but it is unlikely that estrogen elevation is a primary mechanism leading to ascites formation.

ALTERATIONS IN RENAL HEMODYNAMICS. A decreased glomerular filtration rate (GFR) has been found in most patients actively forming ascites. In addition, such individuals, as a rule, also have a decreased renal blood flow (RBF) and an increased renal vascular resistance. The decreased GFR leads to sodium retention. It should be pointed out, however, that it is not possible to correlate active ascites formation with a depression of either GFR or RBF.[10] In conclusion it appears that renal hemodynamic factors play only a contributing role in ascites formation.

Indications for Medical Therapy of Ascites

Symptoms produced by ascites and requiring therapy include:

1. Respiratory embarrassment as a result of decreased vital capacity due to diaphragmatic elevation.

2. Subjective discomfort and loss of appetite.

3. Increased intra-abdominal pressure, which leads to the formation of hernias (umbilical or inguinal) and their incarceration.

The vigor with which diuresis is pursued, if at all, depends upon the severity of symptoms.

Rationale of Medical Management

The major argument for the medical management of ascites is the fact that it is effective in the majority of patients.[4, 13] It may take several weeks or more for stabilization or disappearance of ascites. Failure of ascites to respond to adequate medical management is regarded by many as a bad prognostic sign.

Most efforts in medical management are directed toward the elimination of sodium retention by the kidney.[13] The plasma colloid osmotic pressure also can be improved, at least transiently, by intravenous albumin administration.[7] Portal venous pressure can be lowered only for short periods of time by medical means (i.e., Pitressin administration), an ineffective measure in the management of ascites. At present there is no medical method for diminishing the increased hepatic lymph flow, for changing the peritoneal permeability, or for counteracting the action of ADH and estrogens. General supportive measures, such as abstinence from alcohol, rest, and a good diet, improve the overall hepatic function. A very small number of patients do not respond to good medical management, but still have relatively good hepatic parenchymal function. These patients are candidates for surgery. The problem, however, is to select from this group patients who will survive the shunt surgery and benefit from it, without developing serious complications, such as hepatic encephalopathy.

Program of Medical Management of Ascites

The effectiveness of medical management of ascites should be evaluated by objective criteria. Daily weight determinations and accurate measurements of the abdominal girth are by far the simplest way. Accurate measurement of the 24-hour urinary volume and sodium outputs are more complicated, but also more meaningful: while the ascites is developing, cirrhotic patients excrete less than 5 mEq. of sodium per 24 hours, while during diuresis, the urinary sodium output is higher. Serum electrolytes (sodium, potassium, chloride, carbon dioxide) should be measured frequently in patients undergoing active diuresis.

The different modalities of medical management are listed in Table 2, and the recommended therapeutic program is outlined in a step-like fashion in Table 3.

GENERAL SUPPORTIVE MEASURES are of great importance in attempts to halt the progress of the liver disease and improve hepatic function. Abstinence from alcohol is a must. Bed rest or decreased exertion and a well balanced diet are of great importance. In the absence of signs of hepatic coma or precoma, a protein intake of 80 Gm. per day is most beneficial. If signs of hepatic coma or precoma are present, protein intake restriction, cleansing enemas to rid the colon of bacteria or blood, and neomycin (6 to 8 Gm. per day) are helpful. Neomycin therapy may enable some patients to increase their protein intake without causing coma.

SALT RESTRICTION is the most important and effective measure in the treatment of ascites and the prevention of its recurrence. Many cirrhotic patients improve on a regimen of bed rest and salt restriction, without any additional measures. Some patients fare rather well on a diet containing 10 to 22 mEq. of sodium daily (equal to 0.25 to 0.5 Gm. of sodium or 0.5 to 1.2 Gm. of salt), although others will improve only if the sodium intake is even lower.

The effect of sodium restriction is gradual in onset and is usually seen in 10 days, but occasionally may take a number of weeks, even 2 months, before becoming apparent. In many instances it may be difficult to obtain the cooperation of the dietitians, hospital kitchens, and the patients to follow such a regimen; such a diet is not palatable. Hence, it is important not to label sodium restriction as a failure unless a rigid low-sodium diet has been followed for an adequate time. On a good program, nearly 50 per cent of patients lose their ascites.

DIURETICS are very effective in dissipating the ascites. They will augment the diuresis produced by sodium restriction.

The oldest and cheapest diuretic, *ammonium chloride,* has fallen into disrepute because it may precipitate hepatic coma, and also because more effective diuretics are now available. However, this drug is an effective agent, especially when used to augment the effects of mercurials. The recommended dose is 4.0 to 8.0 Gm. in enteric coated tablets, given orally for 3 days prior to mercurial administration.

TABLE 2.   MEDICAL MANAGEMENT OF ASCITES

Modality	Indication	Site and Mode of Action	Dose	Complications	Comments
General supportive measures: Bed rest Good diet	All patients		High-caloric diet with protein—80 Gm.	High protein may lead to hepatic coma	Neomycin 6 to 8 Gm. daily may prevent coma on high-protein diet
Paracentesis	Tight ascites with: Dyspnea Loss of appetite Incarcerated hernias No response to other measures	Mechanical relief Decompression of renal vein		Shock Hypoproteinemia Hepatic coma Electrolyte imbalance Infection Hemorrhage Azotemia	Necessary also for diagnostic purposes to rule out peritoneal infection, tumor; remove only small amount—not more than 3-5 liters at one time
Salt restriction	All patients with ascites	Prevents sodium retention	250 to 500 mg. sodium intake per day	Hyponatremia Diet unpalatable	48% of patients respond
Water restriction	Patients with hyponatremia with cerebral symptoms	Dehydration	Volume to cover urinary output and imperceptible loss	Dehydration Thirst	
Diuretics *Acting on General Sodium Reabsorption*					
Mercurial diuretics		Inhibits reabsorption of sodium	2 ml. I.M. every other day	Mercury toxicity after prolonged use Hypokalemia Metabolic alkalosis	Effect is potentiated by ammonium chloride, Diamox, aminophylline, chlorothiazide; drug of choice in hepatic precoma
Chlorothiazide	} If sodium restriction alone is ineffective	Inhibits reabsorption of sodium	0.25 to 0.5 Gm. p.o. (tablet) every 8 hours	Hepatic coma Hypokalemia Hyperglycemia Pancreatitis } rare Agranulocytosis	⅔ respond
Ammonium chloride		Potentiates mercurials	8.0 Gm. tablets per day (enteric coated) for 2 to 3 days prior to mercurial diuretics	Hepatic coma Gastric irritation Excessive acidosis and azotemia	Effective and cheap, historically first in use. Given if no signs of precoma are present. *Use with mercurials only*
Acetozolamide (Diamox)		Carbonic anhydrase inhibitor Decreases tubular $H+$ production Tubular sodium reabsorption is decreased $K+$ secretion is increased	0.25 to 1.0 Gm. (tablet) per day *intermittently only*	Metabolic acidosis May cause hepatic coma	Counteracts metabolic alkalosis created by mercurials Potentiates mercurials

	Indications	Mechanism	Dose	Toxicity	Remarks
Acting on Distal Tubular Exchange Mechanism					
Aldosterone antagonists (e.g., Aldactone-A)	If other diuretics are ineffective	Blocks aldosterone action at the tubular level	Aldactone-A (tablet) 25 mg. q.i.d.	Hyperkalemia Excessive cost	To be given with diuretics that act on the general sodium reabsorption, preferably with chlorothiazide
Increasing Glomerular Filtration Rate (GFR)					
Aminophylline	To promote action of aforementioned agents	Increases GFR	0.5 Gm. I.V. to be given slowly 2 to 3 hours after mercurials	Hypotension Cardiac arrythmias	To be given only with other diuretics acting on the general sodium reabsorption, especially mercurials
Adrenocorticosteroids		Increases GFR Decreases tubular water absorption ? Decreases aldosterone secretion	Prednisolone 20 to 40 mg. (tablet) per day	Increased susceptibility to infections Hypokalemia Peptic ulcers	To be given only with other diuretics acting on the general sodium reabsorption
Osmotic Diuresis					
Salt-free albumin	When combinations of diuretics listed above don't work	Increases plasma colloid osmotic pressure	25 Gm. I.V. every other day	Pulmonary edema Bleeding from varices Excessive cost	May initiate diuresis in otherwise resistant cases
Mannitol	When diuretics listed above don't work In hyponatremia with water retention	Osmotic diuresis	10% solution, 2000 cc. I.V. every other day		

TABLE 3.   SUGGESTED MEDICAL THERAPY OF ASCITES IN ABSENCE OF AZOTEMIA

First Measure: Bed rest, diet, salt 2.0 Gm. daily
Second Measure: Salt restriction, 0.5 to 1.2 Gm. daily
Third Measure: Chlorothiazide (if no signs of precoma are found) 250 mg. q. 8 h.; if no effect, 500 Gm. q. 8 h. or Mercuhydrin 2 ml. I.M. every other day (recommended in cases of precoma)
 If still no response: Mercuhydrin and chlorothiazide can be given together and also in combination with Diamox and ammonium chloride, if no signs of coma are present
Fourth Measure: Add Aldactone-A 25 mg. (tablet) q.i.d. to chlorothiazide and/or Mercuhydrin
Fifth Measure: Add Prednisolone 20 to 40 mg. (tablet) daily
Sixth Measure: Give Aminophylline 0.5 Gm. I.V. several hours after oral or mercurial diuretics
Seventh Measure: Salt-free albumin 25 Gm. I.V. every other day
Eighth Measure: 10% mannitol 2000 ml. I.V. every other day

Mercurial diuretics inhibit the active sodium transport, mainly in the proximal tubules. Mercuhydrin, or a similar preparation, should be given in doses from 1 to 2 ml. intramuscularly every other day. Diamox as well as ammonium chloride potentiates the effects of these diuretics (see Table 2).

Chlorothiazide and its analogues also block the active sodium transport in the tubules, but they are more potent than mercurials, and they can be given orally. The usual recommended dose is 0.25 to 0.5 Gm., in tablets, every 8 hours. These diuretics as well as the mercurials may cause a significant potassium loss in the urine; hence patients receiving these diuretics should receive potassium supplements, e.g., Kaon Elixir, 1 tablespoon (equals 20 mEq. of potassium) 3 times a day, is usually adequate. The amount of potassium given should be guided, however, by the serum potassium levels.

Chlorothiazide (or its analogues) is the drug of choice in the management of ascites, since about two-thirds of all patients will respond to this treatment alone.[13] Chlorothiazide may induce serious complications, such as hepatic coma, an exacerbation or production of hyperglycemia, and more rarely, pancreatitis and agranulocytosis. If hepatic precoma is suspected or anticipated, mercurial diuretics should be given in preference to chlorothiazide. Mercurial diuretics and chlorothiazide produce a better diuresis when given together than when used separately.

Aldosterone antagonists, which block the effects of aldosterone at the distal renal tubule, are a valuable tool in the management of ascites. When given alone they are rarely effective; however, when combined with a diuretic that acts mainly on active sodium transport in the proximal tubule, i.e., chlorothiazide or mercurials, they produce a good sodium diuresis, which is more pronounced than when either type of diuretic is used alone. Sodium loss will be greater and potassium loss smaller. It takes aldosterone antagonists 24 to 48 hours to exert their effect. Spironolactone (Aldactone) is poorly and inconsistently absorbed when given orally, but its microcrystalline form, called Aldactone-A, is much better absorbed. Aldactone-A, 100 mg. per day orally (25 mg. 4 times a day), together with chlorothiazide, 2.0 Gm., in tablets, per day (0.5 Gm. every 8 hours), are an effective combination. Some patients may require as much as 300 mg. of Aldactone-A per day before diuresis will ensue.[13]

It is important to realize that despite hypoalbuminemia and jaundice, this form of combined therapy is usually effective.[4] In some patients, however, even a combination of chlorothiazide, mercurials, and aldosterone antagonists will not induce diuresis. In such cases additional drugs that increase glomerular filtration rate or increase plasma colloid osmotic pressure may initiate diuresis.

Adrenocorticosteroids that increase the GFR,[9] for example, prednisolone, in amounts of 20 to 40 mg. per day, may be sufficient. However, steroids introduce the potential hazards associated with their use.

Aminophylline, given slowly intravenously in a dose of 0.5 Gm., 2 to 3 hours after mercurial administration, will promote diuresis by increasing the GFR transiently.

Salt-free human albumin, given in doses of 25 Gm. intravenously on alternate days, may prompt diuresis by increasing plasma colloid osmotic pressure. Usually albumin administration is helpful to patients with a serum albumin concentration of less than 2.0 Gm. per cent. However, even if the serum albumin is higher, diuresis may be produced by such therapy. It should be emphasized that administration of albumin can cause esophageal varices to rupture, and this can cause a serious, life-threatening hemorrhage.

Mannitol, another osmotic diuretic, given as a 10 per cent solution in amounts of 2000 ml. I.V. on alternate days, is useful especially after prolonged administration of chlorothiazide-type diuretics combined with aldosterone antagonists. The combination can induce a relatively greater sodium loss than water loss and results in hyponatremia.

WATER RESTRICTION is not usually necessary in the treatment of ascites. However, when hyponatremia is associated with cerebral symptoms, water restriction is beneficial. Extreme thirst limits the extent of water restriction.

PARACENTESIS has fallen into disrepute because of serious complications. It may cause shock, hypoalbuminemia, severe electrolyte disturbances, particularly hyponatremia, intraperitoneal infection, as well as hemorrhage. Nevertheless, paracentesis is indicated under several circumstances:

1. For diagnostic purposes, i.e., in order to rule out peritonitis (due to tuberculosis or other causes) or carcinomatosis. Only small volumes of fluid should be removed in such cases.

2. When patients are dyspneic as a result of diminished vital capacity due to the elevated diaphragm.

3. If an external hernia (umbilical or inguinal) has become or is about to become incarcerated.

4. When the ascites is very tense, and the patient is anorectic, and all other measures have failed to induce diuresis.

5. In the face of azotemia, when diuretics do not work.

The peritoneal cavity must be entered under sterile conditions and no more than 3 to 5 liters should be removed at one time.

Disadvantages of Medical Treatment of Ascites

Medical therapy is symptomatic only. By using all modalities of medical therapy as discussed above, diuresis leading to the disappearance of ascites can be obtained in most cirrhotic patients. Experience, good dietetic control, time, close laboratory supervision, and funds are essential if success is to be obtained. Most patients have to continue on a low-sodium diet and take quite expensive medication for long periods of time. The modern combined diuretic therapy causes, in many cases, severe electrolyte imbalances. Azotemia and progressive renal failure are precipitated in some patients, presumably because renal blood flow is decreased. Patients who develop renal complications are, as a rule, in the terminal phase of liver disease.

Indications for Surgery

If medical therapy fails, if patients refuse to cooperate, if close medical supervision is unavailable, or if the financial problems are prohibitive, the surgical approach should be considered, provided that hepatic function is well preserved. It should be kept in mind, however, that portacaval shunt, which is the most effective procedure, carries a high mortality. In addition, patients who survive this procedure require close medical supervision anyway, because of the high incidence of encephalopathy after the shunt procedures,[11] the high incidence of peptic ulcer, and the persistence of hypoalbuminemia and peripheral edema in many cases.

Summary

Ascites in liver disease is a symptom. It is a manifestation of hepatocellular failure associated with portal hypertension, and is most frequently encountered in cirrhosis. Treatment of ascites is symptomatic only, since it does not change the natural history of the underlying hepatic disease. Such therapy is indicated in order to relieve shortness of breath and loss of appetite, and to prevent hernias. Medical therapy for ascites mainly aims to eliminate the sodium retention by the kidney, which must be present for ascites to form. Bed rest, salt restriction, and diuretics, when used in combination, will cause ascites to disappear in almost all cases, despite the presence of jaundice and hypoalbuminemia. Failure to respond to good therapy is usually a poor prognostic sign. In the presence of azotemia, diuretics are usually ineffective, and small repeated paracenteses are indicated. Water restriction is necessary when hyponatremia is associated with cerebral symptoms. The medical management of ascites, though very effective, requires great skill, close clinical and biochemical supervision, time, money, and above all cooperation of the patient. The surgical approach should be considered for the uncooperative patient or for the one who has failed to respond to adequate medical management. Surgery is associated with a high mortality and morbidity, and does not change the natural history of cirrhosis. Moreover, the patients require close supervision after surgery because of the high incidence of encephalopathy, peptic ulceration, and progression of liver disease in patients with portacaval shunts.

References

1. Atkinson, M., and Losowsky, M. S.: The mechanism of ascites formation in chronic liver disease. Quart. J. Med., 30:153, 1961.
2. Dumont, A. E., and Mullholland, J. H.: Alterations in thoracic duct lymph flow in hepatic cirrhosis: significance in portal hypertension. Ann. Surg., 156:668, 1962.
3. Eisenmenger, W. J., and Nickel, W. F.: Relationship of portal hypertension to ascites in Laennec's cirrhosis. Am. J. Med., 20:879, 1956.
4. Howard, H. H., and Leevy, C. M.: Management of ascites. Arch. Int. Med., 112:116, 1963.
5. Laragh, J. H., and Ames, R. P.: Physiology of body water and electrolytes in hepatic disease. M. Clin. North America, 47:587, 1963.
6. Leger, L., Premont, M., and Devissaguet, P.: Le drainage du canal thoracique dans les cirrhoses ascitiques étude du débit lymphatique. Presse med., 70:1643, 1962.
7. Losowsky, M. S., and Davidson, C. S.: The source of ascitic fluid in cirrhosis of the liver. Arch. Int. Med., 110:279, 1962.
8. Losowsky, M. S.: Local factors in ascites formation in chronic liver disease. Editorial. Gastroenterology, 45:429, 1963.
9. Morrison, R. S., and Chalmers, T. C.: Combined diuretic and steroid therapy in cirrhosis with ascites. Ann. New York Acad. Sc., 88:907, 1960.
10. Papper, S.: The role of the kidney in Laennec's cirrhosis of the liver. Medicine, 37:299, 1958.
11. Read, A. E., Laidlow, J., and Sherlock, S.: Neuropsychiatric complications of portacaval anastomosis. Lancet, 1:961, 1961.
12. Sherlock, S.: Diseases of the liver and biliary system. Charles C Thomas, Springfield, Ill., 1955, p. 110.
13. Sherlock, S., and Sheldon, S.: The aetiology and management of ascites in patients with hepatic cirrhosis: a review. Gut, 4:95, 1963.

Portal Decompression

As a Means of Controlling Ascites

C. Stuart Welch

Albany Medical College

Introduction

The surgical treatment of ascites associated with cirrhosis of the liver is indeed a controversial one, if the stand is taken that portacaval shunts are competitive with medical treatment for this complication of liver disease. Medical treatment should always be given first priority. It is usually successful until the disease is far advanced and intractable. We have never advocated the use of portacaval shunts extensively in this disease, but have confined the surgery to cases of medical failure. There are fewer medical failures in the treatment of ascites today than in 1956, when we first employed side-to-side shunts in a small group of patients. Nevertheless, we are convinced that side-to-side portacaval shunts can relieve ascites and has some place in treatment.

Cirrhosis of the liver is a serious disease, and as a cause of death among men in the productive age group it ranks in third or fourth place. It causes about as many deaths as do accidents. Cirrhosis is probably on the increase owing to two factors: hepatitis of serum origin is increasing and the consumption of hard liquor is also on the increase. The United States now ranks first in the per capita consumption of spirits.

Both esophageal varices and ascites are caused by the same fibrotic changes in the liver. When varices exist without ascites, the disease probably is only in a less advanced stage. Almost everyone understands the genesis of esophageal varices from portal hypertension in the splanchnic portal bed and the relation of subsequent hemorrhages into the gastrointestinal tract. Not so many physicians and fewer surgeons have a working knowledge of how ascites comes about. While the mechanism of ascites has been a subject of some debate, there is more general agreement about its cause today. First, then, let us consider the pathologic physiology of the liver and its relation to ascites formation before we take up the results of treatment of ascites by shunts. It is thus that the rationale for shunt employment becomes clearer.

Mechanism of Ascites; Rationale of Portacaval Shunts in Its Treatment

The destruction of hepatic tissue with reduced cellular function of course plays a part in the morbidity and mortality of cirrhosis but we know that there is great functional reserve in this area. Long before complete cellular destruction, there are extensive changes in the vasculature that cause complications such as portal hypertension and ascites, which can be treated with considerable success resulting in extension of the patient's life span and usefulness. Of the three vascular components in the liver—the hepatic arterial system, the portal venous system, and the hepatic venous system, it is the last that is most extensively damaged by fibrosis. The hepatic veins are thin walled and more vulnerable. In morphologic studies of livers removed from patients who died with advanced cirrhosis and ascites, we have found that the hepatic venous system was reduced by one half on the average. This means that there are insufficient hepatic veins to adequately drain the liver of the blood supplied by its two supplying systems, the hepatic arteries and portal veins. An *outflow block* is thus created, and this hemodynamic deficit is the basic difficulty. It results in portal hypertension and ascites, depending upon the degree of involvement and the stage of the disease. High pressure is created in the hepatic venous sinusoids, causing the transudation of plasma and, finally, the formation of an excess of hepatic lymph. The liver lymphatics become enlarged, and lymph actually leaks from the surface of the liver and from its hilum into the peritoneal cavity. Lymph also leaks into the peritoneal cavity from the splanchnic lymphatics. The amount of lymph so produced is greater than can be returned to the blood via the thoracic duct in a given time. Substantial evidence that there is increased hepatic lymph production in cirrhosis and in experimental outflow block has been obtained by measuring thoracic duct lymph production. It is increased over normal in both these derangements.

There are other correlative clinical conditions that produce the same effect; thrombosis of the hepatic veins (Budd-Chiari syndrome) and adhesive pericarditis are two such entities. Experimental surgical procedures in dogs—constriction of the vena cava above the diaphragm and ligation of the hepatic veins—similarly produce ascites. The common denominator is *hepatic outflow block* in all these lesions.

As mentioned above, this outflow block causes leakage of lymph into the peritoneal cavity, where it produces ascites by virtue of its high oncotic pressure. Fluid and electrolytes are thus drawn from the tissue spaces of the internal environment and held there in the peritoneal sac, in equilibrium with the body fluids but in reality outside the body's internal environment.

The familiar picture of low blood volume, low serum albumin, and low serum electrolyte (sodium in particular) results.

Since preservation of water in the body is a fundamental homeostatic mechanism, and since the preservation of sodium is the sine qua non of this feat, the adrenal cortex produces an excess of aldosterone, which holds sodium in the body by stopping its excretion in the urine. Patients with severe, intractable ascites will be found to excrete as low as 3 or 4 mEq. of sodium per day. This hyperaldosteronism is a secondary protective mechanism and not a primary one, as had been thought by some investigators. The medical treatment of ascites has been discussed; it remains to elucidate what surgical intervention might be able to do in remedying outflow block.

It occurred to us that decompression of the liver might be accomplished if a reverse flow in the portal vein was possible, and if this retrograde blood flow could be directed into the inferior vena cava. Considerable evidence exists that reverse flow can and does occur in the portal vein in cases of cirrhosis of the liver.

The fact that the collateral routes for the portal blood to reach the right heart are enlarged and produce varices is prima facie evidence of reverse flow in the portal system. Other measurements have shown reverse flow in the portal vein in cirrhosis.

Anastomosis of the portal vein to the vena cava, performed tangentially (side-to-side), results in retrograde flow from the liver into the vena cava, and thus decompression of that organ. In both human and laboratory subjects, we found that ascites can be relieved by side-to-side portacaval shunt, and have now had seven years' experience in the use of this operation in selected cases. Its success is determined by the decompression of the hepatic sinusoidal area and thus the prevention of excess hepatic lymph production and ascites.

Results of Side-to-Side Shunts

During the past seven years we have performed 40 side-to-side shunts in patients with severe ascites. The hospital death rate was 32.5 per cent and the 1-year mortality rate was 50 per cent. Eleven patients are surviving 1 to 7 years inclusive (27.5 per cent). In Table 1 these data are recorded. We

TABLE 1. PORTACAVAL SHUNTS FOR ASCITES (7 YEARS' EXPERIENCE)

	Number	Per Cent
Total cases	40	
Hospital deaths	13	32.5
Late deaths	16	40
Surviving	11	27.5

TABLE 2. TREATMENT OF ASCITES

	Medical		
Author	*Year*	*Number of Cases*	*Death within 1 Year* *(Per Cent)*
Cates	1943	53	62
Patek et al.	1948	115	35
Douglass and Snell	1950	212	63
Justin-Besancon and Caroit	1959	108	73
Welch, Welch and Carter	1964	90	54.2

	Surgical				
Author	*Year*	*Number of Cases*	*Death within 1 Year (Per Cent)*	*Method*	*Operative Mortality (Per Cent)*
Cates	1943	38	68	Omentapexy	42
Chalmers and Davidson	1949	41	78	Cooney button	35
Neumann	1957	10		Ileo-entectropy	50
Welch, Welch and Carter	1964	40	45	Side-to side shunt	32.5
McDermott et al.	1961	17		Side-to-side shunt	12

believe that these data show some accomplishment in the treatment of ascites by shunts for two reasons. In the first place, the 1-year survival rate of 55 per cent favorably compares with published results of medical and other types of surgical treatment. Second, the patients we selected had, for the most part, advanced liver disease, making them less favorable than the cases given medical treatment. Some collected data on medical and surgical treatment are shown in Table 2. It can be seen that the 45 per cent death rate within one year resulting from shunts is less than for other forms of medical and surgical therapy.

In patients who have a favorable response to side-to-side shunt, hyper-aldosterone manifestations disappear. The sodium output in the urine goes up, ascites disappears, and a normal diet can be resumed.

The high mortality rate of 32.5 per cent is largely the result of liver failure postoperatively. The selection of patients who might reasonably be offered a shunt procedure for cirrhotic ascites is admittedly difficult, and has been in the experimental stage. Preoperative studies are helpful but not decisive. The better the cellular liver function in the presence of a stubborn ascites, the better the outlook with a shunt procedure. The younger the patient, the better the prognosis with surgery. Patients with clinical icterus are usually unacceptable candidates for shunt. The temptation to operate upon patients as a last resort must be restrained, or the hospital mortality rate after surgery will be high. In our present series there are a number of such cases done in our early experience. Today we operate upon fewer than we did five years ago. The results in some cases, however, have been so good that we are convinced of the value of side-to-side portacaval shunts in the treatment of intractable ascites.

References

1. Carter, J. H., Welch, C. S., and Barron, R. E.: Changes in the hepatic blood vessels in cirrhosis of the liver. Surg., Gynec. and Obst., *113*:133, 1961.
2. Cates, H. B.: Surgical treatment of cirrhosis. Arch. Int. Med., *71*:183, 1943.
3. Chalmers, T. C., and Davidson, C. S.: A survey of recent therapeutic measures in cirrhosis of the liver. New England J. Med., *240*:449, 1949.
4. Douglass, B. C., and Snell, A. M.: Portal cirrhosis: an analysis of 444 cases. Gastroenterology, *15*:407, 1950.
5. van der Heyde, M. N., O'Keefe, D., and Welch, C. S.: Thoracic duct lymph flow with variations in hepatic hemodynamics. Surgery, *56*:1121, 1964.
6. Justin-Besancon, L., and Caroit, M.: Prognosis of alcoholic ascitic cirrhosis. Semaine hôp. Paris, *35*:200, 1959.
7. McDermott, W. F., Patozzi, H., Nardi, G. L., and Mondet, A.: Elective portal systemic shunt: analysis of 237 cases. New England J. Med., *264*:419, 1961.
8. Neumann, C.: The absorption of ascitic fluid by means of ileo-entectropy in patients with advanced cirrhosis. Ann. Surg., *146*:700, 1957.
9. Patek, A. J. Jr., Post, J., Ratnoff, O. D., Mankin, H., and Hillman, R. W.: Dietary treatment of cirrhosis of the liver. J.A.M.A., *138*:543, 1948.
10. Welch, C. S., Attarian, E., and Welch, H. F.: The treatment of ascites by side-to-side portacaval shunt. Bull. New York Acad. Med., *34*:249, 1958.
11. Welch, C. S., Welch, H. F., and Carter, J. H.: The treatment of ascites by side-to-side portacaval shunt. Ann. Surg., *150*:428, 1959.
12. Welch, H. F., Welch, C. S., and Carter, J. H.: Prognosis after surgical treatment of ascites: results of side-to-side shunt in 40 patients. Surgery, *56*:75, 1964.

Management of
Duodenal Ulcer

Introduction

In the first volume of Current Surgical Management, equally distinguished authors championed vagotomy with pyloroplasty, or gastroenterostomy and 70 per cent gastric resection as the ideal treatment of the intractable duodenal ulcer.

In Volume II, the controversy included the addition of vagotomy to a lesser resection and discussions of the method of restoring gastrointestinal continuity. Two of the distinguished contributors favored supra-antral or segmental resection of the stomach, and some attention was paid to the importance of antral denervation.

Finally, roentgen irradiation was proposed as a nonsurgical adjunct in the treatment of duodenal ulcer, aimed at the reduction of the acid-producing parietal cells of the stomach.

Debate continues, and equally distinguished surgeons are now supporting additional and novel approaches for the control of acid peptic disease, based upon a dissatisfaction with the secondary phenomenon resulting from either extensive resection or truncal vagotomy, such as malnutrition and diarrhea. Selective vagotomy with antrectomy or gastric drainage is designed to preserve all extragastric vagal influences in an attempt to avoid the so-called "postvagotomy," syndrome, which includes an urgent diarrhea. Gastric freezing is proposed as another nonoperative method of reducing the secretion of acid from the parietal cells of the stomach, while preserving the normal gastric reservoir with normal emptying.

As pointed out previously, only time and careful objective evaluation of long-term results will resolve the current controversies in the management of duodenal ulcer.

E. H. E.

Selective Vagotomy with Billroth I Antrectomy

Henry N. Harkins

University of Washington School of Medicine

The operation of *selective vagotomy with Billroth I antrectomy* as a definitive technique for the surgical treatment of duodenal ulcer has been the basic standard procedure in our clinic since April 1, 1961. We term it the "revised combined operation" in contradistinction to the "combined operation" (conventional Dragstedtian truncal vagotomy with Billroth I antrectomy), which was standard from September 1, 1955, to March 31, 1961. Prior to this latter date, beginning in 1948, measured (average 70 per cent) radical subtotal gastric resection *ad modum* Billroth I (without vagotomy) was our standard procedure. Previous to 1948, I had never done a Billroth I, and used only the Billroth II with an *unmeasured* subtotal resection.

The term *standard* procedure does not signify that this operation is performed in our hospitals to the exclusion of all others. It merely denotes our preferred and most usual operation. As individual circumstances dictate in particular patients we may do otherwise. For example, in massive hemorrhage from bleeding ulcer, we prefer vagotomy with Heineke-Mikulicz pyloroplasty (the Weinberg operation) with suture ligation of the bleeding vessel. If the patient's condition is not too precarious, and the additional 20 minutes required to perform a selective gastric vagotomy are not too important, even in the presence of bleeding, we may modify the Weinberg operation to spare the extragastric branches of the vagi. Other indications for diverging from our standard procedure will occur, depending on the body habitus of the patient, extensive phlegmon in the region of the ulcer, etc.

Before we discuss why we do what we do, possibly a brief discussion of why we no longer prefer what we used to do would be in order. To facilitate and simplify the discussion, I will refer, in the first person, to my own experiences and beliefs.

Page 299

Evolvement of Technique

Phase I. Billroth II Unmeasured Subtotal Gastrectomy

Prior to 1948, I had never performed a Billroth I operation and had seen only one (by Prof. Gunnar Nyström in Uppsala, Sweden, in 1939). I had done about 50 Billroth II unmeasured subtotal resections. There was dumping in some of these patients. The dumping syndrome, first named by Andrews of Chicago in 1920 (*not* first by Mix, as is generally stated, in 1922), was just beginning to be discussed.

Phase II. Billroth I Measured Subtotal Gastrectomy

To obviate dumping I decided to try the Billroth I subtotal resection (see Table 1). Unfortunately, our hopes for preventing the dumping syndrome by the Billroth I were not fully realized. We obtained some improvement in this respect, but actually not as much as that reported by some others who used the Billroth I. This was possibly because our quantitatively *measured* resection, worked out in conjunction with Dr. Horace Moore,[16] was more radical than those performed by the other surgeons; this difference in extent of resection is the most probable explanation for our relative lack of stomal ulcer development following the Billroth I operation for duodenal ulcer. As reported by Savage et al.,[19] in 157 Billroth I operations (70 per cent resections) followed for at least one year (average follow-up of 42.3 months), there were two proved recur-

TABLE 1.   PERSONAL EXPERIENCE IN FOUR PHASES OF PREFERRED
OPERATION FOR DUODENAL ULCER

Phase	Operative Procedure	Years	Number of Cases	Morbidity		
				Dumping	Secondary Stomal Ulcer	Postvagotomy Diarrhea
I	Billroth II—70% resection	1936–1948	50	Fair	Fair	—
II	Billroth I—70% measured resection	1948–1955	350	Fair	Fair	—
III	"Combined operation": truncal vagotomy + Billroth I antrectomy	1955–1961	225	Good	Excellent	Fair
IV	"Revised combined operation": selective gastric vagotomy + Billroth I antrectomy	1961– present	135	Good	Excellent	Excellent

rences and two possible recurrences, an over-all inclusive recurrence rate of 2.5 per cent. The entire subject of why our stomal ulcer incidence was lower than that reported by some other surgeons is a fascinating—but to us academic—question, since we now rarely perform a Billroth I except in combination with vagotomy. Other possible explanations for this difference in stomal ulcer incidence are discussed by Harkins.[7]

Phase III. Standard Truncal Vagotomy with Billroth I Antrectomy

Suffice it to say that our switch to the third phase of technique (see Table 1) was *not* based on a high rate of stomal ulcer development with the Billroth I technique, but rather was based on: (1) our dissatisfaction with *any* radical subtotal resection for duodenal ulcer from the standpoint of dumping and other postgastrectomy difficulties; (2) the suggestive results of our animal studies;[17, 18] and (3) the promising results of the "combined operation" in a pilot series of patients.[10]

We were quite pleased with the results of the "combined operation" (truncal vagotomy with Billroth I antrectomy) from the standpoint of dumping, and were surprised at its astonishingly good outcome from the standpoint of stomal ulcer.[9, 19]

In 1961, Dr. Charles A. Griffith finally persuaded me that selective gastric vagotomy was worthy of a clinical study. It is of interest that I had collaborated with Dr. Griffith on an animal experimental study of selective vagotomy some 4 years before,[6] but had been afraid to apply the procedure clinically because of a possible danger that the all-important *gastric* portion of the vagotomy might not be complete. This fear was partly due to Dr. Griffith's unfortunate use of the word "partial" in the title of our 1957 paper, when he actually was using the word in another connotation. I am now convinced that selective gastric vagotomy is *at least* as apt to completely vagotomize the stomach as is standard truncal vagotomy. Therefore, even though the positive reasons for doing the selective operation may remain to be proved, this objection to the procedure is, in my opinion, not valid.

Furthermore, as Burge,[2] Griffith,[4] and others began to write about postvagotomy diarrhea, steatorrhea, and other complications, we noticed them in some of our patients. Therefore, on April 1, 1961, we set up a plan to study Phase IV.

Phase IV. Selective Gastric Vagotomy with Billroth I Antrectomy (The "Revised Combined Operation")

This phase of our studies now involves anatomic and physiologic investigations as well as operations on some 90 patients. It will be discussed only relative to the new feature introduced into it, namely selective gastric vagotomy, under the following headings:

HISTORY. Selective gastric vagotomy was introduced by Franksson of Stockholm and Jackson of Ann Arbor in 1947, working independently. Shortly afterward, Moore of Boston also reported the operation.[15] All three of these pioneers did the procedure without drainage of the stomach, in conformity with common practice of that time. Possibly for this reason, the operation fell into desuetude, and it remained for Griffith and Harkins,[6] Griffith,[4] and particularly Burge,[2] to revive it, this time with drainage, or as we do it, with antrectomy. Currently, Kraft, Fry and Ransom,[13] Smith and Farris,[20] and a few other groups are studying the operation.

ANATOMIC BASIS. The left vagus gives off gastric rami and a hepatic branch, the latter coursing laterally to the right in the gastrohepatic omentum. The hepatic branch innervates the entire biliary tract and pylorus. Similarly, the right vagus gives off gastric rami and a large celiac branch coursing posteriorly to the right in the omental fold, which carries the coronary vein and left gastric artery. The celiac branch innervates the pancreas, all of the small intestine, and the right half of the colon.

PHYSIOLOGIC BASIS. It is postulated that control of gallbladder tone, common duct motility, flow of bile and pancreatic secretions, intestinal motility, and other similar functions are subject to extragastric vagal influences. Stavney et al. have studied especially the effects on the intestine.[21]

CLINICAL BASIS. Certain symptoms are believed to be a part of the "postvagotomy syndrome," especially a type of urgent diarrhea. The advocates of selective gastric vagotomy believe that such diarrhea can be in large part obviated by preserving the extragastric branches of the vagus nerves. In our own series, using very strict but comparable criteria as to what is diarrhea, the incidence was reduced from 68 to 29 per cent. Especially interesting is the fact that if the complaints of diarrhea are divided into those associated with and those independent of dumping, the former were not reduced at all in incidence, whereas the latter dropped from 38 to 2 per cent.

POSTVAGOTOMY HOLLANDER TESTS. Whereas some say that in truncal vagotomy, as it is performed throughout the country, the incidence of positive Hollander test is over 35 per cent (one writer says over 75 per cent!)— if the test is ever done; even in the better clinics it may be over 25 per cent. In a series of 30 cases of our selective gastric vagotomies, in which the test has been performed, only two (both weak tests) have shown a positive result, 7 per cent. This is at least as good as figures for the truncal technique. The Hollander insulin test is a difficult one to perform, and must be done carefully to be of significance. When properly used, it is the best indication we have of the completeness of vagotomy.

BRIEF COMMENT ON "ANTISELECTIVE VAGOTOMY." Advocates of selective gastric vagotomy soon observed the possibility pointed out by Griffith,[5] that the hepatic and celiac branches lie right in the path of conventional dissections for subtotal—or total—gastrectomy. Thus, in the past surgeons have undoubtedly inadvertently cut these branches, in some cases routinely, with no thought about doing or not doing a vagotomy. Thus, many of the symptoms that allegedly are part of the "postgastrectomy syndrome" may not be at all, and may be due to the cutting of these nerves. Even today, probably not one in 100 abdominal surgeons knows where these nerves are, or in some instances, even that they exist.

STOMAL ULCER INCIDENCE. In 135 cases of selective gastric vagotomy (most of which were combined with antrectomy), in which the follow-up in some cases goes back over 7 years (although in most it has been much shorter), there have been no stomal ulcers.

Summary

Selective gastric vagotomy was introduced as an independent procedure without gastric drainage by Franksson and by Jackson in 1947. It was revived, this time with pyloroplasty or antrectomy, by Griffith, beginning in 1957, and reported by him and by Burge in 1960. This operation vagotomizes the stomach but spares the hepatic (from the left vagus) and celiac (from the right) branches which innervate much of the remainder of the intestinal tract. This type of vagotomy, used by us in the majority of cases in conjunction with Billroth I antrectomy (i.e., the "revised combined operation"), was compared with truncal vagotomy, also plus Billroth I antrectomy (i.e., the "combined operation"). The selective technique resulted in: (1) a probably lower incidence of postoperative positive Hollander tests; (2) a lower incidence of postvagotomy diarrhea; and (3) no recurrences of (stomal) ulceration.

References

1. Andrews, E. W.: "Dumping stomach" and other results of gastrojejunostomy: operative cure by disconnecting old stoma. S. Clinics of Chicago, 4:883, 1920.
2. Burge, H. W.: Vagotomy in the treatment of peptic ulceration. Postgrad. M. J., 36: 2, 1960.
3. Franksson, C.: Proceedings of Meeting of Svensk kirurgisk förening. Stockholm. October 24, 1947.
4. Griffith, C. A.: Gastric vagotomy vs. total abdominal vagotomy. Arch. Surg., 81: 781, 1960.
5. Griffith, C. A.: Selective Gastric Vagotomy. In Harkins, H. N., and Nyhus, L. M.: Surgery of the Stomach and Duodenum. Boston, Little, Brown and Company, 1962.
6. Griffith, C. A., and Harkins, H. N.: Partial gastric vagotomy: an experimental study. Gastroenterology, 32:96, 1957.
7. Harkins, H. N.: Gastric Resection: Billroth I. In Harkins, H. N., and Nyhus, L. M.: Surgery of the Stomach and Duodenum. Boston, Little, Brown and Company, 1962
8. Harkins, H. N., Chapman, N. D., Nyhus, L. M., Condon, R. E., Stevenson, J. K., and Jesseph, J. E. Combined operation: vagotomy, antrectomy, and gastroduodenostomy. Arch. Surg., 85:936, 1962.
9. Harkins, H. N., Jesseph, J. E., Stevenson, J. K., and Nyhus, L. M.: The "combined" operation for peptic ulcer. Arch. Surg., 80:743, 1960.
10. Harkins, H. N., Schmitz, E. J., Harper, H. P., Sauvage, L. R., Moore, H. G., Jr., Storer, E. H., and Kanar, E. A.: A combined physiologic operation for peptic ulcer (par-

tial distal gastrectomy, vagotomy and gastroduodenostomy); a preliminary report. Western J. Surg., *61:*316, 1953.

11. Harkins, H. N., Stavney, L. S., Griffith, C. A., Savage, L. E., Kato, T., and Nyhus, L. M.: Selective gastric vagotomy. Ann. Surg., *158:*448, 1963.

12. Jackson, R. G.: Anatomic study of the vagus nerves, with a technic of transabdominal selective vagus resection. Univ. Hosp. Bull., Ann Arbor, *13:*31, 1947.

13. Kraft, R. O., Fry, W. J., and Ransom, H. K.: Selective gastric vagotomy. Arch. Surg., *85:*687, 1962.

14. Mix, C. L.: "Dumping stomach" following gastrojejunostomy. S. Clin. North America, *2:*617, 1922.

15. Moore, F. D.: Follow-up of vagotomy in duodenal ulcer. Gastroenterology, *11:*442, 1948.

16. Moore, H. G., Jr., and Harkins, H. N.: The Billroth I Gastric Resection: With Particular Reference to the Surgery of Peptic Ulcer. Boston, Little, Brown and Company, 1954.

17. Sauvage, L. R., Schmitz, F. J., Storer, E. H., Kanar, E. A., Smith, F. R., and Harkins, H. N.: The relation between the physiologic stimulatory mechanisms of gastric secretion and the incidence of peptic ulceration: an experimental study employing a new preparation. Surg., Gynec. and Obst. *96:*127, 1953.

18. Sauvage, L. R., Schmitz, E. J., Storer, E. H., Smith, F. P., Kanar, E. A., and Harkins, H. N.: A new operative preparation for production of peptic ulcer in the dog. Proc. Soc. Exper. Biol. Med., *79:*436, 1952.

19. Savage, L. E., Stavney, L. S., Harkins, H. N., and Nyhus, L. M.: Comparison of the combined operation and Billroth I gastrectomy in the treatment of chronic duodenal ulcer. Am. J. Surg., *107:*283, 1964.

20. Smith, G. K., and Farris, J. M.: Some observations upon selective gastric vagotomy. Arch. Surg., *86:*716, 1963.

21. Stavney, L. S., Kato, T., Griffith, C. A., Nyhus, L. M., and Harkins, H. N.: A physiologic study of motility changes following selective gastric vagotomy. J. Surg. Res., *3:*390, 1963.

Gastric Freezing*

J. P. Delaney, R. L. Goodale, R. C. Doberneck, J. Engle,
F. A. Largiader, *and* O. H. Wangensteen

University of Minnesota Medical School

The variety of medical regimens and surgical procedures aimed at alleviating the ulcer diathesis attests to the fact that no treatment currently available is uniformly satisfactory. The introduction of gastric freezing to this number has engendered considerable controversy. Both the safety and the efficacy of the procedure have been questioned. Although gastric freezing is still in the developmental stage, enough information is now available to draw some useful inferences.

The concept of gastric freezing as a definitive treatment for peptic ulcer evolved from our earlier use of local intragastric hypothermia to control massive upper gastrointestinal bleeding. Attending cooling of the stomach, peptic activity was found to be suspended, diminution in gastric blood flow was observed, and acid secretion was suppressed. With these observations in mind, an attempt was made to allow ulcers to heal by putting them at rest by means of prolonged local hypothermia. The extreme discomfort to the patient and the transient duration of the effect, however, combined to make protracted gastric cooling impractical. With the experimental use of progressively lower temperatures for shorter periods of time, it soon became apparent that the canine stomach could, within certain limits, tolerate actual freezing without necrosis. Further studies demonstrated that: (1) isolated canine gastric pouches could be rendered achlorhydric to all stimuli by means of freezing; and (2) freezing the intact stomach of dogs provided definite protection against peptic ulcer, induced either by histamine or by gastrin, the latter released from an antral pouch anastomosed to the colon.

After the limits of freezing tolerance were delineated in the dog, the procedure was introduced in October, 1961, for treatment of patients suffering from the various manifestations of the ulcer diathesis.

* Supported by the U.S.P.H.S., the John A. Hartford Foundation, Inc., and the Donald J. Cowling and Jay and Rose Phillip Funds for Surgical Research.

Page 305

Technique

The majority of patients were treated according to the following protocol: The patients accepted for therapy had intractable or complicated manifestations of ulcer disease and were, in general, candidates for surgery. Each patient had upper gastrointestinal x-ray studies. Each had gastric secretory studies, an 8-hour unstimulated overnight collection, followed by Hollander and peptone tests. These studies were made both before and after gastric freezing. More recently, gastric secretory assessment has been confined to collection of a one-hour fasting basal specimen and another one-hour collection following the administration of 50 mg. of Histalog. These studies are made before and two days after the freeze, and at periodic intervals thereafter.

A hypothermia unit was used to circulate cold 80 per cent alcohol solution via a coaxial tube into a latex balloon, shaped to fit the stomach. Currently we employ a silicone fluid (Dow-Corning 200) as the perfusant instead of alcohol, to avoid ethanol poisoning should the balloon rupture, an occurrence we have not observed. Inflow temperatures have ranged in the area of $-18°$ to $-22°$ C., while the return temperatures from the balloon were usually recorded in the $-10°$ to $-12°$ C. range. Flow rates were in the order of 1400 cc. per minute, the balloon volumes about 1000 cc. (700 to 1400 cc.), and duration of the perfusion was 50 to 60 minutes.

Indications and Contraindications

At this clinic to date, 615 patients have undergone 872 episodes of gastric freezing. The most frequent indication for gastric freezing has been longstanding duodenal ulcer disease, resistant to medical management and frequently associated with prior complications, bleeding, or perforation. Other important indications have been postgastrectomy stomal ulcer and esophagitis, with or without stenosis. We have come to regard gastric outlet obstruction as a contraindication to freezing. The edema following a freeze tends to render a partial obstruction complete. Our experience with freezing for primary gastric ulcer has been very limited. Table 1 enumerates the indications for the patients who have undergone the gastric freezing procedure at our hands.

TABLE 1.   INDICATIONS FOR GASTRIC FREEZING

Total number of patients	615
Duodenal ulcer	502
Stomal ulcer	58
Gastric ulcer	25
Esophagitis	15
Miscellaneous	15

Results of Gastric Freezing

Of the 615 patients so far treated, 502 had duodenal ulcer. Of this group, 189 had their initial freezing episode more than a year ago. Some have now been followed as long as 28 months. Table 2 provides an analysis

TABLE 2. FINDINGS IN 189 PATIENTS MORE THAN ONE YEAR AFTER GASTRIC FREEZING FOR DUODENAL ULCER (MARCH, 1964)

	Patients	Per Cent
Asymptomatic	66	35
Improved	34	18
Not improved	47	25
Operated on for ulcer	27	14
Deaths from unrelated causes	7	3.8
Defectors from freezing program	6	3.2
*Late ulcer deaths	2	1

* 1 late death from bleeding esophageal varix; 1 late death from perforated ulcer in patient on continued cortisone therapy for rheumatoid arthritis.

of the current status of this latter group of patients. The severity of the problems dealt with is apparent by the circumstance that 14 per cent of the original group have subsequently undergone operation. Of the 189 patients, about one-fourth underwent more than a single freeze.

Convincing objective evidence for the efficacy of the procedure was the observation by our roentgenologists that in most instances in which an unequivocal ulcer crater was radiographically identified before the freeze, no crater could be found at the next follow-up, 6 to 12 weeks later. It is important to point out that healing occurred without the benefit of special diet or any ulcer medications. The only dietary restrictions imposed on the post-freeze patients were abstinence from caffeine and alcohol-containing drinks. Crater healing was observed in 75 per cent of cases following a single freeze.

Immediate post-freeze depression of acid secretory values exceeding 50 per cent was observed in the majority of patients. However, by the end of six months, the secretory levels quite uniformly returned to the pre-freeze levels. The occurrence of protracted symptomatic relief in many patients with only relatively brief periods of secretory suppression remains unexplained.

The dangers of the freezing procedure have proved to be small; we have had no deaths due to gastric freezing. The few deaths reported in the literature were due, in general, to technical errors. Occult bleeding, as reflected by a routine guaiac test, undoubtedly occurs in every patient subjected to gastric freezing. However, bleeding serious enough to necessitate hospital observation was seen in only 3.8 per cent of the patients treated by the protocol described above. In a few of these, the post-freeze bleeding necessitated transfusion. When significant hemorrhage occurred, an around-the-clock drip of ice-cold milk sufficed to control it. We have come to look upon melena as a benign type of complication.

A more worrisome problem has been the occasional occurrence of gastric ulcer secondary to freezing. This complication has occurred in 3 per cent of the patients treated to date, most of these in the earlier group. Two such ulcers perforated and required surgical closure. For the occasional penetrating post-freeze gastric ulcer, the intensive Winkelstein skim milk drip has been successfully employed. Our experience has been that such lesions heal quite readily and, in contrast to primary gastric ulcers, do not tend to recur.

New Techniques

The occasional complication and the unpredictable recurrence of symptoms have stimulated experimental efforts to improve the freezing technique. Low molecular weight dextran, given intravenously prior to the freeze, was shown in dogs to provide significant, although not complete, protection against post-freeze gastric ulcer. This observation has led to the clinical use of dextran, and it is now employed routinely just prior to freezing (1.5 Gm. per kg. body weight).

The balloon mucosal interface temperature is monitored by means of four thermocouples attached to the outer surface of the latex balloon. Data obtained in this manner provided convincing evidence that the protocol initially employed generally failed to depress mucosal temperatures below 0° C. in man.

Blood flow is the most significant source of heat to the stomach. Of the pharmacologic agents evaluated for reducing mucosal blood flow, Pitressin proved to be the most effective, the reduction in flow to the gastric mucosa of the dog attending its use being about 75 per cent. Our freezing routine now includes the intravenous administration of Pitressin before and during the procedure, 0.01 clinical unit per kg. body weight per minute, until one of the thermocouples attached to the balloon surface registers —4° C. As yet, we have been unable to secure uniform depression of the mucosal temperature as registered by all four thermocouples.

The current clinical freezing technique includes the adjuncts dextran, Pitressin, and mucosal balloon interface temperature monitoring. At present the policy is to keep the mucosal temperature at —4° C. for 20 to 25 minutes, and below 0° for a total of 40 minutes. To date 53 patients have undergone gastric freezing according to this protocol. This group of patients has obtained uniform relief of ulcer symptoms, but the follow-up period is still too brief to determine whether this new technique will provide more prolonged relief than the original method. Even with these profound mucosal temperature reductions, complete unresponsiveness to secretory stimulants has been seen in but a few patients.

Future of Gastric Freezing

Certain observations made in the dog are encouraging with regard to the possibility of inducing prolonged secretory depressions in patients. Isolated gastric pouches, Heidenhain or Pavlov, were in most instances rendered achlorhydric to all gastric secretory stimuli when frozen for one hour at an inflow temperature of −20° C. Some of these pouches remain refractory to histamine stimulation as long as 30 months after the freeze. Currently under investigation is the question of the minimum temperature reduction and duration of cold necessary to produce prolonged achlorhydria.

With the use of dextran, Pitressin, and lower mucosal temperatures, we are succeeding frequently, though not consistently, in producing histamine-fast achlorhydria in the intact canine stomach, lasting in some for intervals of two months or longer. We are hopeful that the use of larger balloons and better dispersion of the coolant will be followed by more uniform patterns of mucosal freezing.

Studies in the intact canine stomach indicate that mucosal temperatures below −6° C. sustained for ten minutes or longer invite necrosis. In addition to simple temperature depression, bacteria may also play a role in the development of post-freeze necrosis. Use of antimicrobial agents as a preventative measure is being experimentally assessed. The protective role of continuous neutralization of gastric acidity and consequent inactivation of pepsin by buffering agents for short periods following the freezing injury also is being evaluated.

Anatomic Changes

Repetitive freezing of canine stomachs using the original temperature-time criteria, twice a week or once a week, for eight episodes, has resulted in profound changes in the mucosal cell population. Table 3 enumerates these alterations. The parietal cell and chief cell reductions closely paralleled one another. The cell count depressions tended to return toward normal with the passage of time. The effect of a single episode of freezing in the intact canine stomach with gastric mucosal temperature in the −4° to −8° C. range has been studied for histologic alterations, but so far only three weeks after the freeze. The numbers of nerve cells in Auerbach's and Meissner's plexuses have also been found to be decreased following freezing. Shown in Table 3 are the relative cell counts in biopsies taken from achlorhydric Heidenhain pouches followed for as long as two years after the initial freeze.

TABLE 3.   CANINE MUCOSAL CELL COUNT CHANGES ATTENDING
GASTRIC FREEZING

	Average Per Cent			
	Mucus Neck Cells	Parietal Cells	Chief Cells	Auerbach's Plexus
I. 16 intact stomachs 3 weeks after 1 freeze	+81.9	−58.5	−61.6	−27.8
II. 7 intact stomachs 3 months after 8 freezes (2 per week)	+85.7	−61.4	−53.1	−26.4
6 months after 8 freezes (2 per week)	+46.4	−34.5	−38.8	−26.4
12 months after 8 freezes (2 per week)	+84.9	−33.0	−32.9	
III. 6 Heidenhain pouches 7 months to 2 years after a single freeze	+42.4	−74.0	−74.6	−56.1

Summary

Clinical gastric freezing is still in the study and development stage. Experience would suggest that the procedure will find a useful place in the management of some manifestations of the peptic ulcer diathesis, including duodenal ulcer, stomal ulcer, and esophagitis.

Gastric freezing has proved to be quite safe in experienced hands. Relief of pain and healing of duodenal ulcer craters have been observed with regularity. Depressions of gastric secretory activity have been short-lived and the symptomatic relief has been of unpredictable duration. Future improvement in therapeutic results is contingent largely on the development of techniques to induce more uniform depression of mucosal temperatures, and thereby more protracted depression of secretory responses. Only further laboratory experimentation and clinical trial will determine the final usefulness of gastric freezing.

References

1. Allcock, E. A., Carpenter, A. M., Bernstein, E. F., Peter, E. T., and Wangensteen, O. H.: Structural changes following gastric freezing. Surgery, 53:764, 1963.
2. Bernstein, E. F., Goodale, R. L., Jr., McFee, A. S., Madsen, A. J., Allcock, E. A., and Wangensteen, O H.: Rationale and results of gastric freezing for peptic ulcer. Am. J. Surg., 107:268, 1964.
3. Wangensteen, O. H., Root, H. D., Jenson, C. B., Imamoglu, K., and Salmon, P. A.: Depression of gastric secretion and digestion by gastric hypothermia: its clinical use in massive hematemesis. Surgery, 44:2, 1958.
4. Wangensteen, O. H., Peter, E. T., Bernstein, E. F., Walder, A. I., Sosin, H., and Madsen, A. J.: Can physiological gastrectomy be achieved by local gastric cooling? Ann. Surg., 156:579, 1962.

Acute Hemorrhage
from Duodenal Ulcer

Introduction

In the first volume of Current Surgical Management two direct surgical approaches were presented for the control of massive hemorrhage from duodenal ulcer, i.e., direct suture control of the bleeding point with delayed definitive ulcer surgery and an immediate three-quarter gastric resection. Initial mortality following direct suture control was said to vary from 1 to 8 per cent, depending upon the age of the patient. Experience across the country has indicated that rebleeding in these patients is a constant threat, and that the majority eventually require either emergency or elective gastrectomy for control of the ulcer diathesis. Available data therefore makes it difficult to determine the actual overall mortality for this method of management. The operative mortality for immediate subtotal gastrectomy at that time and as reported by Hale and Stewart was 12.9 per cent.

The scope of the problem has now broadened, and the necessity of reoperation in the first instance and problems of postoperative nutrition and unpleasant symptomatology (dumping) attributable to more extensive gastric operations have altered both of these approaches. Finally, a general concern over the end results of surgery for bleeding duodenal ulcer has led a number of investigators to study and evaluate an additional non-operative technique applicable not only to control of hemorrhage, but also aimed at inhibiting the acid-peptic secretory activity of the stomach, namely, gastric freezing.

One of the most popular surgical treatments for bleeding duodenal ulcer at the present time embodies the principle of direct suture control of the bleeding point and includes steps to control both the cephalic and gastric phases of gastric secretion by vagotomy and pyloroplasty. Mortality is reported to be only 4.4 per cent (4 deaths out of 90 patients). A second contributor concerned with the overall end result following operation for acute hemorrhage from duodenal ulcer continues to advocate subtotal gastrectomy, however, with a lesser resection and combined with truncal vagotomy,

Page 311

thus avoiding most of the sequelae of extensive gastric resection. This author also compares the results following hemigastrectomy and vagotomy as compared with vagotomy and pyloroplasty in the same institution: four out of 22 patients succumbed following vagotomy and pyloroplasty; in three of these bleeding had recurred, leading to renal and cardiovascular problems with uremia and cardiac arrest in two and aspiration in one. The mortality following hemigastrectomy and vagotomy in 38 patients was 7.8 per cent. The average age for both groups of patients was only 50.7 years and makes one wonder if some adjunctive treatment was not in vogue or under study at the time.

A third approach includes gastric cooling either with or without subsequent operation. Excluding three moribund patients, Nicoloff reports on 27 patients with massive hemorrhage from duodenal ulcer and with a hospital mortality of 15.1 per cent (5 of 27). The hemorrhage was not controlled by gastric cooling in 22.6 per cent. Seven of the patients controlled by gastric freezing came to elective operation at a later time with one death (14.3 per cent). Sixteen of 23 have not required surgical intervention. Hemorrhage was not controlled in 7 of the 27 patients. All of them were operated upon with 4 deaths (57.2 per cent).

In considering the evidence for and against each method, it should be remembered that variations in the reported results may represent the degree of adherence to a strict criteria for surgical intervention and the incidence and severity of associated conditions, rather than the merits of the treatment per se.

E. H. E.

Suture Ligation, Pyloroplasty, and Vagotomy in the Treatment of Acute Hemorrhage from Duodenal Ulcer

Joseph A. Weinberg

University of California, Los Angeles

Rationale

It is only in recent years that surgical therapy has been generally accepted as the preferred method of dealing with the emergency of acute massive hemorrhage complicating duodenal ulcer. Up to the middle of the century, the results with surgical therapy were so poor that it was used mostly as a last resort measure after nonsurgical methods had failed.

With recent surgical improvements, including better anesthesia and better preoperative and postoperative care, the general attitude regarding therapy for the massively bleeding ulcer has changed, and surgical therapy, usually in the form of partial gastric resection, is now widely accepted in preference to medical therapy. But even with its advantages over non-surgical methods, partial gastric resection is far from being a satisfactory answer to the problem. The patient is usually of advanced age and is poorly prepared to withstand the ordeal of a difficult dissection. He is often afflicted with associated chronic debilitating disease. Chronic alco-holism, cirrhosis, cardiac impairment, pulmonary emphysema, and gen-eralized arteriosclerosis are common associated disorders.

Resective surgery in the presence of massive hemorrhage from duode-nal ulcer is hazardous, not only because of the poor condition of the patient resulting from immediate massive blood loss and chronic debilitating disease, but even more because of the technical difficulties imposed by the pathologic changes peculiar to the profusely bleeding chronic duodenal ulcer. The pylorus and first part of the duodenum are fixed and indurated by scar tissue. Neighboring structures, including the common bile duct

Page 313

and the blood vessels that supply the area, are often obscured by congestion and edema, and there is usually deep penetration of the ulcer into the adjacent pancreas. These pathologic alterations make resection a prolonged difficult procedure, and its successful completion is often little less than a surgical feat. Under these conditions, gastric resection can hardly be accepted as a suitable procedure if the emergency can be controlled with a less hazardous procedure.

The favorable experiences reported for vagotomy and pyloroplasty in dealing with other complications of duodenal ulcer, and the relative ease with which ligation of the bleeding vessel is added, led us to adopt this method of treatment beginning in 1949. The theoretical advantages have been confirmed by practical application in 91 patients. The crucial pyloroduodenal area is little disturbed during ligation and pyloroplasty. Mobilization of the duodenal segment by the Kocher maneuver is not only unnecessary, but is contraindicated because of possible injury to the obscured common duct and other adjacent structures.

Technique

The operation of ligation, pyloroplasty, and vagotomy does not require special skill, but it does require adherence to prescribed technical details. This applies particularly to the ligation of the bleeding vessel.[4, 5] Details that are of special importance are described in the paragraphs that follow.

1. Preparation for the operation is started when the patient is first seen and a tentative diagnosis of massively bleeding duodenal ulcer is made. The timing of the operation is as important as the operation itself. There should be no delay if the bleeding is unremitting. It is our policy to operate immediately if bleeding continues after three transfusions in 12 hours or six transfusions during one hospitalization. The patient with rebleeding after arrest for several days is in the same category as the patient with continuous bleeding. Adequate transfusions are given during the preparation and are continued during the surgical procedure. A reduced volume of circulating blood may lead to cardiac arrest, especially in the patient with chronic cardiac disease.

2. If the diagnosis is not already established, an emergency gastroduodenal radiologic examination with barium or Diodrast contrast medium is made while the operating room is being prepared.

3. A nasogastric tube is inserted and remains in place during the operation to afford easy identification of the esophagus in performing the vagotomy. It is also a means of estimating bleeding before the operation.

4. Gauze packing is placed in the mouth around the endotracheal anesthesia tube as a precaution against fatal aspiration of vomited blood.

5. An abdominal incision is made which gives adequate exposure of the pyloroduodenal and esophageal hiatal areas. A high transverse abdomi-

nal incision serves well for this purpose, but the choice between transverse and longitudinal is best determined by the surgeon's personal experience.

6. The bleeding vessel is exposed through a pyloroplasty incision, 7 or 8 cm. in length, which crosses the pyloric sphincter on the anterior aspect of the pyloroduodenal segment. Allis forceps are placed around the thickened edge of the ulcer or around the pyloroplasty wound to improve exposure for the ligation.

7. The needle for suture ligation of the bleeding point must be small enough for easy manipulation in the limited working space, yet large enough to encompass the bleeding site. It must be stout enough to resist breakage in its passage through the indurated ulcer bed. A No. 5 half-circle Mayo needle fulfills these requirements. The ligation is made with No. 20 surgical cotton suture or other nonabsorbable suture material of similar tensile strength. Gut suture material is definitely contraindicated because of its susceptibility to weakening by the lytic action of the digestive juices. A single deep figure-of-eight suture is usually sufficient to arrest the bleeding.

8. The pyloroplasty wound is closed in the Heineke-Mikulicz manner, except that a single row of interrupted nonabsorbable sutures is used instead of multiple rows. This is to avoid infolding, which impairs the lumen and defeats the purpose of the pyloroplasty.

9. A truncal vagotomy is performed according to the Dragstedt principle. It is unwise to postpone the vagotomy for a later stage, as bleeding may recur before it is accomplished.

Results

Experience with ligation, pyloroplasty, and vagotomy has proved its effectiveness in arresting the bleeding and healing the ulcer in acute massive hemorrhage complicating duodenal ulcer. We have now performed 91 operations on patients who meet the requirements for inclusion in the massive hemorrhage group. The basic requirements are: (1) evidence of massive bleeding at the time of operation, (2) hemorrhagic shock or impending shock manifested by sudden drop in blood pressure, rapid pulse and a low hematocrit reading, generally less than 30 mg. per cent, (3) multiple transfusions prior to the time of operation, and (4) passage of gross blood per rectum.

There have been four surgical deaths.[6] Surgical deaths are those occurring at any time in the hospital during the postoperative period, and those occurring after discharge from the hospital within 30 days after the operation. The deaths were in severely debilitated patients past the age of 60. Two suffered from chronic alcoholism and were in delirium tremens during the surgical period. There were others in comparable serious condition who survived the operation. Other surgeons, using similar criteria for massive hemorrhage and using the same principle of treatment, have reported similar experiences.[1-3] This is in contrast to the generally reported mortality of 10 to 25 per cent or higher with partial gastric resection in cases of corresponding severity.

Regarding surgical complications attributable to operative technique, these have been rare and relatively minor. There have been no occurrences of gastric or intestinal wound disruption, common bile duct injury, or traumatic pancreatitis, all of which are hazards with resection. Rebleeding occurred in two of the fatalities mentioned above. Except for these cases, rebleeding has not been a problem.

Summary

The combination of ligation, pyloroplasty, and vagotomy is an effective means of dealing with life-threatening acute massive hemorrhage complicating chronic duodenal ulcer. It is a relatively simple procedure compared to partial gastric resection, as it avoids the hazards of a traumatizing dissection in a field of induration, penetrating ulceration, and edema in a patient weakened by sudden depletion of blood.

The operation does not require special skill, but it demands adherence to prescribed technical details for its success.

References

1. Brizzolara, L. G.: Discussion of presentation by Weinberg on treatment of massively bleeding duodenal ulcer by ligation, pyloroplasty and vagotomy. Am. J. Surg., *102*:164, 1961.
2. Farris, J.: Discussion of presentation by Weinberg on treatment of massively bleeding duodenal ulcer by ligation, pyloroplasty and vagotomy. Am. J. Surg., *102*:164, 1961.
3. Foster, J. H., Hickok, D. F., and Dunphy, J. E.: Factors influencing mortality following emergency operation for massive upper gastrointestinal hemorrhage. Surg., Gynec. and Obst., *117*:257, 1963.
4. Weinberg, J. A.: Treatment of massively bleeding duodenal ulcer by ligation, pyloroplasty and vagotomy. Am. J. Surg., *102*:158, 1961.
5. Weinberg, J. A.: Ligating the vessel in the bleeding duodenal ulcer. West. J. Surg., *70*:291, 1962.
6. Weinberg, J. A.: Pyloroplasty and vagotomy for duodenal ulcer. Current Problems in Surgery. April, 1964, Monthly Clinical Monographs. Year Book Medical Publishers, Chicago.

Hemigastrectomy
with Vagotomy for Acute
Hemorrhage from Duodenal Ulcer

Roger D. Williams *and* George N. Grant

Ohio State University Hospitals

The surgical treatment for acute hemorrhage from duodenal ulcer should stop the bleeding immediately, prevent rebleeding, and have a low ulcer recurrence rate. The magnitude of the procedure is significant only if it increases mortality. Since recurrent hemorrhage will require further surgery with its attendant serious risk, one procedure should suffice. To properly select this procedure requires early surgery, with careful preoperative management of acute hemorrhage and attention to the associated diseases that significantly affect morbidity and mortality.

The Operation Is Not the Major Cause of Mortality

Associated diseases, procrastination that allows prolonged or repeated hemorrhages, and omission of the details in preparation or postoperative care are the significant factors affecting surgical morbidity and mortality. The results of an elective procedure cannot be compared with the same operation when it is used to control hemorrhage. There is no real correlation between hemoglobin values and the presence of shock,[1, 2] unless surgery becomes necessary to control hemorrhage. Therefore, blood loss exceeding 3 liters in 24 hours, repeated hemorrhages while under observation and medical treatment, and bleeding beyond 48 hours become more important considerations than the specific surgical procedure.[3]

With the exception of postoperative rebleeding, associated diseases cause more deaths than complications directly related to the surgical procedure.[1, 4, 5] Since the patient with duodenal ulcer hemorrhage is usually past 50,[6] several factors affect the operative risk. Renal, cardiac, cerebrovascular, and pulmonary lesions account for the majority of postoperative deaths. The prolonged need for a nasogastric tube, bed rest, or vomiting with possible aspiration compound the tendency of these patients to develop atelectasis and pneumonia. Repeated hypotensive episodes, blood in the intestinal tract, and both overtransfusion and undertransfusion add to the incidence of azotemia, cardiac failure, and cerebral or coronary artery occlusion.

Arguments for Hemigastrectomy and Vagotomy

The operation combining hemigastrectomy and vagotomy is the simplest way to stop immediate hemorrhage, and to prevent early rebleeding and most late recurrent ulcers. Its selection is based on these criteria, which are emphasized by the disappointments encountered with lesser procedures.

Excision of the ulcer is important in the prevention of early postoperative rebleeding. This can be accomplished in most cases without great difficulty when hemigastrectomy is performed. When the ulcer involves the second or third portion of the duodenum, it may be oversewn, and a Billroth II procedure will prevent further acid-peptic digestion. Ligating the bleeder or oversewing the ulcer is difficult because of the severe induration and friability, which prevents prolonged control of bleeding if acid-peptic activity continues.

Excision of the antrum is important in the prevention of both early rebleeding and late ulcer recurrence. It is well established that the incidence of recurrent ulceration is less than with vagotomy and pyloroplasty or gastroenterostomy.[7, 8] Although free acid may exist for a short while after hemigastrectomy and vagotomy,[9] the dangers of prolonged gastric distention, slow emptying, and consequently greater acid production exists when the antrum is not excised.

Hemigastrectomy is not technically difficult, a factor important to low mortality with elective as well as emergency surgery. The reported mortality of 2 or 3 per cent with elective hemigastrectomy and vagotomy, although higher than that with vagotomy and pyloroplasty, is relatively insignificant when compared with the total mortality with upper gastrointestinal bleeding.[1, 4, 5] Since other factors are so important in the high mortality with acute duodenal hemorrhage, hemigastrectomy cannot be condemned as too radical. It is not associated with the late sequelae of extensive gastric resection.

Management and Technique

Early surgery in the patient with continuous bleeding from a duodenal ulcer depends upon detailed records with careful observation. A specific hemorrhage sheet is used to record response to therapy every 4 hours.[3] Initial studies must include bleeding and clotting time, platelet count, prothrombin, and BSP retention to eliminate a hemorrhagic disorder as a cause of continued bleeding. A nasogastric tube is inserted, the stomach washed with saline, and continuous mild suction applied. This serves to decrease the acid reaching the ulcer, prevent gastric distention and vomiting, and permit monitoring of new or continued bleeding. In addition to frequent checks of pulse, a plan of action based on blood loss is established.

Assuming that the cause of bleeding is known or will be established by emergency upper gastrointestinal radiography, the requirements of blood replacement determine the time or need for surgery.[3, 10] Six units (3000 cc.) of blood are kept constantly available in the hospital blood bank. The hemoglobin and hematocrit are brought to 11 Gm. and 35 per cent respectively, based upon the estimated blood deficit. Patients who require over 6 units in the first 24 hours, more than 500 cc. per 8-hour period, transfusions beyond a 48-hour period, or transfusions for a second hemorrhage while in the hospital are candidates for emergency surgery. While gastric cooling may decrease the number requiring surgery in the first 48 hours, it will not permit procrastination in the continued bleeder or after rebleeding.

The Billroth I procedure is preferred with vagotomy because of technical simplicity and fewer sequelae. A midline incision allows rapid entrance into the abdomen, pressure control of hemorrhage, and ready access to the esophagus and vagi after the left lobe of the liver is separated from its diaphragmatic attachment. Removal of the omentum from its colonic attachments widely to the left, a liberal Kocher maneuver, and section of the posterosuperior peritoneum, which binds spleen and upper stomach to the diaphragm, prevent tension on the suture line. The gastric mid-point is determined by the third gastric vein down on the lesser curvature and the closest proximity of gastroepiploic vessels and gastric wall on the greater curvature.[11] In rare cases the Billroth II procedure, which consists of turning in the duodenal stump after suturing the ulcer base, may be required.

Results

Over the past 13 years several procedures have been utilized to control acute hemorrhage from duodenal ulcer. In more recent years vagotomy and pyloroplasty have been used in the hope that a lesser procedure would improve these results. The results of hemigastrectomy and vagotomy are compared with those of vagotomy and pyloroplasty in Table 1. This small series includes only those with duodenal ulcer in whom surgery was performed to control acute hemorrhage. The lower mortality with hemigastrectomy and vagotomy is significant. There is little difference in the average age of the two groups. Of greater importance is the fact

TABLE 1. ACUTE HEMORRHAGE FROM DUODENAL ULCER (1950–63)

	Hemigastrectomy and Vagotomy	Vagotomy and Pyloroplasty
Total	38	22
Ulcer excised	33	1
Oversewn	5	21
Mortality	3(7.8%)	4(18.1%)
Rebled	1	3*
Average age	52.2 yrs.	48.8 yrs.

* 2 deaths

that in three patients there was rebleeding following vagotomy and pyloro-plasty. This complication also occurred in one of those patients in whom the ulcer was not excised when hemigastrectomy and vagotomy were per-formed. These results emphasize the need for ulcer excision.

The type of operation did not contribute significantly to the three deaths after hemigastrectomy and vagotomy. Renal and cardiovascular problems with uremia and cardiac arrest caused two deaths. Both patients were considered "poor risks," and, because of pre-existing uremia and poor cardiac status, were permitted to bleed beyond the time usually per-mitted before emergency surgery is indicated. In the third patient, there was rebleeding soon after surgery from the remaining ulcer bed; he vom-ited and aspirated some material. A small suture line leak causing local peritonitis was another complication in this patient.

Rebleeding was a significant factor in two of the four deaths following vagotomy and pyloroplasty. In a third patient there was leakage from the suture line. In the fourth patient, perforation of another duodenal ulcer in the postoperative period followed failure of vagotomy and pyloroplasty to control the ulcer diathesis. Autopsy did not show an endocrine tumor, although there was hyperplasia of the parathyroid glands.

Summary

Hemigastrectomy with vagotomy is the preferred operation in the treatment of acute hemorrhage from duodenal ulcer because it stops hem-orrhage immediately, prevents early rebleeding, and prevents most recur-rent ulcers. A lesser procedure can be justified only if it is associated with a lower morbidity and mortality. Because of frequent recurrent hemorrhage after vagotomy and pyloroplasty, our mortality has been higher than with hemigastrectomy and vagotomy. Associated diseases play a major role in mortality regardless of the surgical procedure. The safer, and often easier, method of controlling hemorrhage is by excision of the ulcer. Hemigas-trectomy, technically less difficult than subtotal gastrectomy, has a low incidence of late sequelae or recurrent ulceration.

References

1. Mitty, W. F., Breen, F. J., Wallace, R., and Grace, W. J.: Factors influencing mortality in bleeding peptic ulcer. Am. J. Digest. Dis., 6:389, 365, 400, 1961.
2. Bennett, J. M., and Whiteside, W.: Acute upper gastrointestinal hemorrhage in patients over 65 years of age. Arch. Surg., 81:504, 1960.
3. Elliott, D. W., Hartle, R., Marshall, F., and Zollinger, R. M.: Response to transfusion as guide in management of upper gastrointestinal hemorrhage. Arch. Surg., 77:386, 1958.
4. Kelley, H. G., Grant, G. N., and Elliott, D. W.: Massive gastroduodenal hemorrhage. Arch. Surg., 87:6, 1963.
5. Darin, J. C., Polacek, M. A., and Ellison, E. H.: Surgical mortality of massive hemorrhage from peptic ulcer. Arch. Surg., 83:71, 1961.
6. Palumbo, L. T., and Sharpe, W. S.: Partial gastrectomy for chronic duodenal ulcer with hemorrhage. Surgery, 49:585, 1961.
7. Scott, H. W., Jr., Herrington, J. L., Jr., Edwards, L. W., Shull, H. J., Stephenson, S. E., Jr., Sawyers, J. L., and Classen, K.: Results of vagotomy and antral resection in surgical treatment of duodenal ulcer. Gastroenterology, 39:590, 1960.
8. Farmer, D. A., Harrower, H. W., and Smithwick, R. H.: Hemigastrectomy and vagotomy for duodenal ulcer: an evaluation. Am. J. Digest. Dis., 7:195, 1962.
9. Bauer, A. R., Elliott, D. W., and Zollinger, R. M.: Free gastric acid following hemigastrectomy with vagotomy. Ann. Surg., 154:281, 1961.
10. Hoerr, F. O., Dunphy, J. E., and Gray, S. J.: The place of surgery in the emergency treatment of acute massive upper gastrointestinal hemorrhage. Surg., Gynec. and Obst., 87:338, 1948.
11. Zollinger, R. M., and Williams, R. D.: Considerations in surgical treatment for duodenal ulcer. J.A.M.A., 160:367, 1956.

Gastric Cooling: A Method for
Control of Massive Gastric Hemorrhage*

Demetre M. Nicoloff, Robert L. Goodale, Jr., *and*
Owen H. Wangensteen
University of Minnesota Medical School

The numerous articles written each year on the management of patients with massive gastrointestinal hemorrhage, and the large mortality attending care of this emergency suggested the need for a new look at the problem.[1-3]

In 1952, hemorrhage was reported as responsible for 46 per cent of the deaths from peptic ulcer in Minnesota.[4] Massive hemorrhage from stress ulcer, esophageal varices, and postoperative bleeding continue to have an even higher mortality. Any method used to control bleeding under the circumstance of massive gastric hemorrhage should make its impact felt upon the problem. At the University of Minnesota, since May 1958, local gastric hypothermia has been employed in the management of gastric bleeding. It appears to offer an effective method for control of hemorrhage in a high proportion of patients bleeding from duodenal ulcer, and with lesser regularity in patients bleeding from gastric ulcer, steroid ulcer, and esophageal varices. "Control of hemorrhage" means that bleeding was completely stopped for at least 24 hours, vital signs recovered, and the hemoglobin attending transfusion was sustained at a satisfactory level (12 Gm. or more).

Rationale

Experimental evidence supporting the clinical use of gastric hypothermia has shown that local gastric hypothermia (1) decreases the acid-peptic activity of gastric juice, (2) inhibits the secretion of hydrochloric acid from the parietal cells, (3) inhibits the release of pepsinogen granules from the chief cells, (4) reduces considerably gastric and duodenal blood

* This work was supported by Grants from the U.S.P.H.S., the Hartford Foundation, and the Donald J. Cowling Fund for Surgical Research.

flow, and (5) decreases greatly gastric motility.[5, 6] All these factors play an important role in the treatment of massive gastrointestinal bleeding.

It is well known that the mortality rate of patients undergoing emergency surgery for gastrointestinal hemorrhage is much higher than in patients whose operations are elective procedures.[7, 8] With hemorrhage controlled by local gastric hypothermia, one can replace the patient's blood volume, correct fluid and electrolyte disturbances, and begin treatment of any other coexistent diseases, such as heart failure, diabetes, or liver disease. Such correction ensures better tolerance of operation, should it be necessary, and should also diminish the incidence of postoperative complications.

The site of bleeding, which may be a matter of conjecture during early management, also may be difficult to determine when emergency surgery is performed. If gastric hypothermia succeeds in controlling the hemorrhage, studies can be done to ascertain the nature and location of the lesion and more effective definitive therapy planned and executed. Also, there are patients whose general condition is such that they are very poor risks for operation.

Indications

Patients accepted for this mode of management are those who failed to respond to the usual corrective methods of treatment, which include sedation, anticholinergic drugs, milk drip, nasogastric suction, and transfusions. The criteria we have employed as guides to using local gastric hypothermia have been (1) shock, manifested by blood pressure of less than 90 mm. Hg and tachycardia, (2) continuing hemorrhage with hemoglobin less than 10 Gm., and (3) necessity to continue transfusion in order to support a falling blood pressure.

Present Apparatus

Gastric hypothermia units are commercially available and consist essentially of a refrigeration unit, reservoir, and water pump. A suitable valvular system is used so that fluid can be pumped into the balloon and replaced by a similar volume from a reservoir. The patient is put on a warming blanket to maintain body temperature at the level desired. Since the technique of using gastric hypothermia is described in detail elsewhere, it will not be discussed here.[9]

Results

Since 1958, we have treated 122 cases of massive gastrointestinal hemorrhage with local gastric or esophagogastric cooling. The results are

given in Tables 1 and 2. Because the achievement differs in the various
groups, each will be discussed separately.

Duodenal Ulcer

Twenty-four of 31 patients (77.4 per cent) with the established diagnosis of duodenal ulcer and massive hematemesis were controlled with
local gastric hypothermia. Seventeen (54.8 per cent) were 60 years old
or older. Fourteen patients (45.3 per cent) subsequently had surgery, with
five patients dying in the postoperative period, giving an overall postoperative mortality rate of 35.6 per cent. However, there was only one
postoperative death in the seven patients in whom hemorrhage was controlled with local gastric hypothermia, whereas there were four deaths
in the seven patients in whom hemorrhage was not controlled. The mortality rates in these two groups were 14.3 per cent and 57.2 per cent
respectively. Beyond the obvious decrease in operative mortality, 17 patients (54.7 per cent) did not need surgery. Of these 17 patients, seven later
accepted gastric freeze when it became available, and only one of the seven
subsequently required surgery.

Of the 31 patients in the group, eight died, of which five were postoperative deaths. The remaining three were not operated upon. Hemorrhage was controlled in each of these three patients, but death was due
to complications existing prior to treatment for the bleeding episode.
One patient died of staphylococcal pneumonia, one of severe emphysema
and pneumonia, and the third of respiratory insufficiency due to obesity
(450 pounds). If all eight are counted as deaths due to bleeding duodenal
ulcer, the mortality rate is 25.8 per cent. If one excludes the three dying
from pre-existing disease, the mortality rate is 16.1 per cent.

Gastric Ulcer

Of the 21 patients seen with hematemesis and a diagnosis of gastric
ulcer verified by x-ray or operation, bleeding was controlled with local
gastric hypothermia in 11 (52.4 per cent). Fifteen of the patients (71.4
per cent) were more than 60 years of age. Sixteen patients underwent
surgery. In 6 of that number, hemorrhage was controlled by cooling.
In the remaining 10, cooling failed to control bleeding. Only one patient
in the group in which hemorrhage was controlled died in the postoperative
period (16.7 per cent mortality). In the group of 10 patients in whom
cooling failed to control hemorrhage, 7 died in the postoperative period
(70 per cent mortality). This mortality rate is higher than that which
is usually reported.[1, 3] Twelve of this entire group expired while in the
hospital (a mortality rate of 57.2 per cent). However, at the time of
cooling, four of these patients were moribund from pre-existing disease.
If these patients are excluded, the mortality rate would then be 38.1
per cent.

TABLE 1. RESULTS OF GASTRIC COOLING SINCE 1958

Diagnosis	Number Patients	Average Age	Avg. Amt. Blood Given Prior to Cooling (ml.)	Patients Controlled		Patients in Shock		Hospital Mortality		Number Patients Moribund Prior to Cooling	Corrected Hospital Mortality	
				Number	Per Cent	Number	Per Cent	Number	Per Cent		Number	Per Cent
Duodenal ulcer	31	66	3600	24	77.4	24	77.4	8	25.8	3	5	16.1
Gastric ulcer	21	68	4000	11	52.4	16	76.2	12	57.2	4	8	38.1
Esophageal varices	21	48	4500	13	61.9	17	81	15	71.5	6	9	42.8
Postoperative bleeding	24	57	6500	15	62.5	23	95.8	14	58.3	8	6	25
Steroid ulcer	5	29	2500	3	60	5	100	4	80	2	2	40
Erosive gastritis	7	57	3500	5	71.4	7	100	4	57.2	0	4	57.2
Gastric carcinoma	6	56	5000	4	66.6	5	83.3	4	66.6	2	2	33.3
Hemorrhagic dyscrasia	5	58	2900	4	80	5	100	3	60	1	2	40
Esophageal ulcer	2	65	2500	2	100	2	100	2	100	1	1	50
										Per Cent		
Total	122	56	3900	81	66.4	104	85.4	66	54.2	27	22.1	39	32.1
All cases in 1963	23	—	——	14	60.8	20	87	6	26.1	2	22.1	4	17.4

TABLE 2. OPERATIVE MORTALITY FOLLOWING GASTRIC COOLING SINCE 1958

Diagnosis	Patients Operated on		Overall Operative Mortality		Number Patients Controlled Prior to Surgery	Operative Mortality of Controlled Patients		Number Patients Not Controlled Prior to Surgery	Op. Mortality of Patients Not Controlled	
	Number	Per Cent	Number	Per Cent		Number	Per Cent		Number	Per Cent
Duodenal ulcer	14	45.3	5	35.7	7	1	14.3	7	4	57.2
Gastric ulcer	16	76.2	8	50	6	1	16.7	10	7	70
Esophageal varices	18	85.8	12	66.7	11	7	63.6	7	7	100
Postoperative bleeding	9	37.5	5	55.6	3	—	—	6	5	83.3
Steroid ulcer	1	20	1	100	1	1	100	—	—	—
Erosive gastritis	5	71.4	3	60	3	1	33.3	2	2	100
Gastric carcinoma	2	33.3	0		2	0		—	—	—
Hemorrhagic dyscrasia	2	40	1	50	2	1	50	—	—	—
Total	67	54.9	35	52.3	35	12	34.2	32	25	78.2
All cases in 1963	14	60.8	3	21.4	6	1	16.7	8	2	25

Esophageal Varices

Bleeding was controlled by local esophagogastric cooling in 13 (61.9 per cent) of the 21 patients seen with the established diagnosis of esophageal varices and massive hematemesis. Five patients (23.8 per cent) were 60 years of age or older. In five patients, the Sengstaken-Blakemore tube was unsuccessful. Three of these were subsequently controlled by local esophagogastric hypothermia. Even so, 15 of the 21 patients expired during hospitalization with an overall mortality rate of 71.5 per cent. Comparing the mortality rates of the group in which hemorrhage was controlled with the group in which it was not, one finds that the mortality rates were 69.2 per cent and 75 per cent respectively. In the group in which hemorrhage was controlled, four of the nine deaths were due to hemorrhage. In one of these four patients a shunt was not technically possible, and two patients expired from hemorrhage after the shunt was established. In one patient rebleeding occurred and he expired before cooling could be reinstituted. In the group in which hemorrhage was not controlled all deaths were due to hemorrhage. It is apparent that the ultimate prognosis of patients with cirrhosis and bleeding varices is poor, even though esophagogastric cooling effectively controls bleeding in many instances. Many other problems determine the patient's ability to survive, the severity of the liver disease playing the major role in the ultimate prognosis of these patients. In two of the patients, initially controlled, rebleeding occurred within 24 hours, an occurrence suggesting that one would do well to weigh the consideration of performing a portacaval shunt or splenorenal shunt immediately on discontinuance of cooling.

Since the operative mortality rate is high in both the controlled and uncontrolled groups, an attempt is being made to minimize the need for surgery in this group by freezing the esophageal mucosa in patients who have recently had severe varix bleeding. The present experience, though small, is encouraging. It is believed that multiple episodes of esophageal freezing may toughen the mucosa and provide better cover for the varices.

Postoperative Bleeding

Twenty-four patients developed massive hematemesis following severe trauma or in the postoperative period. Ten of these patients (41.7 per cent) were 60 years old or older. Bleeding was controlled in 15 (62.5 per cent) of these patients. The lesions responsible for the bleeding varied: gastric ulcer, 6 patients; gastric erosion, 8 patients; diffuse erosive gastritis, 5 patients; and hemorrhagic gastritis, 5 patients.

Three patients in the controlled group and six in the uncontrolled group underwent surgery. Five patients died following the surgical procedures, giving a post-surgical mortality rate of 55.6 per cent. All of these deaths occurred in patients who did not respond to local gastric hypothermia. The mortality rates for the controlled group as compared to the noncontrolled group were 46.6 per cent and 77.8 per cent respectively, the mortality rate of this entire group being 58.3 per cent. Of the 14 patients who expired in this group, 8 were moribund from a desperate postoperative surgical situation. Several of these patients had severe sepsis and bacteremia. If these are excluded the hospital mortality rate would be 25 per cent. The above figures indicate that gastric hypothermia does improve the prospects for this group of patients, whose condition often strikes the observer as virtually hopeless.

Steroid Ulcer

Five of the patients were on steroid therapy just prior to or during the episode of hematemesis. Hemorrhage was controlled in three (60 per cent) of these patients. This group of steroid ulcers demands special consideration. It would appear that the steroid ulcer represents a special entity somewhat apart from the usual peptic ulcer. Two patients experienced rebleeding two days after the control of the initial hemorrhage. These experiences have led us to advise operation in the immediate post-cooling period in such patients. Rebleeding is much more probable in this type of ulcer than after cooling for a chronic duodenal or gastric ulcer.

Erosive Gastritis

In seven patients whose ages ranged between 26 and 74 years (average 57), hemorrhage was controlled in 5 (71.4 per cent) by local gastric cooling. Operations were performed on five of these patients; 2 with uncontrolled hemorrhage and 3 with hemorrhage controlled by gastric hypothermia. Only one of the patients in the controlled group died following surgery, whereas both patients in the uncontrolled group died in the postoperative period.

Gastric Carcinoma

Control was achieved in 4 of these patients (66.6 per cent). If the immediate outlook from the extent of the cancer in these patients is very poor, we do not advocate the use of cooling. If the patient has a potentially operable lesion, once control of hemorrhage has been achieved, the patient should be taken to the operating room for resection without delay.

Bleeding Dyscrasia

In this group gastric hypothermia is principally a palliative procedure, since the disease itself is life-threatening. At the same time patients in this group have a very strong contraindication to surgery. Therefore, any means that would prevent the necessity of surgery is helpful in their management. In four of the five patients the hemorrhage was controlled.

However, three of the patients died of their disease and complications unrelated to gastric hemorrhage.

Complications

One disastrous complication during cooling has occurred in these five and one-half years. While cooling a cirrhotic patient with esophageal varices an undetected air leak developed which displaced the fluid from the reservoir machine into the balloon. This allowed 1400 cc. of fluid to enter the balloon and burst the stomach. The patient was taken to the operating room but because of poor liver function, general condition, and ensuing postoperative complications, the patent expired. Steps were taken immediately to preclude the recurrence of such overfilling of the balloon by installation of a safety switch, which automatically shuts off the entire unit when 75 cc. of fluid is lost or displaced by air in the main reservoir. It is always necessary to observe caution in positioning and inflating the balloon. Moreover, during cooling these patients are watched closely by a physician to ensure their comfort and to note that the apparatus is working normally and optimally at all times.

Discussion

The results of gastric cooling for massive hemorrhage have been presented for a 5½-year period at the University of Minnesota (May 1958 to January 1964). There is no doubt that the operative mortality rate is lessened by controlling the hemorrhage prior to surgery in all the groups represented except esophageal varices (15.5 per cent for gastroduodenal ulcers). This conclusion is supported also in the results reported by others.[10, 11] Kelly, Grant, and Elliott at the University of Ohio have not only shown a decrease in the mortality, but also state that whereas emergency operations were necessary in 40 per cent of the patients prior to local gastric cooling, such procedures are now required in only 20 per cent.[11] In addition to converting the operative procedure from an emergency to an elective procedure and decreasing the operative mortality rate, we have been gratified to observe that 55 patients, or 45.1 per cent, did not require surgery. In other words, if these 55 patients had been submitted to emergency procedures, published mortality figures suggest that a mortality in the area of 25 per cent might have been anticipated in this group.[1, 3, 8, 11–13]

In Table 1 are listed the overall mortality rates in each of the groups. The patients moribund from another disease existing prior to hemorrhage and the institution of gastric cooling are listed in a special column. A large fraction of the mortality is accountable to this group, examples of which are to be noted especially in massive hemorrhage from gastric ulcer, steroid ulcer, esophageal varices, and the postoperative hemorrhage group. All patients must be considered in evaluating the efficacy of any method in controlling hemorrhage. The failure rate will always be high in patients whose plight is almost beyond hope and in whom any therapy at the time carries overtones of heroic and desperate efforts. The salvage rate in this group is low, but justifies the effort.

It is a very chastening experience to observe how high the operative mortality is in patients with massive hemorrhage when gastric cooling failed to control bleeding. However, a review of the literature serves to indicate that it is a common and universal problem. Welch of Boston, in two recent papers, reports the experience of the Massachusetts General Hospital with 335 patients, admitted because of upper gastrointestinal hemorrhage. The overall mortality was 16.4 per cent[14]; in patients presenting with massive hemorrhage, the mortality was 26.4 per cent. The operative mortality in the group of patients with massive hemorrhage (31 per cent) was observed to be four times that occurring in patients with mild or moderate hemorrhage.[15] All patients in our series reported upon herein fall in the category of massive hemorrhage as defined by Welch. Too often, these are frightening and desperate situations in which it is not easy for the clinician to attain satisfying results. Our own results suggest that increased experience in gastric cooling is making its impress felt. During the past year, the overall hospital mortality has decreased considerably (see Tables 1 and 2). In this accomplishment, the following items have played a role:

1. Realization that in some instances cooling only slows hemorrhage, and surgery should be performed as soon as it becomes apparent that cooling will not suffice. The operative mortality rate is increased by protracted unsuccessful efforts to control hemorrhage with gastric cooling. From past experience, it is now our practice to discontinue cooling and resort to surgery if control with gastric cooling is not attained within 2 to 4 hours.

2. Familiarization of the resident staff with the technique of cooling and the prevention of pulmonary complications, which are known to accompany any gastric intubation and prolonged use of cooling. These circumstances require constant and vigorous care and clearance of the tracheobronchial tree during the entire period of cooling and maintenance of the patient in a semisitting position.

Pitressin has enjoyed extensive trial in the management of bleeding from esophageal varices in many hands.[16, 17] Recent studies suggest very definitely that Pitressin reduces gastric blood flow, and it is recommended for all patients with massive gastric hemorrhage.[18, 19, 20]

Summary and Conclusions

Local gastric hypothermia has been shown experimentally to reverse many of the factors responsible for hemorrhage in the peptic ulcer diathesis. It is an especially effective agent in the management and control of massive hemorrhage from a variety of manifestations of the peptic ulcer diathesis. Massive gastric hemorrhage occurring postoperatively in patients is essentially a stress ulcer phenomenon. In five instances the massive hemorrhage following operation in which sepsis had intervened was found to be caused by hemorrhagic gastritis. Massive hemorrhage occurring from gastric ulcer, steroid ulcer, and gastric carcinoma, even though controlled by local gastric cooling, has a strong tendency to recur. Operation, therefore, is to be recommended if the patient's condition permits. Use of local gastric hypothermia in patients suffering from blood dyscrasia seldom offers permanent cessation of hemorrhage. Although the mortality of massive hemorrhage from bleeding esophageal varices remains defiantly high, several patients have survived who would have succumbed if local gastric hypothermia were not available.

Local gastric hypothermia is an additional helpful tool for the surgeon or the physician to use in the management of massive gastric hemorrhage. In some patients operation can be avoided through the use of this expedient. If operation is necessary, the lag phenomenon accompanying shock will have been partially overcome, providing the surgeon with a better operative risk. When four hours of gastric cooling proves unsuccessful in arresting hemorrhage, prompt surgery is strongly advised, since protracted unsuccessful efforts to control hemorrhage with cooling leads to a higher mortality rate. Pitressin reduces gastric blood flow and merits clinical trial in all patients with massive hemorrhage, it also may prove to be a very helpful adjunct to local gastric cooling.

References

1. Kozell, D. D., and Meyer, K. A.: Massively bleeding gastroduodenal ulcers. Arch. Surg., 86:445, 1963.
2. Fraser, K. W., and West, J. P.: The management of bleeding duodenal ulcers. Ann. Surg., 129:209, 1949.
3. Stewart, J. D., Sanderson, G. M., and Wiles, C. E.: Blood replacement and gastric resection for massively bleeding peptic ulcer. Ann. Surg., 136:742, 1952.
4. Casey, J. H.: Deaths from peptic ulcer in Minnesota during 1952. Minnesota Med., 3:488, 1954.
5. Wangensteen, O. H., Salmon, P. A., Griffen, W. O., Patterson, J. R. S., and Fattah, F.: Studies of local gastric cooling as related to peptic ulcer. Ann. Surg., 150:346, 1959.
6. Sosin, H., Bernstein, E. F., Madsen, A. J., Fusino, K., and Wangensteen, O. H.: The mechanism of control of hemorrhage from duodenal ulcer by gastric hypothermia. J.A.M.A., 186:219, 1963.
7. Heuer, G. J.: The surgical aspects of hemorrhage from peptic ulcer. New England J. Med., 235:777, 1946.
8. Gardner, B., and Baronofsky, I. D.: The massively bleeding duodenal ulcer. Surgery, 45:389, 1959.
9. Nicoloff, D. M., Griffen, W. O., Salmon, P. A., Peter, E. T., and Wangensteen, O. H.: Local gastric hypothermia in the management of massive gastrointestinal hemorrhage. Surg., Gynec. and Obst., 114:495, 1962.

10. Wangensteen, S. L.: Intragastric cooling for upper gastrointestinal hemorrhage. S. Clin. North America, 42:1171, 1962.

11. Kelly, H. G., Grant, G. N., and Elliott, D. W.: Massive gastroduodenal hemorrhage. Arch. Surg., 87:6, 1963.

12. Darin, J. C., Polacek, M. A., and Ellison, E. H.: Surgical mortality of massive hemorrhage from peptic ulcer. Arch. Surg., 83:55, 1961.

13. Ivy, A. C., Grossman, M., and Bachrach, W. H.: Peptic Ulcer. Philadelphia, The Blakiston Co., Division of McGraw-Hill Book Co., 1950.

14. Welch, C. E.: The treatment of upper gastrointestinal hemorrhage. Am. Surgeon, 23:900, 1957.

15. Leape, L. L., and Welch, C. E.: Late prognosis of patients with upper gastrointestinal hemorrhage. Am. J. Surg., 107:297, 1964.

16. Kehne, J., Hughes, F., and Gompertz, M.: The use of surgical Pituitrin in control of esophageal varix bleeding. Surgery, 39:917, 1956.

17. Davis, W. D., Gorlin, R., Reickman, S., and Slorassli, J. P.: Effect of Pituitrin in reducing portal pressure in the human being. New England J. Med., 256:108, 1957.

18. Peter, E. T., Nicoloff, D. M., Sosin, H., Bernstein, E. F., and Wangensteen, O. H.: Observations upon portal hemodynamics during vasopressin (Pressin) administration in dogs. J. Surg. Res., 2:370, 1962.

19. Madsen, A. J., Goodale, R. L., Delaney, J. P., Engle, J. C., and Wangensteen, O. H.: Unpublished observations.

20. Wangensteen, O. H., Goodale, R. L., Jr., Delaney, J. P., Doberneck, R. C., Engle, J. C., and Largiader, F. A.: Gastric freezing for duodenal ulcer: potentiation with vasopressin. Ann. Int. Med., 61:4:636, 1964.

Treatment
of Gastric Ulcer

Introduction

There has always been some controversy over the question of whether patients with gastric ulcer should have surgical treatment (immediately or after a trial of medical management) or medical treatment, and, indeed, there has also been disagreement among surgeons as to the best operative treatment for these patients. The latter controversy was presented in the first (1957) volume of *Current Surgical Management*. Now, however, a relatively new issue in the surgical management of gastric ulcer has been presented, that is, treatment by vagotomy and pyloroplasty. This compounds the pre-existing controversy, which seemingly had begun to be resolved.

All surgical methods of treatment of gastric ulcer at the present time take cognizance of the presently accepted pathogenesis of benign gastric ulcer—that of antral stimulation of gastric acid–peptic activity due to gastric stasis. Thus removal of the antrum (with or without removal of the gastric ulcer) as well as pyloroplasty for the decreasing of stasis and antral stimulation both have theoretical justifications as satisfactory treatment. The role of vagotomy seems to have less justification unless one takes into account the fact that the vagus nerves play a part in the antral phase of gastric secretion.

Whichever type of surgical operation one chooses to perform in patients with benign gastric ulcer, it is still the primary obligation of the surgeon to determine, if at all possible, whether the ulcer is malignant or benign. The difficulty in making this differentiation, by present clinical methods (even surgically and pathologically at times), and the reliability of diagnostic techniques are discussed in the following two presentations. It should be realized that if the ulcer proves to be malignant, the chances for long-term survival by resection are better than for patients with frank, clinically diagnosed gastric cancer. Furthermore, if the ulcer proves to be benign, surgical treatment has been reported to yield more satisfactory results than medical treatment. Now the questions seem to be: Which surgical operation is better for the patient with a gastric ulcer that is proved to be benign, and should one perform a biopsy of the ulcer at the time of operation?

S. R. F.

Treatment of Gastric Ulcer
(in Situ) by Vagotomy and
Pyloroplasty: A Clinical Study*

Jack Matthews Farris,
University of California at Los Angeles,
and Gordon Knight Smith,
University of Southern California

Although subtotal gastrectomy is a satisfactory operation for most benign gastric ulcers, the possibility exists that a more conservative procedure, namely pyloroplasty, may give results just as satisfactory, without sacrificing a major portion of the stomach. This is particularly true when the ulcer is located near the esophagus.

We believe that antral stimulation due to stasis is an important factor in the genesis of gastric ulcer. The relief of gastric stasis by pyloroplasty will nullify the role of the antrum in the formation of gastric ulcer just as effectively as antrectomy, and will result in prompt healing of a gastric ulcer when left in situ.

Biopsy of the gastric ulcer may be done at the same time and, in fact, we suggest that biopsy should be done in *all* cases promptly after the roentgenologic diagnosis has been established. There is no place for the so-called *medical treatment*. Even if the ulcer heals, only one of four patients will remain symptom free, one of six will die from cancer of the stomach, and one of five will present the urgent indications for operation.

This approach allows an appropriate *cancer type* operation to be done in the 10 per cent (or less) of gastric ulcers that prove to be malignant. More important, it allows conservative *stomach-saving* operations to be performed in the 90 per cent that prove to be benign.

* Adapted by permission from Annals of Surgery, *158*:461, 1963.

Rationale for Pyloroplasty in Treatment of Benign Gastric Ulcer

I. Resection of the Pyloric Canal will Result in Prompt Healing of a Proximal Gastric Ulcer Left in Situ

Kelling, in 1918, and Madlener, in 1923, demonstrated that distal resection of as little as 5.0 cm. of the pylorus results in prompt healing of a benign gastric ulcer left at a higher level. Of 77 gastric ulcers reported in 1929, 17 were treated by the Kelling-Madlener principle, usually because of a position near the cardia. A Billroth I reconstruction was followed by complete recovery, and all 17 patients achieved an excellent long-term result.

Smoler, another German surgeon, corroborated these experiences in 1934, and again emphasized that simple excision of the pyloric canal (only 5.0 cm.) was sufficient to nullify the "chemical and motor performance" of the stomach responsible for the hypersecretion associated with gastric ulcer. He stated "the essence of the operation is removal of the pylorus" and reported excellent results in 15 consecutive patients.

Maurer, in 1951, reported 55 cases treated by the Kelling-Madlener operation and enthusiastically recommended it for all gastric ulcers that could not be removed with ease by the usual distal gastrectomy.

Failure to realize the effectiveness of pyloroplasty in the treatment of high lying gastric ulcers will obviously lead to either total gastrectomy or transthoracic resection of the cardia and esophagus—both much less desirable anatomic rearrangements than pyloroplasty.

These considerations have suggested, furthermore, that the success of gastrectomy is not related to removal of the gastric ulcer and/or antrum, but to the destruction of the integrity of the pyloric canal, with relief of gastric stasis. Removal of the ulcer is incidental. Therefore, pyloroplasty (which also destroys the integrity of the pyloric canal) should accomplish the same thing.

II. Wedge Resection of Gastric Ulcer

Corollary information comes from experiences with wedge resection of gastric ulcer, particularly of the lesser curvature, which as originally employed was regularly followed by a high incidence of recurrence. However, if one adds pyloroplasty to wedge resection to prevent stasis, success is achieved in almost 100 per cent of cases. Fifty-seven such operations at the Long Beach Veterans Hospital resulted in one recurrence. These experiences suggested that removal of the ulcer may be incidental, and that pyloroplasty alone is all that would be necessary.

III. Gastric Ulcer as a Sequel to Resections of the Esophagus

Delayed gastric emptying may follow esophagectomy for cancer because of incidental division of the vagus nerves. Some of these patients develop gastric ulcer as reported by Smith, Moulder and Adams.

This gastric ulcer may be prevented or cured by any surgical maneuver (i.e., pyloroplasty) designed to ensure gastric emptying.

IV. Vagotomy Alone for Duodenal Ulcer May be Followed by Gastric Ulcer Paradox

Some of the first vagotomies—without drainage procedures—cured the duodenal ulcer, but a new gastric ulcer appeared. This paradoxic effect was a result of gastric stasis and antral stimulation, and it was later found that it could be nullified by antrectomy, pyloroplasty, or gastroenterostomy. Delayed gastric emptying, either organic or functional, from any cause has been regarded as a cardinal roentgenologic sign associated with gastric ulcer.

V. Gastric Ulcer May Develop as a Sequel to Duodenal Ulcer

At least 20 per cent of patients with gastric ulcer will show evidence of duodenal ulcer—usually old—with pyloric stenosis and stasis. The new gastric ulcer is more imposing, and the old duodenal ulcer—sometimes burned-out—may be overlooked. Relief of the stenosis will cure the gastric ulcer, but may awaken the hypersecretion associated with the duodenal ulcer diathesis unless vagotomy is added. When they coexist, treatment of the duodenal ulcer will cure both.

Clinical Study

With these considerations in mind, in 1959 we began to examine the effect of pyloroplasty and vagotomy upon benign gastric ulcer (in situ).

Originally this operation was used in those patients who were poor risks or in those in whom excision of the ulcer would require an extensive formidable gastrectomy for removal. (Approximately 50 other patients with gastric ulcer have been subjected to conventional gastrectomy.) As confidence has increased in this maneuver, however, gastric ulcers in all locations have been treated in situ by pyloroplasty.

The most attractive feature of this rationale is the opportunity for gastric biopsy. One may view *all* gastric ulcers with the same suspicion as solid tumors of the breast, and can then undertake appropriate extensive operations with conviction, when there is cancer, by removing omenta, spleen, pancreas, and lymph nodes because of an established clear-cut indication. On the other hand, if biopsy shows the ulcer to be benign, operations of lesser magnitude are clearly indicated and may be done with confidence. Zollinger's observation that "transection of tumor-involving lymphatics should not be deleterious when followed by prompt wide-block dissection" supports this plan.[6]

In the past, when operation is undertaken for a roentgenologically diagnosed gastric ulcer (which has not healed), there has unfortunately been an implied obligation to carry out a *cancer* operation, assuming the worst is true until proved otherwise. Fulfillment of this assignment occasionally requires a formidable and sometimes incapacitating operation for an ulcer that ultimately proves to be benign. The theoretic benefits that might accrue to the occasional patient in whom the primary assumption proves correct are open to serious question, and are clearly outweighed by the disadvantages, in terms of mortality and morbidity, that accrue to the others.

We have now had a continuing experience with over 20 patients, all with a preoperative diagnosis of gastric ulcer. Over half showed some evidence of duodenal ulcer, usually pyloric obstruction. There was an initial suspicion of malignancy in two or three patients, but this proved unjustified. Those patients with a preoperative diagnosis of benign gastric ulcer who ultimately proved to have cancer are not included in this experience.

When the gastric ulcer was in the fundus or cardia, biopsy was done through a separate gastrotomy incision. When the frozen section showed the ulcer to be benign, the gastrotomy was closed. A new 10-cm. gastroduodenotomy incision was then made and converted to a pyloroplasty. During the latter maneuver, evidence of pyloric stenosis was almost invariably demonstrated.

Most of the patients have also had either a total or a selective vagotomy. While we were initially interested in determining the effect of pyloroplasty alone on the healing of gastric ulcer, we soon began to perform some type of vagotomy in all cases for these reasons: At least 20 per cent of patients with gastric ulcer have an old duodenal ulcer. Patients with old duodenal ulcer possess a hypersecretory potential and, although not demonstrable in the presence of pyloric obstruction, it may return when the latter is corrected. Furthermore, evidence of old duodenal ulcer diathesis may be unrecognized in the presence of the new imposing gastric ulcer.

The addition of vagotomy adds little or nothing to the magnitude of the operation, and particularly when patients are carefully selected, there are few significant undesirable postoperative effects.

Also, there is evidence that hypersecretion of antral origin may be under cephalic as well as hormonal control. A large dilated stomach that shows little or no acid upon recovery may secrete high levels.

It is safer to add than to omit it, although the pyloroplasty alone would undoubtedly suffice in practically all cases.

In this clinical experience with pyloroplasty for gastric ulcer, there has been one death. A 62 year old man was discharged on the seventh day after operation for pyloric ulcer with uneventful recovery. Approximately one week later he vomited some thick undigested food, which was aspirated followed by asphyxiation and sudden death. Autopsy showed gastric dilatation and superficial minute multiple gastric ulcers, but no anatomic complications of healing pyloroplasty or healing chronic ulcer.

All the remaining patients have had complete postoperative roentgenologic studies, and all but one have had current critical personal interviews. The exception has been followed by detailed questionnaire. There are no recurrences.

These follow-up studies indicate that the results of pyloroplasty (usually combined with vagotomy) are as good or superior to any similar group of our patients who have been subjected to conventional gastrectomy. The outstanding feature of the pyloroplasty patients, when compared with our gastrectomy patients, has been their favorable nutritional status and physical well-being. All patients are classified as an excellent subjective result, with two exceptions. A 56 year old man has complaints which appear to be functional in origin. X-ray and secretory studies have repeatedly been negative. Another patient has intermittent symptoms of indigestion. However, she is only five months postoperative and appears to be improving. Roentgenologic studies show no evidence of ulcer.

Two illustrative case reports, with appropriate photographs, follow:

E. M., a 79 year old man, operation performed April 29, 1960. Operation for pyloric obstruction associated with large, 2.5-cm., gastric ulcer near the cardia. After biopsy proved the ulcer to be benign, the gastrotomy incision was closed followed by Heineke-Mikulicz pyloroplasty and total vagotomy and temporary gastrostomy. There was an excellent recovery. Roentgen examination two months later showed complete disappearance of the ulcer crater and a good functioning pyloroplasty, and follow-up Feburary 19, 1963, revealed excellent result with a 15-pound gain in weight (Fig. 1).

M. S., a 53 year old man, operation performed July 19, 1959. A giant ulcer crater high on the lesser curvature measured 5.0 cm. in diameter. There was advanced cirrhosis of the liver. Frozen section of the ulcer was benign, Pyloroplasty alone followed by closure of the gastrotomy with ulcer in situ was followed by prompt recovery. The patient has been well for 45 months. Figure 2 shows pre- and postoperative x-ray and status of patient's nutrition (Feburary 21, 1963).

Comments

These are patients in whom gastrectomy has apparently been successfully avoided. The incidence of dumping, malabsorption syndrome, and other undesirable symptoms is just as frequent after gastrectomy for gastric ulcer as for duodenal ulcer. To accomplish wide excision of the ulcer, total gastrectomy would have been necessary in a number of these patients, with resultant undesirable effects upon nutrition. It has been obvious from our follow-up studies that the excellent nutrition of these patients is one of the outstanding features of this method of treatment.

There may be some reluctance to rely upon frozen section for the diagnosis of cancer in a gastric biopsy. Problems in this connection, however, rarely arise. In the first place, certain cases of gastric cancer are immediately apparent to the experienced surgeon *without* biopsy. Secondly,

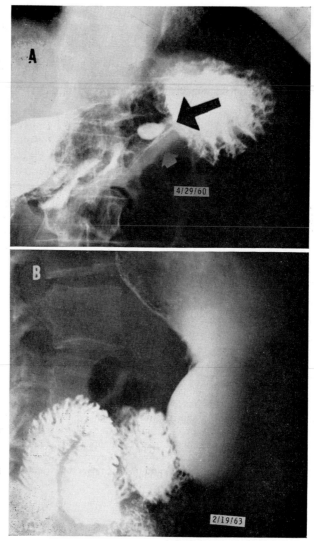

Fig. 1. *A,* High mid-body gastric ulcer. *B,* Disappearance following pyloroplasty alone—6 weeks later. (From Farris, J. M., and Smith, G. K.: Ann. Surg., *158*:461, 1963.)

as experience is gained with mucous membrane lesions, the confidence and cooperation of pathologists generally improves. At our Veterans Hospital in Long Beach, there was initial reluctance to adopt this method of frozen-section diagnosis, but skill was rapidly developed and there were 83 consecutive biopsies where frozen-section diagnosis was in agreement with the paraffin section. On the eighty-fourth, an occult early carcinoma in the base of a gastric ulcer was overlooked, necessitating re-operation. This hazard, however, is infinitely less than the hazard of being misled by apparent healing of an ulcer (as viewed by x-ray examination), which ultimately proves to be cancer.

This experience thus seems to indicate that gastric ulcer can be effectively treated by pyloroplasty and vagotomy. This relatively simple operation spares the patient the nutritional sequelae that so often follow in the wake of more extensive procedures. In the rare patient in whom biopsy at the time of pyloroplasty misses an occult cancer, a more extensive, cancer type operation can then be done. When visual inspection or biopsy indicates that the gastric ulcer is malignant, a more radical operation can be done, with the assurance that this procedure has been rightly reserved for those patients who warrant it.

Gastric biopsy, as herein described, allows immediate histologic diagnosis of gastric ulcer as soon as it is roentgenologically diagnosed, and provides an implement that should destroy the last citadel of those who treat gastric ulcer with an initial medical program.

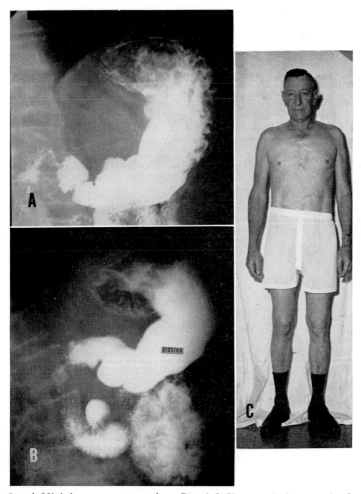

Fig. 2. A, High lesser curvature ulcer. *B* and *C*, X-ray and photograph of patient 45 months following pyloroplasty. (From Farris, J. M., and Smith, G. K.: Ann. Surg., *158:* 461, 1963.)

Summary and Conclusions

Eighteen cases are reported in whom pyloroplasty, usually combined with some type of vagotomy, has been used as a treatment for gastric ulcer in situ. The majority of these patients have achieved an excellent subjective result, and a follow-up study, including roentgenologic studies, fails to reveal evidence of recurrence.

Therefore, pyloroplasty may nullify the role of the antrum in the genesis of gastric ulcer just as effectively as antrectomy, and the success of the latter, for that matter, may well be due to excision of the pyloric canal with correction of stasis, rather than to removal of the antrum and/or ulcer itself.

It is suggested that this discipline provides a plan for biopsy of all gastric ulcers soon after roentgenologic diagnosis is established, with appropriate "cancer-type" operation in those that prove to be malignant and a conservative (stomach-saving) operation in those that prove to be benign.

Reference

1. Kelling, G.: Ueber die Operative Behandlung des Chronischen Ulcus Ventriculi. Arch. klin. Chir., *109:*775, 1918.
2. Madlener, M.: Uber Pylorektomie bei pylorusfernem Magengeschwur. Zentralbl. Chir., *50:*1313, 1923.
3. Mauer, H.: Die Operation nach Madlener und ihre Ergebnisse. Bruns Beitr. klin. Chir., *182:*266, 1951.
4. Smith, C. A., Moulder, P. F., and Adams, W. E.: Gastric ulcer following esophagogastric anastomosis. Trans. Am. Surg. Assn., *75:*326, 1957.
5. Smoler, F.: Uber Dauer Folge nach Madlener Pylorektomie. Med. Klin., *30:*1027, 1934.
6. Zollinger, R. M., Watman, R. N., and Denkewalter, F.: Should all gastric ulcers be treated surgically? Gastroenterology, *35:*521, 1958.

Gastric Resection for Gastric Ulcers

J. E. Strode

Straub Clinic, Honolulu, Hawaii

Until comparatively recently, the surgical treatment of most benign ulcers of the stomach was accepted by most surgeons as being subtotal gastric resection. Farris and Smith and others have recently suggested pyloroplasty alone, or combined with vagotomy; and they have demonstrated rapid healing of such ulcers following this method of approach.[1] At present, I still believe that the vast majority of benign ulcers of the stomach are best handled by gastric resection. An attempt will be made in the following discussion to substantiate this conclusion.

The Case against Medical Treatment

After many years of observing ulcerating lesions of the stomach, it has become my firm conviction that all such lesions should be removed without submitting such individuals to a trial of medical therapy. It is realized that this approach to this problem is not acceptable to most internists and gastroenterologists, but is endorsed by a fair percentage of surgeons. The advisability of removing all ulcerating lesions of the stomach—exceptions being made for the poor risk individual, the very rarely encountered ulcer of the stomach in infancy and childhood, or those thought to be of drug origin—was stimulated by the fact that in Hawaii a large percentage of our population is Japanese, and in this race, cancer of the stomach occurs approximately two and one-half times more frequently than in any other race. Results of surgical treatment of cancer of the stomach are universally poor, except in very early cases while the lesion is still localized. In these cases, it is practically impossible to decide preoperatively whether the ulcer is benign or malignant.

In our hands, and in the published statistics of most others, this remains around 10 per cent. Treating early malignancy of the stomach medically may result in symptomatic improvement and apparent diminution, or, even at times, complete disappearance of any visible ulcer crater on x-ray examination. Meanwhile, if the ulcer ultimately proves to be malignant, the

Page 343

golden opportunity of curing the patient, in all likelihood, has been lost. I am sure that the constant peristaltic activity of the stomach accounts for such early metastasis so commonly seen in this condition.

In our Clinic, we have no statistics to offer on the medical treatment of ulcerating lesions of the stomach, but those who have reported on an appreciable number, subscribe to the conclusion that results, for the most part, are disappointing; recurrences are frequent, an appreciable number of such ulcers perforate, severe hemorrhage is not an infrequent complication, and the more frequently that recurrences take place, the higher the incidence of associated cancer. A report from the Mayo Clinic[2] in which 664 patients were treated medically and followed for 5 to 10 years, or until this form of treatment was abandoned, revealed that only 21.7 per cent remained free of symptoms. The mortality from treating such ulcers medically, in the long run, had been found to be higher than from treating such ulcers surgically. Complications following surgery are few, and end results, usually, are most gratifying. In 500 consecutive gastric resections for benign gastric ulcer at the Straub Clinic, the mortality has been approximately 0.5 per cent in elective operations.

Gastric Resections vs. Biopsy and Pyloroplasty or Vagotomy

It has been suggested that pyloroplasty, perhaps combined with vagotomy, if the biopsy of the ulcer shows no evidence of malignancy, be substituted for subtotal gastric resection. Our results have been so satisfactory with gastric resection that I hesitate to discard this method for one, so far, relatively untried and which, I believe, has a few definite drawbacks.

The vast majority of ulcers of the stomach occur in the lesser curvature and can be readily removed without sacrificing more than the antrum, or, at most, 50 per cent of the stomach. A Billroth I reconstruction can almost always then be accomplished. Many believe that this is more desirable than a Billroth II anastomosis, but of this I have not been entirely convinced. The removed specimen with the entire ulcer and immediate surrounding lymph nodes is then available for study by the pathologist. I have been surprised over the years at how many early carcinomas of the stomach have been found when least expected.

It has long been taught, and I believe clinical experience indicates, that gastric ulcers result from irritation of the antral mucosa resulting in the production of the hormone, gastrin, which stimulates the acid secreting cells of the body of the stomach. It has been the feeling of most investigators that the vagus nerves are important in the genesis of duodenal ulcers, but play an unimportant role in the production of gastric ulcers. An antrectomy or hemigastrectomy has been followed by so few recurrent ulcers that I am encouraged to believe that this observation is correct. I believe that this conclusion is further strengthened by the fact that gastric ulcers have shown rapid healing following pyloroplasty. This operation permits more rapid emptying of the stomach, thus less irritation of the antral mucosa by the gastric contents. It has also been recognized clinically that pyloric obstruction is prone to be followed by the development of a gastric ulcer.

It has long been my belief that opening the stomach to obtain a biopsy from an ulcerating lesion is not a wise thing to do. It delays the operation, further contaminates the operative field, and if the lesion proves to be malignant, there is the possibility of seeding the peritoneal cavity with malignant cells. More important is the fact that examination of several biopsy specimens of an ulcer wall may fail to reveal a small area of malignancy. Even when the pathologist has the resected stomach containing the ulcer in his hands, he may miss a small area of carcinoma by frozen section, which is later picked up by more careful examination. This, in my opinion, is not a reflection on the ability of the pathologist, but emphasizes the fact that no one can make an early clinical diagnosis, with but few exceptions, of cancer of the stomach. Unfortunately, the only type of cancer of the stomach one can hope to cure with any assurance is the one where the microscope, unexpectedly, reveals the true nature of the lesion. When the pathologist confirms the clinical preoperative diagnosis of gastric cancer, arrived at by any of our present methods of diagnosis, the chances of the patient's five-year survival become small indeed. So, it is my conclusion that opening the stomach to obtain a biopsy from the wall of an ulcer that appears to be benign is an inadequate examination to rule out malignancy.

It has been my experience that I can do a 50 per cent gastric resection and a Billroth I anastomosis as quickly and with as little trauma to the patient, as I can do a gastrotomy and biopsy of an ulcer followed by a pyloroplasty. In my hands, at least, it is not a simple matter to do an adequate vagotomy, and if this is added to a biopsy of the ulcer and pyloroplasty, it is a more formidable procedure than partial gastrectomy alone. Certainly, an excision of the ulcer adds considerably to the magnitude of such a procedure.

No doubt there are benign ulcers that lie so high that their removal will result in compromising the esophageal outlet. I have never been confronted with this dilemma. To date, I have been able, by properly mobilizing the stomach and structures around the ulcer, to gain sufficient room to perform a resection and satisfactory reconstruction of the gastric outlet. I would never subscribe to doing a total gastrectomy for a benign gastric ulcer that I could not resect. If it ever falls to my lot to deal with such a problem, I will, under these circumstances, obtain a biopsy from several areas of the ulcer, and if no malignancy is found, I will consider doing either a high gastric resection or possibly a pyloroplasty. At the moment, I do not believe that a sufficient number of pyloroplasties have been done from which to draw conclusions as to their effectiveness in curing benign gastric ulcers. Unless there was evidence that the patient had an active duodenal ulcer, or residual evidence of a previous duodenal ulcer, I would not advise a bilateral vagotomy.

Summary

To briefly summarize my present attitude regarding the treatment of ulcerating lesions of the stomach:

I consider all such ulcers malignant until proved benign by a competent pathologist after adequate microscopic study of the entire ulcer area. My experience, and the experience of most observers with the greatest familiarity with this problem, is that 10 per cent of such ulcers will ultimately prove to be malignant, regardless of how benign they may appear to be by any present method of investigation.

I do not believe in any trial of medical treatment of such ulcers because (1) comparatively few gastric ulcers are cured by medical treatment; (2) medical treatment of even a malignant ulcer may result in temporary symptomatic improvement during which time malignant cells may spread beyond the area of subsequent resectibility (no one can predict when this may occur; no one believes in treating a fire conservatively); and (3) conservative treatment of such ulcers may result in perforation, hemorrhage, pyloric obstruction, and long periods of physical incapacitation.

I believe in gastric resection, with few exceptions, for all benign ulcers of the stomach because (1) the surgical mortality has been shown to be lower than mortality following medical therapy, and (2) results, in general, have been much more satisfactory than by medical treatment.

I believe in gastric resection for ulcerating lesions of the stomach in preference to what has been termed more conservative operations because (1) mortality from gastric resection has been so low, and results so satisfactory, and (2) biopsy of gastric ulcers invites potential complications, and I do not believe it is an adequate method of ruling out malignancy, and (3) these "conservative operations" in my hands have proved to be even more major than gastric resection, and it remains to be shown that they produce any better, or as good, results. I have been so well pleased with the results of gastric resection for benign gastric ulcers that I am very hesitant to adopt any new procedures.

References

1. Farris, J. M., and Smith, G. K.: Treatment of gastric ulcer (in situ) by vagotomy and pyloroplasty: a clinical study. Ann. Surg., 158:3, 1963.
2. Larson, N. E., Cain, J. C., and Bartholomew, L. G.: Prognosis of the medically treated small gastric ulcer. I. Comparison of follow-up data in two series. New England. J. Med., 264:119, 1961. II. Ten-year to nineteen-year follow-up study of 391 patients. New England J. Med., 264:330, 1961.

The Prevention
of Postoperative
Abdominal Distention

Introduction

Not all surgeons would agree that attempts should be made to *prevent* postoperative abdominal distention by some form of gastrointestinal intubation; some wait for distention to develop before using decompression therapeutically. Whenever peritoneal trauma is sufficient to have produced an ileus, resulting gastrointestinal distention due to swallowed air usually can be prevented by two practical means: nasogastric intubation (introduced over 30 years ago) and surgical gastrostomy. The following two presentations point out the advantages and disadvantages of each. No discussion of the recently described electronic stimulation of peristalsis in postoperative ileus is included in this chapter, because the editors feel there has been insufficient application of this technique for the determination of results at this time.

S. R. F.

The Prophylactic
Use of the Nasogastric Tube

Ralph F. Bowers

University of Tennessee College of Medicine and
Veterans Administration Medical Teaching Group Hospital,
Memphis, Tennessee

Historical Considerations

It is a source of wonderment to surgeons who worked in the prenaso-gastric tube era that its use was not conceived and employed much earlier. At one time abdominal operations were followed by intense gas pains, which caused many patients to fear abdominal surgery; many were so discouraged about the discomfort that surgery was reserved for the more dangerous conditions.

The more astute surgeons realizing that paralytic ileus resulted from intestinal trauma, attempted to reduce the trauma; "rough" surgeons were urged by their teachers and confreres to develop a lighter touch. Later in the postoperative course, the ileus began to disappear, the pain lessened, and the patient was grateful to be rid of this torture.

During the period of distress, some dangers are obvious. Distention of the intestine and dilatation of the stomach increase intra-abdominal pressure, which in turn places much stress on suture lines in the abdominal incision, causing wound dehiscence and evisceration. These conditions are attended by high morbidity rates and mortality rates ranging around 20 per cent.

Evisceration, gastric dilatation, and respiratory embarrassment with resultant cardiopulmonary changes are dangerous and warrant attempts at prevention. But another danger threatens the distended patient with paralytic ileus—namely, vomiting in the immediate postoperative period. His less alert reflexes and lowered physical strength cannot prevent tracheal aspiration of the vomitus, which may result in the dangerous aspiration pneumonia. In the early part of this century all surgeons dreaded post-operative pneumonia. With the advent of antibiotics, however, the mortality from postoperative pneumonia was reduced, but antibiotics are not always effective when the pneumonia is due to aspiration of food particles, or gastric, biliary, and duodenal juices.

Perhaps, most importantly, all surgeons dread the consequences of duodenal stump blowouts, rupture of suture lines in the duodenum after operations as simple as sphincterotomy, and rupture of the intestinal suture lines in many small and large bowel operations. Few, indeed, will question the added safety provided by the nasogastric tube in these conditions.

Wangensteen, around 1930, introduced the nasogastric tube in this country, popularized its use, improved the apparatus and gadgets, and provided a simple means of gastric decompression. However, the discomfort of the patient as he tolerates the tube in the nose or mouth has stimulated the profession to seek other, less disagreeable means to accomplish gastric decompression.

Gastric decompression, therefore, is desirable in properly selected cases. The questions arise: (1) When is the tube needed? (2) Is its passage easy? (3) Does it accomplish the desired effect? (4) What are the enumerated dangers? (5) Is there a safer, less distressing method and is this method free of danger and discomfort?

Indications for Preoperative Nasogastric Intubation

For those operations often followed by paralytic ileus, gastric retention, and undue tension on stomach, duodenal, and intestinal sutures, preoperative nasogastric intubation is indicated. These include gastric surgery, colon resection, major traumata such as gunshot wounds and stab wounds, splenectomy, most cholecystectomies, and all cases of peritonitis secondary to ruptured appendix, diverticulitis, etc.

Modern anesthesia sometimes induces sufficient distention of the stomach to interfere with the operation. The tube prevents accumulation of this gas if placed preoperatively. It is not used in operations for nonstrangulated hernia, but is important when strangulation or incarceration with obstruction is present. It is not usually needed in interval appendectomy or appendectomy for early acute nonruptured appendix. Therefore, the use is selective and, in doubtful cases, can be placed postoperatively if necessary.

Technique of Intubation

The introduction of the tube is easy and requires little experience, but the operator improves with practice; it can be passed by doctors, nurses, practical nurses, and in some cases by the patients themselves. The procedure is first performed under the direction of the physician, but he need not be in attendance when his personnel finally acquire the skill. In the management of the tube, particular attention is given to the proper tip location, the prevention of buckling, and the prevention of obstruction by irrigation.

Advantages of Intubation

Nasogastric intubation prevents gastric dilatation and rests the gastrointestinal tract by preventing the intake of air and fluid. Few realize that about 70 per cent of the gas in obstructive distension is due to swallowed air. Obviously a properly functioning tube will not permit air to remain in the stomach and intestine.

It appears to help in paralytic ileus by relieving gastric dilatation, removing some of the intra-abdominal pressure, and perhaps partially decompressing the upper small bowel.

Repeated observations of the vital signs reveal improved physiological activity following intubation. If properly functioning, it will prevent the tracheal aspiration of vomitus. The tube may be passed preoperatively, during the operation, or postoperatively.

Another advantage exists in the use of the long tube, double-lumened if desired. In some cases of intestinal obstruction due to adhesions, the long tube may be brought to the cecum at time of operation and left in place as a splint, which prevents obstruction even though numerous adhesions reform. Some surgeons prefer the long tube for preoperative decompression in intestinal obstruction, but it is doubtful whether this tube accomplishes much more than the ordinary Levin tube. Often when the long tube is used, a second short tube must also be introduced to drain gastric contents, and then one wonders which tube is exerting the most good. The long tube is seldom used in our clinic now.

The nasogastric tube can be used in the nonoperated patient. Operation of course must be done to insert the gastrostomy tube.

Dangers of Intubation

The tube should never be introduced into the trachea. The location of the tube can be determined by stethoscopic examination or by placing the free end of the tube in water. If, when the patient breathes, bubbles are noted in the water, the tube is in the trachea. This catastrophe occurred only once in our experience. Fortunately the patient recovered from the aspiration pneumonia that resulted from irrigation of his tube.

It would be possible to engage the tube in upper or lower esophageal diverticuli, but this has not occurred in our experience. The experienced person soon recognizes these dangers and corrects them or ceases the effort which he knows will be dangerous. Accidents during intubation are extremely rare and almost never occur in experienced hands.

Esophagitis, ulcerated esophagus, and fibrotic esophagus serious enough to require manual or operative interference rarely occur as a result of intubation. Even when varices are known to be present, esophageal bleeding in copious amounts usually indicates the presence of ulceration.

Intubation rarely causes bleeding from hiatal hernia or gastric ulcer. Bleeding from hiatal hernia occurred in only one of our patients, and bleeding stopped as soon as the tube was withdrawn. Mild esophagitis has been seen in an occasional patient in whom a tube has been in place a long time. There have been no reports of fibrotic esophagus or stricture.

Only these few complications occurred in the more than 10,000 patients in whom intubation was performed over a period of 17 years. During these 17 years, only 29 eviscerations occurred in spite of the large percentage of desperately ill elderly patients. Complications do not always contraindicate use of the tube.

Contraindications to Nasogastric Intubation

Conditions that contraindicate nasogastric intubation are:
1. Cardiac failure
2. Extreme respiratory distress (marked emphysema, pulmonary fibrosis, pneumonia)
3. Bleeding esophageal varices
4. Peptic esophagitis
5. Obstructive esophageal lesions
6. Blood dyscrasia

The tube is especially dangerous to the elderly patient who has cardiac disease, emphysema, or pulmonary fibrosis—particularly if the tube is expected to remain in place for more than 48 hours. The average time required for bowel function to return is 30 to 48 hours, depending upon the extent of surgical trauma, whether infection is present, and the unexplained capacity of some patients to recover peristaltic activity sooner than others.

Nasogastric Intubation vs. Gastrostomy Tube

When the surgeon selects a gastrostomy tube, he is not denying the advantages of the decompressive effort. He simply wants to spare the patient the discomfort of the nasogastric tube, and fears the sequelae mentioned above.

Common sense dictates the use of the gastrostomy tube when nasogastric tube cannot safely be employed or the patient's protestations are so vehement that the resulting mental state may be damaging. Here the surgeon's philosophy, common sense, and courage modify his action.

The use of the gastrostomy tube has caused death, usually as a result of leakage, extravasation into the abdominal wall, evisceration, infection, and hemorrhage. When we compare the complications, more can be said against the gastrostomy tube than the nasogastric tube. Also, the gastrostomy tube does not always decompress satisfactorily, and the many variations in types of tubes are evidence of this difficulty.

Nasogastric Intubation vs. No Intubation

One can state that the nasogastric tube can be safely introduced in many postoperative patients, and that most surgeons admit the advantages, even those who are reluctant to use it on account of the patient's discomfort. These same surgeons necessarily impose the discomfort of the operation itself upon patients—but the patient *does not* blame the surgeon, accepting the discomfort as part of the postoperative course.

The surgeon certainly is blamed by the patient for the discomfort of the nasogastric tube. In simpler abdominal procedures, the tube can be introduced at the first sign of trouble postoperatively (gas pain, distention, fast pulse, collapse, etc.); the patient experiences considerable relief when the tube is passed and praises the surgeon for using it. Little does the patient know that if the tube were placed prophylactically either before the operation or by the anesthetist the distress would have been eliminated entirely in most instances.

Those of us who use the tube pass it either immediately before the induction of anesthesia or immediately after induction. The patient must be informed of its purpose, its accomplishments, and the dangers of neglecting to use it. The vast majority of the patients accept it, and do not regard the surgeon to be a torturer. If great apprehension or fear of the tube precedes the operation, it is passed after the patient is anesthetized. Also, if the surgeon studies and knows his patients, he can usually adjudge which condition and which patients should be treated by the gastrostomy tube, or risk using no tube. Conversely, the surgeon who uses the tube, just because there is such a thing, must be condemned.

Any patient who has had severe gas pains without the tube welcomes the tube as being the lesser evil. Perhaps electronic stimulation of the intestine will eventually make obsolete the use of any postoperative tube, nasogastric or otherwise. But until that time arrives, cardiopulmonary complications, electrolytic imbalances, evisceration, intestinal suture leaks and long convalescences can be prevented by the use of prophylactic nasogastric tube, and if that cannot be done, gastrostomy at the time of laparotomy in selected patients. So far, the literature reveals less dangerous sequellae from the use of the nasogastric tube, although it is attended by more discomfort. Prophylactic nasogastric tube placement is desirable in many abdominal, gastrointestinal, mouth, and neck operations.

The proper use of the nasogastric tube saves lives daily—how many, no one knows, but probably more than even its most ardent advocates realize.

References

1. Cantor, M. O.: Mercury—Its role in intestinal decompression tubes. Am. J. Surg., 73:690, 1947.
2. Miller, T. G., and Abbott, W. O.: Intestinal intubation: a practical technique. Am. J. Sc., 187:595, 1934.
3. Wangensteen, O. H.: The early diagnosis of acute intestinal obstruction with comments on pathology and treatment, with a report of successful decompression of three cases of mechanical bowel obstruction by nasal catheter suction siphonage. West. J. Surg., 40:1, 1932.

Temporary Gastrostomy

Gordon Knight Smith *and* Jack Matthews Farris

Los Angeles, California

Indications for Gastrostomy

Although decompression of the gastrointestinal tract following most operations upon the stomach or intestine is unnecessary, it may be life-saving in certain selected instances.

Temporary gastrostomy to implement this decompression has proved to be of value in patients with pulmonary disease (particularly in chronic bronchitis and emphysema), which is associated frequently with duodenal ulcer. Nasogastric tubes are poorly tolerated in patients with cardiac decompensation and in the very aged and young. Additionally, certain patients undergoing major procedures, such as portacaval anastomosis and aortic resections, may require prolonged decompression of the gastrointestinal tract, and temporary gastrostomy may be a good choice here. It is also of value in patients with esophagitis who are operated upon for repair of hiatal hernia combined with vagotomy and pyloroplasty. Other patients in whom prolonged decompression is anticipated, such as those with intestinal obstruction, peritonitis, pancreatitis and abdominal trauma, may be more comfortable with a temporary gastrostomy than with nasogastric suction.

Major complications may occur as the result of the presence of a nasogastric tube. Complications such as laryngeal obstruction, ulceration and late stricture of the esophagus, as well as perforation of the stomach or intestine, are well documented.[1] Additionally, there is an almost universal aversion to the presence of the nasogastric tube, which may long be remembered as an uncomfortable experience associated with recovery from major surgery.

Technique

Careful fusion of the visceral and parietal peritoneal surfaces is most important to prevent leakage. The site for the gastrostomy is selected

Page 355

approximately midway between the lesser and greater curvatures at about the junction of the middle and lower thirds of the stomach. A stab wound is then made with a No. 11 blade, preferably one smaller than the diameter of the tube, with careful attention to hemostasis. A No. 16 Foley catheter is enclosed by a double pursestring suture of catgut. The balloon is inflated with approximately 7 ml. of water. The catheter is brought out through a small stab wound in the abdominal wall, and the site of exit is carefully chosen so that there is no undue tension or distortion of the stomach resulting from traction upon the tube. The visceral and parietal peritoneal surfaces are then approximated with interrupted catgut sutures. Traction is maintained upon the balloon with a modified Hesseltine umbilical clamp. A larger balloon is unnecessary and may be undesirable because of the likelihood of stimulation of the antrum with resultant increased gastric secretion.

Management of the Tube

In contrast to the usually rather large amounts of drainage from nasogastric suction within the first 24 hours, very little drainage can be expected when a temporary gastrostomy is used. Attempts to irrigate the tube will be unavailing. Figure 1 depicts postoperative management. During the first 48 hours the gastrostomy tube is attached to constant suction—either the motor type or the Wangensteen type of water vacuum. If there

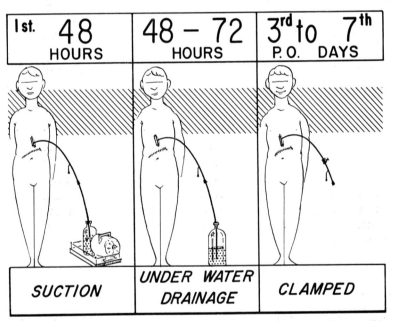

Fig. 1. Postoperative management of gastrostomy tube. (From Ann. Surg., 102:168, 1961. J. B. Lippincott Co.)

is any question as to the patency of the tube, small amounts of water or saline can be instilled through the end of the tube. At the end of 48 hours, the tube is disconnected from the suction and attached to underwater drainage. When this has been tolerated for another day or two, the tube is clamped, to be opened only if the patient shows evidence of gastric retention as manifested by nausea or vomiting. If this occurs, drainage is again instituted.

Early in our experience, the catheter was removed on about the fourth or fifth postoperative day. However, at the present time, our average is about six or seven days from the time of the operation. It is essential that the patency of the gastrointestinal tract be determined prior to removal of the tube. The tube is removed on a fasting stomach. It is first aspirated, and if the volume is greater than 200 or 300 ml., the tube remains in place. If there is any question as to the patency of the gastrointestinal tract, suitable radiopaque substances for roentgenographic examinations may be instilled to establish this fact. When these precepts are followed, removal of the gastrostomy tube is followed by healing within a few hours.

Complications

In our experience,[3] complications of gastrostomy are usually an indictment of the technique or management of the gastrostomy rather than the method itself. The complication of persistent or recurrent drainage through the gastrostomy site after removal is invariably a sequel to premature removal and indicates mechanical or physiologic obstruction distal to the site of the tube. The complication of bleeding from the gastrostomy site has occurred very seldom in our experience. Some authors have been concerned because of so-called nonfunction of the tube as measured by inability to irrigate it. It is obvious that the tip of the tube ventrally placed in a recumbent position selectively removes air and only small amounts of fluid. Data have been accumulated on over 3000 patients in whom temporary gastrostomy has been employed. Distressing major complications rarely occur. Gillesby and Puestow[2] reported a fatality in a patient who removed his gastrostomy tube while asleep with resultant leakage and peritonitis from which the patient expired. In this particular case the visceral and parietal peritoneal surfaces had not been approximated. Spaulding[4] reported that of 300 patients, there were three in whom leakage occurred, requiring re-operation. One of our patients died as the result of error in management. This patient, convalescing from vagotomy, pyloroplasty, and temporary gastrostomy, had the tube removed on about the seventh day and prompt healing occurred. Prior to discharge the following day, during a paroxysm of coughing, the wound dehisced. The wound was closed, but the patient manifested severe cardiovascular collapse and expired. Autopsy revealed that, apparently, during the secondary wound closure, the stomach had been sheared away from the abdominal wall by a retractor and the gastrostomy site reopened, with resultant chemical peritonitis and septic shock. Obviously this is a preventable complication.

Physiologic Considerations

One of the most important aspects of the use of temporary gastrostomy with a Foley bag catheter is that it permits selective removal of air that enters the stomach and still permits fluids to traverse the pyloric canal to physiologic tolerance. Table 1 shows the gastric drainage in 25 consecutive

TABLE 1.   AVERAGE GASTROSTOMY DRAINAGE IN 25 PATIENTS*

Postoperative Day	Intake By Mouth (ml.)	Gastrostomy (ml.)	Balance (ml.)
1st	690	598	+ 92
2nd	652	458	+ 94
3rd	392	80	+312

* Adapted from Smith, G. K., and Farris, J. M.: Am. J. Surg., *102:*168, 1961.

patients undergoing vagotomy, pyloroplasty, and temporary gastrostomy for duodenal ulcer. Small amounts of fluids were given by mouth from the beginning. During the first postoperative day, this group ingested 690 ml. with adequate intravenous fluids, and the average gastrostomy output was about 600 ml. with a positive balance of 92 ml. By the end of the third day the positive balance was over 300 ml. of fluid.

Taylor[5] has shown that when *nasogastric suction* is employed with no oral intake during a 24 hour period, the average yield is 1.83 L. When 3000 ml. of oral intake is allowed, as much as 5 L. will be aspirated. Gillesby and Puestow showed in a series of 15 patients undergoing temporary gastrostomy that the addition of a clamped Levin tube increased the amount of aspirate by 750 ml. per day. This supports the thesis that the presence of an indwelling nasogastric tube increases gastric secretion.

Summary and Conclusions

When prolonged decompression of the gastrointestinal tract is desired, temporary gastrostomy is an acceptable substitute for nasogastric suction. It requires meticulous surgical technique, as well as careful postoperative management and should be used with care and only with clearcut indications.

It is impossible to evaluate the decrease in morbidity or mortality in critically ill patients in whom this method has been used. We are convinced that in certain poor-risk patients the use of this method has been a critical consideration in the ultimate recovery of the patient. We do not advocate routine decompression of patients following gastrointestinal surgery. We believe, however, that when some form of decompression is desirable in patients undergoing gastrointestinal surgery, temporary gastrostomy that is carefully performed with proper postoperative management is as safe, if not safer, than ordinary nasogastric suction, particularly in the chronically ill patient.

References

1. Farris, J. M., and Smith, G. K.: An evaluation of temporary gastrostomy. A substitute for nasogastric suction. Ann. Surg., *144:*475, 1956.
2. Gillesby, W. J., and Puestow, C. B.: Tube gastrostomy in abdominal surgery. Am. Surgeon, *25:*927, 1959.
3. Smith, G. K., and Farris, J. M.: Re-evaluation of temporary gastrostomy as a substitute for nasogastric suction. Am. J. Surg., *102:*168, 1961.
4. Spaulding, K.: Personal communication.
5. Taylor, F. W.: Electrolyte loss by postoperative nasogastric suction (discussion). Arch. Surg., *66:*538, 1953.

The Mechanism of the Dumping Syndrome – Acute Plasma Deficits vs. Humoral Stimulation

Introduction

Too rapid an entrance of food into the upper jejunum, usually resulting from one of several operative procedures upon the stomach, produces a variable symptom complex commonly referred to as the dumping syndrome. The symptomatology is worsened by the ingestion of hyperosmotic foods and includes weakness, sweating, tachycardia, dizziness, and even collapse. Abdominal cramps and diarrhea occur in some patients, and in the past have been attributed to jejunal distention resulting from the outpouring of fluid from the plasma into the intestinal lumen.

The pathogenesis of the dumping syndrome has been the subject of numerous studies and scientific writings, and on occasion was thought to have been the result of a particular operation on the stomach. In turn, many a distinguished surgeon has championed "his" operation as one less likely to result in this unfortunate complication. Cumulated knowledge, however, has led the majority to believe that the symptom complex referred to as "dumping" is a sequel to the loss of pyloric function caused by a variety of operations, ranging from such simple procedures as pyloroplasty to extensive gastric resection and even total gastrectomy.

In 1954, Roberts and co-workers reported acute water shifts from the plasma in gastrectomized patients challenged with oral hypertonic glucose, and related the resulting deficit in blood volume to the dumping syndrome. Objections to this proposal were many, and included the observation that the average mean plasma deficit approximated only 300 cc.

and could hardly result in the exaggerated autonomic response seen frequently during the symptomatic period. Furthermore, the severity of the reaction showed little correlation with the mean deficit in blood volume. Those contributors favoring this explanation, i.e., Lawrence and Randall, have repeated the original studies, using animals challenged with a hypertonic intrajejunal feeding while measuring the blood volume with a constant infusion technique. In this instance, the average decrease in "defective circulating volume" was 23 per cent as compared to a decrease of 9.3 per cent by the indirect Cr^{51} and T-1824 techniques.

The most recent hypothesis proposes that the early symptoms of dumping are the result of the release of a vasoactive hormone from the jejunal mucosa in response to a hyperosmolar stimulus. Those supporting this explanation, i.e., Jesseph and Sloop, implicate 5-hydroxytryptamine or serotonin, which has been found elevated in the portal venous blood of dogs following stimulation of the jejunum with hyperosmolar solutions. In addition, a serotonin antagonist, such as cyproheptadine, is said to have controlled the symptomatology in some patients.

Careful consideration of these proposals is important since the prevention and, in particular, the effective management of those patients suffering from the dumping syndrome will ultimately depend on the mechanism at fault.

E. H. E.

Postgastrectomy Dumping Syndrome:
Role of Acute Blood Volume Change

Walter Lawrence, Jr., *and* Henry Thomas Randall

*Memorial Sloan Kettering Cancer Center
and Cornell University Medical College*

Symptoms of the Dumping Syndrome

Since the symptoms of the "dumping syndrome" were first described by Hertz[2] over 50 years ago, there has been much speculation regarding the cause and treatment of this disturbing symptomatology. It is now generally accepted that this group of symptoms is a sequel to the loss of pyloric function produced by a variety of operative procedures on the stomach, although extensive resection of the stomach is more often the offender than limited resection or gastroenterostomy. The incidence of this disturbing problem varies somewhat with the interest of the author describing postgastrectomy status, as so much of the symptomatology is subjective in nature. After subtotal gastric resection, we believe that definite dumping symptoms of the early postprandial type probably occur in 10 to 25 per cent of the patients.

Abdominal symptoms and signs of "dumping" are those of epigastric fullness, hyperperistalsis, borborygmi, and cramps, with occasional nausea, vomiting, or diarrhea. Many of these symptoms are aptly described by the term "intestinal hurry." In addition to these abdominal complaints, a more striking series of postprandial symptoms suggesting sympathetic discharge are observed, and these include unpleasant warmth, tachycardia, sweating, pallor, weakness, and dizziness, as well as nonspecific electrocardiographic findings. All these "early" dumping symptoms are most marked approximately 15 minutes after the ingestion of foodstuff by the gastrectomized patient. They are quite distinct from those symptoms of hypoglycemia that occur much later in some patients ("late" dumping syndrome).

This complex of symptoms and signs can occur with all degrees of severity. For some patients, these symptoms are only elicited by an abnormal challenge with hypertonic foodstuff, and others experience disabling

Page 363

symptoms with most of their normal meals. There is little wonder that it is difficult to arrive at a specific incidence for the dumping syndrome. There is, however, a relatively close correlation between postgastrectomy malnutrition and the severity of these symptoms, as reducing dietary intake is one solution the patient finds effective for controlling symptoms. This factor emphasizes the seriousness of the dumping syndrome when it does occur.

Evidence of Acute Postprandial Blood Volume Change

For many years various mechanical explanations were given for these symptoms, but none were well substantiated. These concepts of etiology led to frequent comment regarding preference for one method of reconstruction over another. When physiologic evidence for acute postprandial alterations in plasma volume was first offered, it led to a renewed interest in the investigation of the physiology of "dumping." For such a complex series of symptoms presenting so differently in individual patients, it is no small wonder that a unified explanation such as this met with some objections. It is our contention, however, that an acute alteration in effective circulating volume after the ingestion of hypertonic foodstuff by the gastrectomized patient plays a primary role in many of the symptoms associated with the dumping syndrome. What is the evidence to support this theory?

Machella[7] established the fact that a shift of fluid into the bowel occurs after intraluminal introduction of hyperosmolar solution. This situation would occur with the ingestion of many foodstuffs, particularly carbohydrate, by the patient without pyloric function. He attributed most of the symptoms that occur during the dumping syndrome to the local effect of this large fluid shift into the bowel. Using an indirect method of plasma volume determination, Roberts,[11] from our laboratory, then reported the response of gastrectomized patients to standard hypertonic meals of hypertonic glucose. It was found that *water* shifts from the plasma occurred 15 to 30 minutes after ingestion of these test meals, but these shifts were initially described as acute deficits in the circulating blood volume.

One disturbing feature of this explanation of blood volume deficit as the major mechanism for the dumping syndrome was the clinical evidence of exaggerated autonomic response that was noted during the symptomatic period. Others raised objections to this thesis on the basis that there was not a very good correlation between the magnitude of the changes in blood volume measured by this method and the severity of symptoms and signs noted in the patients.[12] Peddie et al.,[9] in a study of 33 patients, found a maximum decrease in plasma volume ranging from 8 to 697 cc. with a mean decrease of only 300 cc. While changes of this magnitude might be accompanied by a marked sympathetic response in some debilitated patients, it seemed unlikely that they could account for the severe cardiovascular changes, sweating, pallor, and weakness so often observed in relatively well nourished patients with the dumping syndrome. Furthermore, the secondary rise in hematocrit that was observed after a test meal of hypertonic glucose was often less than expected from the deficit in plasma volume measured by the indirect technique with either Evan's blue (T-1824) or I^{131}-tagged albumin (RISA). These disturbing features of what initially appeared to be a simple explanation led many of us to further investigation of changes in blood volume associated with hypertonic intrajejunal feedings.

The method for measuring "plasma volume changes" in the studies described above was by measurement of the deviation produced in the late fall-off curve of RISA or T-1824, the so-called "indirect method" described by Gibson and Evans.[1] The increase in concentration of the indicator used, over that expected from extrapolation of the plasma samples drawn prior to administration of the test meal, represents only an increase in concentration of plasma protein, since these indicators are actually tagged to plasma protein. Conversely, this also represents a decrease in concentration of water in the individual plasma samples. We have since considered it more accurate to term the changes detected by this indirect plasma volume method as relative water losses from the plasma, since the actual plasma volume is not measured as it is with simple dilution methods. The total loss of water from the plasma during a dumping episode could be estimated from these figures if they were combined with the plasma volume value determined initially by classic dilution calculations. However, if the circulating blood volume was altered by any means other than plasma water loss during the period of the dumping test, this indirect method of measurement would not be able to reveal the change.

In our own studies in unanesthetized dogs, the degree of cardiovascular alteration that did occur after intrajejunal feeding of hypertonic glucose solution was often quite severe, despite relatively small plasma water losses in some experiments.[6] The change in mean corpuscular volume of the red blood cells during such a test also demonstrated some water loss from the erythrocytes, but the total water loss from plasma and red cells was still far short of that which might be expected to initiate many of the cardiovascular alterations noted during the dumping syndrome. Intestinal water volume increase was measured in these experiments and was found to be consistently greater than the acute water loss from the blood volume, a finding that could be easily explained by some water donation from the interstitial fluid. Although acute fluid influx in the intestine after hypertonic feeding could easily explain many of the abdominal or intestinal symptoms of "dumping," the plasma and red-cell water loss, as measured in these studies, could hardly be considered a reasonable explanation for all of the other early symptoms.

To detect dynamic transient alterations in circulating blood volume

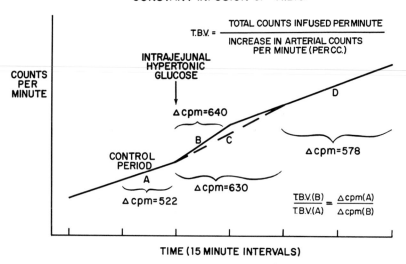

Fig. 1. Schematic representation of data obtained with a constant Cr[51] r.b.c. infusion method in dogs subjected to intrajejunal 50 per cent glucose.

produced by blood or plasma loss, vasomotor changes, or some type of vascular pooling, repeat injections of the indicator used would be necessary to accurately establish the dilution of the indicator in the "new" pool being studied. In other experiments, we utilized this approach to detect changes in what might be best termed "effective blood volume" occurring during the dumping episode.[8] To circumvent some of the disadvantages of accumulated errors from many isolated and repeated injections of an indicator substance, we utilized a method that employed a constant infusion of Cr[51]-tagged red blood cells and constantly monitored blood radioactivity. Using this approach, the rate of increase in blood radioactivity, as estimated from the slope of the graphic representation of this activity, could be related to the administration rate of the isotope to give a value for the circulating blood volume for any desired time interval. Changes in the effective circulating pool, whether produced by extravascular loss, by temporary nonfunction by means of pooling, or by contraction by pronounced vasoconstriction, would all be indicated in such a study by a change in the slope of the graphic representation of the blood radioactivity (Fig. 1). Although not measuring a static blood volume, a slope obtained by this constant injection method would more clearly establish the effective circulating volume during all periods of the study.

The serial change in total blood volume, as measured by the technique described, was most striking in the first 15-minute period after hypertonic intrajejunal feeding and usually had returned to normal in the second 30-minute period. These circulatory changes observed in the experimental animal coincided chronologically with the period when symptoms are ordinarily most marked in patients exhibiting the dumping syndrome. The levels of blood radioactivity required to carry out these experiments in animals made it inadvisable to confirm the results in man, but we have no reason to doubt that the changes would be similar. In contrast to the values obtained by indirect methods of measurements, the mean decrease in total blood volume during the first 15 minutes in this series of 14 experiments was 23.1 per cent (Fig. 2). It seems reasonable to expect that an acute loss of effective blood volume of this degree resulting from the hyperosmolar solution in the intestine would in turn result in significant sympathetic stimulation from various pressoreceptors.

Since the decrease in effective circulating volume observed was considerably greater than could be accounted for by the water losses into the bowel, a consideration of other factors responsible for such an acute and transient decrease must assume a redistribution of the blood volume and flow. A relatively stagnant area of flow or a predominance of flow within a less active circulatory circuit could effect such a transient decrease in effective circulating volume. Confusing alterations in renal blood flow and digital blood flow that have been reported with dumping may also be a manifestation of acute redistribution of flow. Blood flow experiments by Huse and Hinshaw,[3] using the square wave electromagnetic flow meter, have also demonstrated a marked redistribution of blood flow in dogs after hypertonic intrajejunal feeding, as evidenced by a significant increase in mesenteric artery flow, while a marked decrease in flow occurred in the renal, carotid, coronary, and femoral arteries. An average decrease in cardiac output of 20 per cent was observed after intrajejunal challenge with hypertonic glucose in his experiments, and changes of comparable magnitude were observed in studies carried out in our laboratory by

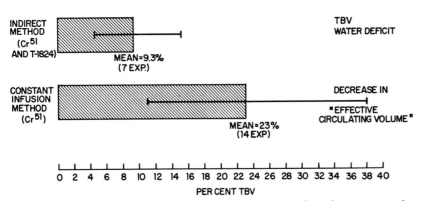

EXPERIMENTAL DUMPING SYNDROME
(INTRAJEJUNAL 50% GLUCOSE)

Fig. 2. Blood volume change after intrajejunal administration of 50 per cent glucose solution. The indirect method, which actually measures only relative water loss from the plasma is compared with Cr[51] r.b.c. infusion method for measuring change in effective circulating volume.

Klauber et al.[5] It is our feeling that this "pooling" in the mesenteric bed produces, in essence, a transient and significant decrease in effective blood volume and a decrease in cardiac output, and these changes play a significant role in initiating many of the symptoms usually associated with the dumping syndrome.

Humoral Factor

Recently Johnson and co-workers[4] have postulated a humoral factor as the underlying initiating agent for the dumping syndrome, and their work has been substantiated by others.[10] That this humoral agent might be serotonin is often suggested due to the similarities between "dumping" and the physiological manifestations produced by an excess of this amine in the peripheral blood. Pretreatment of the experimental animal or patient with so-called serotonin antagonists has been shown to reduce some of the cardiovascular changes that have been associated with hypertonic intrajejunal feeding. Most of these pharmacologic agents have other functions as well and can hardly be considered pure antagonists of serotonin, but the reduction in symptoms experienced by patients, as well as the reduction in some physiologic responses have been most impressive. These studies, plus previous experimental studies demonstrating serotonin release from the small bowel after intraluminal installation of hypertonic solution, make a convincing argument for the role of serotonin in the etiology of the dumping syndrome.

Is Humoral Factor Related to Decreased Blood Volume?

It is quite possible that the marked decrease in effective circulating blood volume, which we have described, and the phenomenon of serotonin release from the small bowel are not mutually exclusive explanations for this complex syndrome. It is quite possible that the acute transient decrease in effective circulating volume is due to a redistribution of blood flow and pooling that is in some way initiated by a humoral mechanism. The question has actually evolved to the point where it bears a certain similarity to the old argument—which appeared first, the chicken or the egg? Without attempting to refute evidence regarding a role for serotonin or a serotonin-like substance which has evolved from studies in several laboratories, we would still like to stress the fact that acute, significant, and sometimes serious postprandial decreases in effective circulating volume do occur in patients with the postgastrectomy dumping syndrome.

References

1. Gibson, J. G., and Evans, W. A.: Clinical studies of the blood volume. I. Clinical applications of a method employing the Azo Dye "Evan's Blue" and the spectrophotometer. J. Clin. Invest., *16*:301, 1937.

2. Hertz, A. F.: The cause and treatment of certain unfavorable after-effects of gastro-enterostomy. Ann. Surg., 58:466, 1913.

3. Huse, W. M., and Hinshaw, D. B.: Blood flow studies in the experimental dumping syndrome. S. Forum, 11:316, 1960.

4. Johnson, L. P., Sloop, R. D., Jesseph, J. E., and Harkins, H. N.: Serotonin antagonists in experimental and clinical "dumping." Ann. Surg., 156:537, 1962.

5. Klauber, L. D., Poppell, J. W., Kahn, R. E., Randall, H. T., and Roberts, K. E.: Alterations in cardiac output following the intrajejunal administration of hypertonic solutions. A.M.A. Arch. Int. Med., 100:255, 1957.

6. Lawrence, W., Jr., and Matthews, D. H.: A study of water shifts in experimental dumping syndrome. S. Forum, 10:180, 1960.

7. Machella, T. E.: The mechanism of post-gastrectomy dumping syndrome. Ann. Surg., 130:145, 1949.

8. Matthews, D. H., Lawrence, W., Jr., Poppell, J. W., Vanamee, P., and Randall, H. T.: Change in effective volume during experimental dumping syndrome. Surgery, 48:185, 1960.

9. Peddie, G. H., Jordan, G. L., and DeBakey, M. E.: Further studies on the pathogenesis of the post-gastrectomy syndrome. Ann. Surg., 146:892, 1957.

10. Peskin, G. W., and Miller, L. D.: The role of serotonin in the "dumping syndrome." Arch. Surg., 85:701, 1962.

11. Roberts, K. E., Randall, H. T., Farr, H. W., Kidwell, A. P., McNeer, G. P., and Pack, G. T.: Cardiovascular and blood volume alterations resulting from intra-jejunal administration of hypertonic solutions to gastrectomized patients: the relationship of these changes to the dumping syndrome. Ann. Surg., 140:631, 1954.

12. Webber, B. M., Bender, M. A., and Moore, G. H.: Dumping syndrome; an evaluation of some current etiologic concepts. New England J. Med., 256:285, 1957.

Dumping Syndrome:

The Humoral Mechanism

John E. Jesseph
Medical Research Center, Brookhaven National Laboratory, Upton, New York and University of Washington School of Medicine,

and Richard D. Sloop
Los Angeles County Harbor General Hospital, Torrance, Calif.

Herein we will present evidence to support the hypothesis that the early postprandial vasomotor and gastrointestinal derangements of "dumping" are initiated and sustained by the release of some substance from the upper intestinal mucosa in response to the hyperosmolar stimulus of eating.

After carefully scrutinizing the reported observations of others, we concluded that while a great variety of physiological derangements occur following ingestion of hyperosmolar substances by such patients (e.g., decreases in blood volume and serum potassium concentration and wide changes in blood glucose concentration), none of these had been shown to be of significant magnitude soon enough after the meal to account for the *earliest* change, that is, vasodilatation. These conclusions motivated us to perform certain experiments in this area. Hinshaw first described this phenomenon,[6] and we were able to confirm it in similar clinical experiments in postgastrectomy patients. Almost without exception, careful observation shows that *increases* in digital pulse amplitude begin either before or at the same time as the subjective visceral and circulatory changes, and may begin as soon as 3 to 5 minutes after ingestion of a test hyperosmolar solution.[8] Read and Swenson[17] likewise noted the incongruity of increasing skin temperature and digital blood flow with decreases in circulating blood volume. The very early appearance of this key change—vasodilatation—caused us to speculate that some strongly vasoactive (and gut active) substance might be released from the intestinal mucosa, and that the early vasomotor and intestinal motor changes are the pharmacologic consequences of its systemic effects. A reflex neurologic mechanism seemed less likely, since such responses usually occur more rapidly. On the other hand, the changes appear too soon to be logically attributable to major fluid shifts. Furthermore, it seemed illogical and paradoxical to us that *vasodilatation* should occur in response to *diminution of intravascular volume*, even if the latter could shrink significantly in less than 5 minutes. In short, the published explanations of the causation of the early changes in dumping were not (to us) convincing.

Experimental Support for Theory

Several reports in the medical literature have hinted at a humoral explanation for the early sequence of events in dumping,[1] but no experimental or laboratory support existed prior to 1961. In that year we reported[7] that a reproducible complex of vomiting, diarrhea, and lethargy could be passively transferred to recipient dogs by transfusion of portal venous plasma from hyperosmolar-stimulated segments of intact dog jejunum. Later, we were able to show that this transferrable stimulus also induced measurable increases in foreleg volume as measured plethysmographically.[9]

Nature of Agent

With the establishment of the humoral hypothesis, it became necessary to determine the nature of the agent released from the mucosa of the gut. The amine serotonin (5-hydroxytryptamine) came under immediate suspicion. It has been shown to be formed in the argentaffin cells, with pharmacologic properties entirely consistent with the major responses in dumping, and probably plays an important role in the autoregulation of gastrointestinal motility.[4, 5, 10, 11, 18]

Role of Serotonin

The investigations of O'Hara and others[13] had suggested that serotonin might play some part in the intestinal phase of dumping. Since our initial report, there have been several investigators who found elevated serotonin levels in the portal venous blood following dumping stimuli. Notable are those of Drapanas[3] and of Peskin and Miller.[16] Recently Warner[20] demonstrated hyperserotoninemia in some patients with "functional" gastrointestinal disease, and in a few, treatment with cyproheptadine (a potent antagonist of both serotonin and histamine) relieved symptoms entirely for prolonged periods. Moore, Norwell, and Eiseman[12] point out that serotonin may, under special experimental circumstances, serve as an intermediary in the release of histamine from the liver and lung, and suggest that this mechanism may be involved in the pathogenesis of dumping. Our own experimental experience agrees with this view indirectly, in that we were never able to demonstrate consistent elevations of serotonin in the peripheral blood of animals with a marked vascular response to hyperosmolar stimulation, even using an exquisitely sensitive bio-assay method.[19] On the other hand, Prof. Aldo Torsoli and his co-workers of the University of Rome have found consistent and striking elevations of peripheral plasma serotonin levels in dumping patients and in normal individuals given hyperosmolar stimuli by upper intestinal intubation.[2] Their detailed studies of changes in blood pressure and pulse rate, and of intestinal motility (cinefluoroscopy), together with the serotonin findings, strongly support the concept of the primary role of serotonin in dumping.

Substance P

Pernow and Wallensten of Stockholm have proposed another agent for the role of humoral intermediate in dumping, Substance P.[14, 15] It has not as yet been shown, however, that Substance P is involved in the vasomotor changes in dumping, or that it is more than a by-product in some complex mechanism within the intestinal wall.

Conclusions

It is our belief that a satisfactory theory of the *genesis* of dumping can be constructed from the clinical and experimental evidence available. Most of the observations that seem not to fit the theory do so if it is accepted that individuals may vary considerably in degree of response to the same stimulus or series of interdependent stimuli. Briefly stated, the theory is as follows:

The loss of gastric outlet regulatory function through removal or bypass of the pylorus allows rapid passage of ingested materials into the proximal small intestine, where there is rapid dilution and hydrolysis by secretions from the digestive glands and by intestinal fluids. The resulting hyperosmolar state of the bolus stimulates the intestinal mucosa in a normal manner, but to an excessive degree, causing it to release excessive quantities of serotonin. This amine then passes into the portal and systemic circulations, and finally acts through target organs to bring about the circulatory and gastrointestinal disturbances characterized as dumping. The later (in sequence) phenomena of hypovolemia, electrolyte imbalance, and wide swings in blood sugar levels are all consequences of the chain-reaction process initiated by intestinal hyperosmolarity.

As here stated, certain implicit features of the theory must be emphasized. First, the entire process is an exaggerated but normal response to the ingestion of normal foodstuffs. Second, the role of serotonin seems to be quite firmly established, but it has yet to be demonstrated whether it acts singly or in concert with other substances, such as histamine, the adrenal secretions, or other as yet unrecognized physiological compounds. Third, the individual variations in pattern and severity of response are explained by the variability among individuals of such factors as argentaffin cell mass, threshold and sensitivity to complex interacting stimuli, and effectiveness of opposing and compensating mechanisms. This theory then, while incomplete, contains all the essential features for a description of the sequence of events known as the early postprandial dumping syndrome.

References

1. Abbott, W. E., Krieger, H., Levey, S., and Bradshaw, J.: The etiology and management of the dumping syndrome following a gastroenterostomy or subtotal gastrectomy. Gastroenterology, 39:12, 1960.
2. Cassano, C., Torsoli, A., Ramorino, M. L., Colagrande, C., Carrutu, R., Caprilli, R., and Arullani, P.: Elementi di Fisiologia e di Fisio-patologia Gastro-intestinale nei Resecati Gastrici per Ulcera Peptica. Presented at a Symposium on "La patologia dei gastroresecati per malattia ulcerosa," during the 64th Congress of the Italian Society of Internal Medicine, Padua, October, 1963.
3. Drapanas, T., McDonald, J. C., and Stewart, J. D.: Serotonin release following instillation of hypertonic glucose into the proximal intestine. Ann. Surg., 156:528, 1962.
4. Haddy, F. J.: Serotonin and the vascular system. Angiology, 2:21, 1960.
5. Hendrix, T. R., Atkinson, M., Clifton, J. A., and Ingelfinger, F. J.: The effect of 5-hydroxytryptamine on intestinal motor function in man. Am. J. Med., 23:886, 1951.
6. Hinshaw, D. B., Joergenson, E. J., Davis, H. A., and Stafford, C. E.: Peripheral blood flow and blood volume studies in the dumping syndrome. Arch. Surg., 74:686, 1957.
7. Johnson, L. P., and Jesseph, J. E.: Evidence for a humoral etiology of the dumping syndrome. Surg. Forum, 12:316, 1961.
8. Johnson, L. P., Sloop, R. D., and Jesseph, J. E.: Etiologic significance of the early symptomatic phase in the dumping syndrome. Ann. Surg., 156:173, 1962.
9. Johnson, L. P., Sloop, R. D., and Jesseph, J. E.: Plethysmographic evidence supporting the concept of a humoral etiology of the experimental dumping syndrome. J. Surg. Res., 2:241, 1962.
10. Johnson, L. P., Sloop, R. D., and Jesseph, J. E.: Serotonin, duodenal hyperosmolarity and the enterogastrone concept of gastric motor inhibition. Rev. Surg., 20:91, 1963.
11. Kaulbersz, J., and Konturek, S.: Comparison of enterogastrone derived from various sections of the intestine. Gastroenterology, 43:457, 1962.
12. Moore, T. C., Normell, L., and Eiseman, B.: Effect of serotonin loading on histamine release and blood flow of isolated perfused liver and lung. Arch. Surg., 87:58, 1963.
13. O'Hara, R. S., Fox, R. O., and Cole, J. W.: Serotonin release mediated by intraluminal sucrose solutions. Surg. Forum, 10:215, 1959.
14. Pernow, B., and Wallensten, S.: The relationship between substance P and the motility of the small intestine in man. In Symposium on Substance P., Proc. Sci. Soc. Bosnia Herzegovina, 1:83, 1961.
15. Pernow, B., and Wallensten, S.: Personal communication.

16. Peskin, G. W., and Miller, L. D.: The role of serotonin in the "dumping syndrome." Arch. Surg., *85:*701, 1962.
17. Read, R. C., and Swensen, D.: Blood pressure and osmolarity changes in the dumping syndrome. Surg., Gynec. and Obst., *112:*488, 1961.
18. Resnick, R. H., and Grey, S. J.: Distribution of serotonin (5-hydroxytryptamine) in the human gastrointestinal tract. Gastroenterology, *41:*119, 1961.
19. Sloop, R. D., Johnson, L. P., and Jesseph, J. E.: Bio-assay of plasma serotonin in the experimental dumping response. Surg. Forum, *13:*243, 1962.
20. Warner, R. R. P.: Hyperserotoninemia in functional gastrointestinal disease. Ann. Int. Med., *59:*464, 1963.

Treatment of the Dumping Syndrome

Introduction

As indicated in the editorial comment of the previous section, it is commonly accepted that the symptom complex referred to as "dumping" is a sequel to the loss of pyloric function leading to rapid emptying of the gastric remnant, so that ingested food enters the jejunum promptly. If such foods are hyperosmotic, then a variety of clinical manifestations occur, either as a result of an acute loss of water from the plasma into the bowel lumen or secondary to the release of a vasoactive amine from the intestinal mucosa. When faced with such a problem, the clinician has several choices, depending on the severity of the symptom complex. In the first place, the dumping manifestations may be prevented by the avoidance of those foodstuffs that could result in hyperosmolarity of the jejunal contents, i.e., control of diet. In addition, as suggested by Johnson and Stevenson, serotonin antagonists, such as cyproheptadine or UML-491, may be employed, and the preliminary results of the effectiveness of these drugs support their usefulness. On the other hand, one might utilize an operative procedure designed not only to increase the capacity of the gastric reservoir, but also to decrease the emptying time of the gastric bag. Our second contributor, Poth, proposes such a procedure, which includes the use of an antiperistaltic segment of jejunum.

E. H. E.

Anti-Serotonin Agents and Diet in the Treatment of the Dumping Syndrome

Lloyd P. Johnson *and* John K. Stevenson

University of Washington School of Medicine, Seattle, Washington

The postgastrectomy "dumping syndrome" of Mix no longer remains a mystifying complex of widely divergent symptoms.[12] It is now possible to separate the various pathophysiologic sequelae of gastric surgery into somewhat distinct clinical entities. The understanding and correct diagnosis of these components of the postgastrectomy syndrome form the basis for a rational treatment program. For example, the postprandial nausea and bilious vomiting of the afferent loop syndrome are believed to represent an obstructive phenomenon at the stoma and are corrected only by surgical means.[10] Similarly, the frequent epigastric bloating and discomfort encountered in postgastrectomy patients following a meal of moderate volume comprise a distinct symptom-complex related to distention of a small gastric reservoir.[1] A third major group of physiologic disturbances is known as the "late" phase of the dumping syndrome, manifest by typical hypoglycemic symptoms occurring two to four hours after meals and relieved by carbohydrate ingestion. None of these postgastrectomy problems can be alleviated by serotonin antagonists. On the contrary, they require surgical correction or other specific symptomatic treatment. Finally, a host of nutritional deficits and anemias may complicate the postgastrectomy syndrome, and may often require specific replacement measures.

Usually, the above mentioned symptoms can be differentiated from the most common postgastrectomy symptoms—those of the "early" phase of dumping—characterized by immediate postprandial warmth, sweating, faintness, weakness, intestinal cramps, and diarrhea, which do respond favorably to serotonin antagonists. These vasomotor and intestinal symptoms have been studied extensively. Measurements of a variety of physiologic parameters have demonstrated widespread changes occurring in multiple organ and metabolic systems. Interest has recently centered around a humoral intermediary as the single unifying link between intestinal hyperosmolarity and the complicated vasomotor and intestinal sequelae.[6–8] Subsequent studies suggest that serotonin plays a predominant role in this humoral mechanism.[3, 11, 14]

This concept constitutes the rationale for the use of anti-serotonin agents in the treatment of the early phase of the dumping syndrome.

Therapy Based on the Diagnosis of Early Phase Symptoms

Unfortunately, the various postgastrectomy symptoms do not usually present in pure form, but rather as composites of several components of the total postgastrectomy syndrome. Since the management of each differs, an effort to differentiate between them and understand them in the individual patient is basic to successful treatment. It is very important to carefully obtain a dietary history with particular attention to the time sequence of symptoms. Various laboratory determinations, including a complete blood count and serial blood glucose levels, should be obtained, and are necessary in the diagnosis of late hypoglycemia and postoperative anemia. Intubation of the efferent loop during the symptomatic period may be diagnostic in the afferent loop syndrome. Radiologic examination should be performed in order to estimate the size of the gastric remnant and its stoma, as well as the functional aspects of gastric emptying and intestinal transit time.

Measurement of plasma volume changes has failed to disclose a correlation between reduction of volume and symptoms, and is of limited clinical value.[2, 16] Conversely, plethysmography has become a reliable objective index of early vasomotor dumping. Hinshaw et al. first used plethysmography as a measure of the clinically apparent increase in peripheral blood flow occurring during the early phase of the dumping syndrome.[5] They were able to predict, by means of preoperative plethysmographic studies, which patients were likely to develop vasomotor symptoms postoperatively.[4] Other studies demonstrating the close relationship in timing and severity between the measurable plethysmographic changes and vasomotor symptoms have further confirmed the diagnostic value of digital plethysmography.[7–9]

In our experience, this test, utilizing a simple mercury strain gauge to monitor digital blood flow during a hypertonic glucose test meal, has become the most significant objective measurement to differentiate early vasomotor dumping from the other symptoms. It is simple and inexpensive, and can be performed in the physician's office by a nurse or other assistant. Asymptomatic postgastrectomy patients and those with very mild early symptoms rarely evidence any increase in peripheral blood flow. An increase in digital pulse amplitude and rate is the rule in patients with true early vasomotor symptoms. Experience with serotonin antagonists in the treatment of these patients has demonstrated a good correlation beween the test and the subsequent response to therapy. Patients with increased peripheral blood flow in response to the test meal usually improved with drug treatment; while those with a negative plethysmographic dumping test did not benefit from anti-serotonin administration.

If plethysmography is not available, a therapeutic trial of an anti-serotonin drug can be of diagnostic value. One of the most interesting features of the drug treatment has been the "sorting out" of the various components of patients' symptoms. The early vasomotor symptoms, cramps, and diarrhea usually diminish or disappear, leaving the late hypoglycemic phase, or the epigastric small reservoir problems in more pure form. Thus, it is possible, by means of therapeutic trial, to determine whether or not the early phase symptoms do exist, and if they account for a major portion of the patient's complaints.

Therapy Based on Severity of Early Postprandial Symptoms

Early experience with serotonin antagonists in studies of both experimental and clinical dumping syndromes readily proved the efficacy of cyproheptadine in reducing symptoms and plethysmographic changes following a hypertonic glucose test meal. Patients with severe early dumping symptoms who were placed on this medication reported marked improvement with prompt reduction of vasomotor symptoms, cessation of diarrhea, and weight gain.[9] Peskin and Miller subsequently reported relief of vasomotor symptoms and diarrhea in eight patients using another serotonin antagonist, l-methyl-d-lysergic acid butamine tartrate (Sansert).[15]

A two-year follow-up study of our patients has revealed that not all individuals with characteristic vasomotor symptoms and increased peripheral blood flow are candidates for drug therapy. Generally the patients can be classified in three groups of graded severity. The first group of patients had mild symptoms, with little or no weight loss and no diarrhea, and did not continue taking the drug, since the severity of the early phase symptoms and the degree of benefit were not sufficient to warrant indefinite medical therapy. They have managed adequately with dietary restriction, including the avoidance of rich carbohydrate and fatty foods, a decrease of liquids with meals, and more frequent, smaller feedings.

The intermediate group are those patients with more intense immediate postprandial symptoms of weakness, weight loss, diarrhea, and moderate to severe late symptoms. Although all the patients in this category experienced relief of early symptoms and some weight gain, two of them had major concomitant epigastric distress and late hypoglycemic symptoms, respectively. These two patients underwent operative procedures to increase gastric reservoir capacity when it became apparent that the early phase symptoms were not the chief component of their postgastrectomy complaints. The remaining patients in this group continued on the drug with gratifying results.

The last group, representing those patients with severe early dumping symptoms and minimal late symptoms, experienced a dramatic response to serotonin antagonist therapy. These patients had profound prostrating vasomotor symptoms, diarrhea, and weight loss of major proportions. Nutritional deficits and anemias were also present in this group. In the latter category, one patient, a 48 year old married female, had severe symptoms with diarrhea and weight loss to the point of cachexia, following a 75 per cent resection with gastrojejunostomy. Each meal was followed by prostrating weakness and sweating, with several episodes of diarrhea and gross steatorrhea. With treatment there was remarkable cessation of diarrhea and steatorrhea, and striking reduction of postprandial symptoms. This patient has continued to gain weight over a two-year follow-up period, and at this time is approaching her preoperative level, representing a weight gain of nearly 50 pounds.

It has become apparent to us that the use of anti-serotonin agents is indicated in patients with moderate to severe early vasomotor symptoms who have significant weight loss or postprandial diarrhea. It can be anticipated that such individuals will be relieved of their vasomotor symptoms and diarrhea, but they should be advised that anti-serotonin drugs will not improve the other manifestations of the postgastrectomy syndrome. In these patients, alleviation of the early symptoms of dumping often "clears the water," as it were, thus making possible the accurate evaluation and effective treatment of late or delayed symptoms.

Treatment

It is questionable whether the added antihistamine action of the anti-serotonin drug that we are presently using is beneficial. Certainly it is conceded that antihistamine drugs alone are of little value in the treatment of dumping. Studies demonstrating histamine release by serotonin infusion into isolated perfused liver and lung preparations suggest that some relationship exists between serotonin and histamine with respect to the dumping syndrome.[13]

Although some newer medication may prove more effective in the future, up to the present time we have found that cyproheptadine obtains the most successful results. We recommend 4 mg. three times a day, taken at least two hours before meals; shorter intervals have proved unsatisfactory. The early drowsiness that sometimes accompanies the onset of treatment is transient and usually disappears within one week. There have been no long-lasting problems encountered with continuing therapy.

The object of drug therapy is to alleviate the early symptoms of dumping and to permit the patient to return to more normal eating patterns. We have, therefore, encouraged patients who are on this drug to try all foods they would normally eat. However, some dietary restriction is generally practiced by these patients who have been long accustomed to harsh penalties for slight indiscretions in their eating habits.

The patients with very mild vasomotor dumping in the absence of significant weight loss or diarrhea are best managed by the usual frequent small feeding regimen, with reduction of liquids at mealtime and the avoidance of rich foods. Similarly, patients with severe postgastrectomy problems, in whom the early phase symptoms are of minor importance, are not candidates for drug therapy. These patients should be managed by diet and other appropriate medical means or by surgical procedures.

Summary

1. The postgastrectomy dumping syndrome includes a number of pathophysiologic processes of various etiologies. One of these, the early postprandial vasomotor and intestinal reaction, is probably mediated in part by serotonin.

2. Only these early phase symptoms of dumping are benefited by anti-serotonin therapy. Thus, an accurate diagnosis and differentiation of postprandial symptoms becomes essential to successful therapy. The plethysmographic "dumping test" is a useful objective tool in the diagnosis of early phase dumping, and is a reliable guide to therapy.

3. Patients having moderately severe early vasomotor and intestinal symptoms and associated diarrhea or weight loss are candidates for anti-serotonin therapy. The improvement, which is sometimes dramatic, is usually proportional to the severity of the dumping problem.

4. Conversely, those patients having mild early phase symptoms without weight loss or diarrhea are not improved by drug treatment, nor are those patients in whom the early phase symptoms are not predominant. Dietary restriction of rich carbohydrates, decreased food intake, and limitation of liquids with meals have proved most effective in the management of these patients.

References

1. Amdrup, E.: Variations in food tolerance after partial gastrectomy. Acta chir. scandinav., *120:*410, 1961.

2. Butz, R.: Dumping syndrome studies during maintenance of blood volume. Ann. Surg., *154:*225, 1961.

3. Drapanas, T., McDonald, J. C., and Stewart, J. D.: Serotonin release following instillation of hypertonic glucose into the proximal intestine. Ann. Surg., *156:*528, 1962.

4. Hinshaw, D. G., Joergenson, E. J., and Stafford, C. E.: Preoperative "dumping" studies in peptic ulcer patients. A.M.A. Arch. Surg., *80:*738, 1960.

5. Hinshaw, D. G., Joergenson, E. J., Davis, H. A., and Stafford, C. E.: Peripheral blood flow and blood volume studies in the dumping syndrome. A.M.A. Arch. Surg., *74:*686, 1957.

6. Johnson, L. P., and Jesseph, J. E.: Evidence for a humoral etiology of the dumping syndrome. S. Forum, *12:*316, 1961.

7. Johnson, L. P., Sloop, R. D., and Jesseph, J. E.: Plethysmographic evidence supporting the concepts of a humoral etiology of the dumping syndrome. J. Surg. Res., *2:*241, 1962.

8. Johnson, L. P., Sloop, R. D., and Jesseph, J. E.: Etiologic significance of the early symptomatic phase in the dumping syndrome. Ann. Surg., *156*:173, 1962.
9. Johnson, L. P., Sloop, R. D., Jesseph, J. E., and Harkins, H. N.: Serotonin antagonists in experimental and clinical "dumping." Ann. Surg., *156*:537, 1962.
10. Jordan, G. L., Jr.: The afferent loop syndrome. Surgery, *38*:1027, 1955.
11. Lawrence, W., Jr., Khentigan, A., Hudoch, J., and Vanamee, P.: The effect of intra-duodenal administration of hypertonic glucose solution on external pancreatic secretion. Surgery, *49*:666, 1961.
12. Mix, C. L.: "Dumping stomach" following gastrojejunostomy. S. Clin. North America, *3*:617, 1922.
13. Moore, T. C., Nowell, L., and Eiseman, B.: Effects of serotonin loading on histamine release and blood flow of isolated perfused liver and lung. A.M.A. Arch. Surg., *87*:42, 1963.
14. Peskin, G. W., and Miller, L. D.: The role of serotonin in the "dumping syndrome." A.M.A. Arch. Surg., *85*:701, 1962.
15. Peskin, G. W., and Miller, L. D.: The use of serotonin antagonists in postgastrectomy syndromes. Am. J. Surg., *109*:7, 1965.
16. Weber, B. M., Bender, M. A., and Moore, G. E.: Dumping syndrome: an evaluation of some current etiologic concepts. New England J. Med., *256*:285, 1957.

Treatment of the Dumping
Syndrome by the Use of an
Antiperistaltic Segment of Jejunum

Edgar J. Poth

University of Texas Medical Branch

The purpose of this treatise is to deal with the "dumping syndrome," one of the several undesirable physiologic phenomena following gastric operations. While "dumping" may be the sequel of almost any gastric procedure, it occurs most frequently and in its most severe form following extensive gastrectomy, by which the volume of the remaining stomach is greatly reduced, precluding the taking of a normal sized meal without forcing the food into the jejunum.

It is commonly observed that "dumping" results when the major portion of the small bowel mucosa is bathed with a hyperosmolar solution. The use of an antiperistaltic segment of jejunum will slow this process. However, the indications for such a "valve" must be recognized. This procedure should be resorted to only after dietary and medical measures fail. Definition of these limits and indications divides these "dumping" patients roughly into three groups.

Classification of Patients with Dumping Syndrome

First Group. These individuals present the syndrome in greater or lesser severity as soon as they begin to take adequate amounts of food postoperatively. They respond readily to dietary management, which consists primarily of forcing fluids between meals, administering at least 250 cc. of fluid 20 to 30 minutes before eating, and giving a diet that includes carbohydrates impregnated with fats and proteins. The fats and proteins are slowly digested and prevent intimate contact between the water soluble digestive ferments and the impregnated carbohydrates, thereby slowing the speed of carbohydrate splitting to prevent hyperosmolarity of the bowel contents. The syndrome disappears after a short time and the dietary restrictions are relaxed. Gastric and small bowel motility should be studied by cinefluorography.

SECOND GROUP. These individuals cannot relax the above dietary restrictions and will occasionally experience "dumping" in spite of medical and dietary control, but the episodes are sufficiently infrequent to preclude operative intervention. They can maintain essentially normal weight and activity.

THIRD GROUP. These patients cannot be managed satisfactorily by diet and medication. Almost invariably the muscular emptying mechanism of the stomach extending from the incisura to the pylorus has been lost. Usually insufficient stomach remains to serve as a pouch to receive an adequate meal and hold it for any length of time. They are essentially "gastric invalids."

Diagnosis

The following additional study is imperative for proper evaluation. The patient is given a normal diet simultaneously with the rapid administration of 10 per cent glucose intravenously. Under these circumstances, "dumping" should not occur. Nausea, abdominal pain, diarrhea, syncope, sweating, nervousness, etc., should not develop. This procedure is both diagnostic and therapeutic. If the administration of glucose intravenously does not prevent "dumping," one must rule out some other cause for the postgastrectomy syndrome.

Operative Procedure

If 50 per cent or more of the stomach remains, the procedure presented by the author in 1957 may be utilized. The length of the antiperistaltic segment, while not critical, should be determined by the gastric emptying and peristaltic activity as demonstrated by cineofluorographic studies. The operative procedure referred to above permits the use of relatively long segments of jejunum while only a limited segment is reversed. This technique ensures a good blood supply. A short segment of jejunum, with only a single mesenteric artery, is highly vulnerable to thrombosis and necrosis or may develop sustained spasm and fail to function properly.

Usually little or none of the stomach remains in these individuals. If no stomach remains, the technique is altered to provide an isoperistaltic inlet to protect the esophagus from regurgitation.[2] If any stomach remains, as much as 10 per cent can be converted into a tube to serve as an isoperistaltic inlet to the pouch and protect the esophagus against regurgitation.[4] All pouches have a true antiperistaltic outlet. They empty in small amounts over a prolonged period of time by dilution. A normal diet of regular meals is tolerated well without "dumping." Snacks between meals and at bedtime are usually desired. Normal weight is regained and maintained; overweight has occurred. Appetite is restored to normal.

These operative procedures are indicated in a small percentage of individuals, and when they are applied, the severest forms of "dumping" are regularly corrected, apparently because large surfaces of small bowel mucosa are no longer exposed to excessive quantities of hyperosmolar solutions, which in turn cause extensive shifting of fluid into the lumen of the bowel.[3]

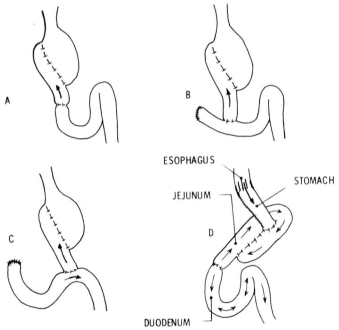

Fig. 1. Application of the principle of the antiperistaltic segment of jejunum. *A, B,* and *C* illustrate the use of an isolated segment of jejunum, appliqued by suture to the entire cut end of the gastric remnant in such fashion as to result in an antiperistaltic outlet, the distal end of which is anastomosed to the end of the duodenum (*A*), or to other sites on the duodenum (*B* and *C*) should the proximal end of the duodenum be unsuited. If 10 per cent or less of stomach remains, the gastric remnant is converted into a tube and a substitution pouch fashioned as shown in *D*. (See Fig. 3, in Ann. Surg., *160*:493, 1964, for a variety of possible procedures including those for instances when no stomach remains.)

The length of the antiperistaltic outlet segment, which is functioning as the "valve," should be approximately equal to and not greater than half the circumference of the jejunum at that site.

References

1. Poth, E. J.: The dumping syndrome and its surgical management. Am. Surg., *23*:1097, 1957.
2. Poth, E. J.: The substitution gastric pouch (A). Texas Rep. Biol. Med., *17*:238, 1959.
3. Poth, E. J.: Surgical correction of severe "dumping" and postgastrectomy malnutrition. Ann. Surg., *160*:488, 1964.
4. Poth, E. J., and Cleveland, B. R.: A functional substitution pouch for the stomach (B). Arch. Surg., *83*:42, 1961.

The Management

of Mesenteric

Arterial Occlusion

The editors have sought in vain for someone to oppose Shaw's management of superior mesenteric arterial occlusion. In view of such widespread acceptance, we have chosen to include his paper, "The 'Second Look' after Superior Mesenteric Arterial Embolectomy or Reconstruction for Mesenteric Infarction," as originally submitted.

The Editors

The "Second Look" After Superior Mesenteric Arterial Embolectomy or Reconstruction for Mesenteric Infarction

Robert S. Shaw

Harvard Medical School

The specific clinical problem under discussion becomes defined in the operating room when exploratory laparotomy demonstrates infarcted bowel and absent or reduced pulsation in the superior mesenteric artery. My specific therapeutic objective is to restore circulation to the gut and salvage as great a length of gut as possible. This objective is defensible only as far as its pursuance augments rather than compromises the more basic objectives of patient survival and rehabilitation.

Two clinical subdivisions of this problem may be encountered and should be discussed separately. In the first, 50 per cent or less of the small bowel may be frankly infarcted, inviting argument for the older conventional operation of resection and enteroenterostomy without reopening the obstructed superior mesenteric artery. In the second instance, ischemia involves all or almost all of the small bowel, demanding reconstruction of the superior mesenteric artery for survival of the patient. Here the argument revolves around methods of handling the bowel which, after revascularization, does not return to immediate and unquestioned viability.

Limited Infarction

In the presence of obstruction in the main superior mesenteric artery, the extent and need for resection of an apparently infarcted segment of intestine cannot be evaluated until this artery is reopened. Even where a frankly gangrenous segment seems well demarcated from adjacent pink bowel, primary resection should not be performed without restoring normal flow in the main artery, since to do this would be to invite ischemic impairment of healing of the anastomosis. Complications such as small bowel fistula are common in old experience with limited resection.

Page 389

After reopening the superior mesenteric artery, a previously cyanotic segment may become bright and hyperemic before the eyes of the surgeon. Here, primary resection obviously is not indicated. On the other hand, the segment may show return of circulation only in the mesenteric side of the bowel or not at all, with obvious full thickness death of the bowel wall. When this is the case, primary resection is clearly indicated. Problems in judgment arise when the bowel shows some improvement, but remains a little cyanotic, with circulation which is still questionable. This problem is identical to that encountered in the evaluation of bowel viability after release of a strangulated hernia. The same judgment should apply, and when serious doubt of viability remains, bowel should be resected, since resection will not be so extensive as to result in a severe short bowel syndrome. It might be possible to salvage short segments of bowel with very severe ischemic injury by returning them to the peritoneal cavity and re-exploring the patient after twelve to twenty-four hours of vigorous supportive therapy, at which time the viability or nonviability of the bowel segment would have more clearly declared itself. However, the penalty for preserving seriously injured bowel segments may be the occurrence of late cicatricial stenosis or chronic ulceration and bleeding.[7]

Thus primary resection should be performed as required in the case showing a limited and discrete segment of infarcted bowel, and a routine "second look" is not indicated.

Extensive Infarction

When the circulation of the entire small bowel is found severely compromised at operation, restoration of circulation through the superior mesenteric artery may again be followed by immediate return of the entire small bowel to bright hyperemia and unquestionable viability. In these instances there would appear to be no reason for routine re-exploration in the absence of specific signs indicating further trouble in the abdomen. Such patients may have melena postoperatively, and often show diarrhea for several days after they recover peristalsis, but should show a falling white blood count and no more evidence of postoperative peritonitis on physical examination than follows the ordinary laparotomy.

The "second look" is indicated in the more usual response in which the bowel will become pink in some segments and remain blue in others, and resection of all questionable bowel would involve multiple suture lines or a major loss of gut length. During the interval between the initial exploration and the "second look" it is most important to do everything possible to encourage the return and maintenance of good bowel circulation in order that the "second look" not be too commonly disheartening. I have closed the abdomen on bowel that showed a fairly good return of circulation with only a few spotty areas in doubt, and on re-exploration have found extensive infarction involving not only the entire small bowel, but the large bowel and stomach as well, all in the presence of open major visceral vessels. Understanding of the mechanisms at work here is essential and requires further discussion.

It is now well documented that frank infarction of the small bowel can occur in the absence of major vessel occlusions from prolonged and severe reduction in cardiac output, as in uncorrected hypovolemic shock or severe heart disease.[1, 5] Both mechanisms are apt to be operating full force in a patient with intestinal infarction, with the result that restoration of mesenteric arterial patency may be followed by little improvement in bowel circulation. In such a case, the importance of splanchnic vasospasm, occurring as a compensatory response to low cardiac output, can be graphically demonstrated on the operating table by injecting the root of the mesentery with procaine, producing bright hyperemia in the segment of the bowel thus denervated.

It is essential for the maintenance of a good cardiac output to recognize and treat the profound and increasing hypovolemia secondary to ischemic injury of the gut. There are losses of large volumes of plasma and whole blood into the wall of the bowel from reverse flow down the portal venous system during the period before revascularization. Following revascularization and restoration of high pressure to the arterial side, there are major losses of whole blood into the submucosa, mucosa, and bowel lumen.[6] These losses will be measured in terms of liters. They are usually incompletely corrected in practice, either from failure to recognize them or from timidity due to fear of producing congestive failure. Adequate and safe replacement therapy requires either monitoring and maintenance of an adequate central venous pressure or periodic measurement of blood volume. The use of vasopressors to maintain central blood pressure is to be condemned, because it acts to reduce splanchnic blood flow.

There is cogent argument for the use of some method of splanchnic nervous block during this interval,[4] but as yet clinical tests have not been sufficient to state its effectiveness. The reason for the failure of immediate return of bowel circulation following reconstructive vascular surgery should not be residual thrombus or obstruction in major vessels, since distal thrombosis is exceedingly rare in the smaller vessels of the mesenteric arterial tree,[2] and such thrombus as exists can be milked back manually from the mesentery at the time of the initial operation.

Essential to the rationale of efforts to salvage bowel with severe ischemic injury is the knowledge that repair and regeneration will occur in such bowel following revascularization, even where the mucosa has been almost completely devastated.[3] Chronic ulceration or cicatricial stenosis has not been a common late problem in these cases. Severe postoperative malabsorption has been seen, but eventual regeneration of a normally functioning bowel occurred after several months.[8]

The purpose of the "second look" then, is not just to allow a clear definition between dead and live bowel to take place, but also to allow time for the institution of supportive measures, which may render more of the bowel viable.

Summary

In cases with obstruction in the main superior mesenteric artery and discrete and limited infarction of intestine, primary resection is justified, but only when the viability of the bowel segment still appears doubtful after the restoration of continuity in the main vessel.

If the major portion of the small bowel is ischemic and does not return to unquestioned viability immediately following the restoration of flow in the superior mesenteric artery, maximal bowel salvage may result after 12 to 24 hours of intensive therapy, directed at increasing cardiac output and decreasing splanchnic vasospasm, followed by re-exploration and resection of bowel that is noted to have irreversible full-thickness ischemic injury.

References

1. Ende, N.: Infarction of bowel in cardiac failure. New England J. Med., 258:879, 1958.
2. Glotzer, D. J., and Shaw, R. S.: Massive bowel infarction. New England J. Med., 260: 162, 1959.
3. Glotzer, D. J., Villegas, A. H., Anekamaya, S., and Shaw, R. S.: Healing of the intestine in experimental bowel infarction. Ann. Surg., 155:267, 1956.
4. Liang, H., Bernard, H. R., and Dodd, R. B.: Effect of epidural block upon experimental mesenteric occlusion. Arch. Surg., 83:409, 1961.
5. Lillehei, R. C.: Intestinal factor in irreversible hemorrhagic shock. Surgery, 42:1043, 1957.
6. Marston, A. B. M.: Causes of death in mesenteric arterial occlusion. I. Local and general effects of devascularization of the bowel. Ann. Surg., In Press.
7. Rosenman, L. D., and Gropper, A. N.: Small intestine stenosis caused by infarction: unusual sequel of mesenteric artery embolism. Ann. Surg., 141:254, 1955.
8. Shaw, R. S., and Rutledge, R. H.: Superior mesenteric artery embolectomy in the treatment of massive mesenteric infarction. New England J. Med., 257:595, 1957.

Management

of Rectal Segment

in Familial Polyposis

Introduction

It probably is fair to say that everyone agrees that there is such a strong potentiality of malignant change in familial polyposis of the colon and rectum that a total colectomy, at the least, is indicated in these patients. A *bona fide* controversy exists, however, in the surgical management of the rectum (with polyps and without carcinoma) when such patients have their total colectomy. There are three alternatives: (1) total colectomy with ileoproctostomy and fulguration of rectal polyps; (2) pancolectomy (total colectomy with complete excision of the rectum) and abdominal ileostomy; or (3) total colectomy with excision of rectal mucosa and anal ileostomy. One can find good arguments, and proponents, for each of these alternative approaches. Certainly the most positive means of preventing the development of cancer is pancolectomy (total excision of colon and rectum), particularly in those patients who are not likely to remain under careful observation. This method of treatment requires an abdominal ileostomy, to which there has been an abhorrence, but which now is more easily managed than previously. In those patients with polyposis in whom there is no cancer of the rectum at the time of colectomy, the temptation is great to advise preservation of the rectum, or at least its musculature and anal sphincters. If the rectum is preserved *in toto*, with ileoproctostomy, the mucosa requires regular, almost continuous, observation for polyps, which must be removed as soon as they are noted.

In some of these patients, one of the most interesting facets of the phenomena of new growth has been observed: Spontaneous regression of the polyps of the rectum has been reported to occur (1) after colectomy, or (2) after second-look removal of all metastatic cancer some time after colectomy. This phenomenon suggests an immune mechanism in the colon-polyps-cancer relationship. This occasional spontaneous regression is uncommon and should not be depended upon; it should not preclude active removal of the polyps by one means or another in any case, at least until more is learned about such phenomena. The probability of success of the third alternative, that of removal of the rectal mucosa and submucosa, with preservation of the rectal sphincter musculature by anal ileostomy, depends much on the technical considerations of the operation. Both good and bad functional results have been reported with the various sphincter-saving operations, but in evaluating such results the reader must be cognizant of the type of sphincter-preserving operation being reported before he passes judgement on all the operations that have been described. Meticulous attention to operative details and experience portend better results.

Additionally, careful observation of the progeny of patients with familial polyposis is an obligation of the patient and of the physician, because of the mendelian dominance of this hereditary characteristic.

The following sections present opposing views on what to do with the rectum at the time of colectomy; cogent reasons for each of the alternatives are clearly documented.

S. R. F.

Preservation of the Rectum in the Surgical Management of Familial Polyposis

Jack W. Cole

Hahnemann Medical College and Hospital,
Philadelphia, Pennsylvania

Background

Familial polyposis is a hereditary disease characterized by the development of adenomatous polyps in the colon and rectum. It is transmitted as a mendelian dominant by either afflicted parent and may be expected to occur in one-half the offspring.

In most cases the adenomas do not appear before puberty or after the fifth decade of life. The number of adenomas may vary in any afflicted individual from a few to so great a number that they completely obscure the normal mucosa.

Although patients with the disease may find the associated symptoms of diarrhea, abdominal pain, and anemia distressing, if not incapacitating, it is the risk of the development of cancer, if the disease is untreated, that poses the greatest threat to life and a challenge in the management of these patients. In a recent study of 83 patients with familial polyposis at St. Mark's Hospital, 38 (45 per cent) were found to have one or more adenocarcinomas of the large bowel. Eighteen (21 per cent) of the 83 patients had more than one cancer at the time of surgery. One patient had 5 independent carcinomas of the colon. A total of 69 adenocarcinomas were found in the 83 patients with familial polyposis.[5]

There is general agreement that once the diagnosis of familial polyposis has been established, prompt surgical intervention is indicated to avoid the risk of the patient's developing a malignancy. The major decision confronting the responsible surgeon is the type of surgical procedure to perform. A total coloproctectomy, a total colectomy and ileoproctostomy, or ileo-anal anastomosis are the choices.

The rectum should be removed in those instances in which a carcinoma is present, or in those patients who, for various reasons, cannot be relied upon to submit faithfully to periodic examination of the retained rectal segment if an ileoproctostomy is performed. Some surgeons feel that the presence of large numbers of adenomas in the rectum is also an indication for removal of the rectum, but this opinion is not shared by the author.

It is our opinion that, with the above exceptions, most patients with familial polyposis are best managed by total colectomy and ileoproctostomy, making certain that the anastomosis between the ileum and the rectum is within easy reach of the examining sigmoidoscope (8 to 10 cm.) to facilitate removal of the adenomas within the retained rectal segment, and to permit easy periodic examination every three months for the remainder of the patient's life.

The following considerations have led us to adopt this form of therapy as the procedure of choice in most patients with familial polyposis.

The Risk of Cancer in Retained Rectum Not Excessive

Although there is an ever-present risk of cancer in the retained rectal segment, we do not feel that it is prohibitive in cooperative intelligent patients. Its occurrence does not preclude a possible cure if careful periodic examinations are performed and prompt excision of the rectum carried out when the diagnosis is made. In a recent review of 62 patients treated at St. Marks Hospital from 1926 to 1962, in whom the rectum had not been removed, only 3 patients developed carcinoma in the retained rectal segment. In these 3 patients, carcinoma of the rectum was diagnosed 6 years, 4 years, and 2 years following colectomy and ileoproctostomy. Two of the 3 patients are dead. One died during the immediate postoperative period following proctectomy; without evidence of metastasis, one died of cancer 3 years following proctectomy; and the third patient is alive without evidence of disease four years following proctectomy for carcinoma.

Eight of the 62 patients are dead from unrelated causes. Fifty-one patients are alive and well, one patient with rectum intact after 37 years.

To properly evaluate these data in the selection of appropriate surgical therapy for this disease, one must weigh them against the operative mortality and morbidity associated with the technically more difficult procedures. The late mortality with permanent abdominal ileostomy is approximately 3 per cent. To the best of our knowledge insufficient experience has been obtained with ileoanal anastomosis or ileal, sphincter-sparing, pull-through procedures as described by Ravitch to adequately assess the long-term risk. However, the complications associated with procedures in which the rectum is removed are well known, i.e., bladder dysfunction, sexual impotence, infections, and fistulas, and can be expected to occur in a substantial number of cases undergoing total coloproctectomy and ileostomy. Bacon, in 604 pull-through procedures, reported sexual impotence in 12.2 per cent and bladder dysfunction of various types in 41.8 per cent.

There is some possibility of minimizing these complications by limiting the dissection, as in the management of non-malignant disease, but some complications are inevitable in a significant number of cases when all or a major portion of the rectum is removed.

Lastly, and perhaps the most important consideration of all, has to do with the problem of fecal continence associated with the various sphincter-saving procedures currently being advocated in the treatment of familial polyposis. Wide differences of opinion exist as to the incidence of this complication with sphincter-sparing operations, but suffice it to say that it is a real and most distressing problem in a substantial number of patients so treated.[2] It is not a complication of colectomy and ileoproctostomy.

Procedure Does Not Result in Disability

Another argument for the use of colectomy and ileoproctostomy is the natural revulsion of patients to a permanent abdominal ileostomy or a malfunctioning ileoanal anastomosis. If the responsible physicians and surgeons are to discharge their obligations to the patients with familial polyposis, they must make known to the patient the fact that they have a hereditary disease and emphasize to them the absolute necessity for careful and periodic examinations of all the relatives and any children they may bear. The success of these efforts will depend in a large measure on the type of therapy that is offered. Greater numbers of afflicted patients will doubtlessly come to surgery *earlier*, before cancer develops, if they know that the disease can be treated in a manner that allows for restoration of the continuity of the bowel and fecal continence. This may be of the utmost importance in the management of patients in the younger age groups from a social and psychological point of view. Furthermore, as the medical profession becomes more keenly aware of the disease and appreciates its hereditary nature, we will be charged with caring for more patients in the younger age groups where these factors are of prime importance. It is our opinion that surgery should be undertaken once the diagnosis has been firmly established.

Decision Influenced by Phenomenon of Spontaneous Regression of Adenomas

During recent years attention has been focused on the phenomenon of spontaneous regression of rectal adenomas that occasionally occurs following total colectomy and ileoproctostomy.[3, 4, 7, 8] Although no satisfactory explanation of this regression has been forthcoming, there is no doubt that it occurs and adds additional support to the choice of colectomy and ileoproctostomy.

It is not known how frequently this may be expected to occur. However, in 45 patients undergoing colectomy and ileoproctostomy at St. Marks Hospital, and who have been followed three or more years, 10 patients have had no recurrent adenomas develop since the rectum was cleared. The period of observation in the group ranges from 3 to 13 years. These data suggest that colectomy and ileoproctostomy may inhibit the development of adenomas of the rectum in some cases and have a bearing on the choice of operative procedure. It has been the impression of the St. Marks group that once the colon has been removed, fewer adenomas tend to develop in the rectum, and the propensity for adenomatous polyps to appear is further reduced with advancing age.[6] Certainly, this phenomenon has led us to modify our previous thoughts that the presence of a great many adenomas in the rectum is an absolute indication for total coloproctectomy. It is our practice to remove only those adenomas from the rectum immediately adjacent to the anastomotic site and leave the remaining adenomas intact for several months during the postoperative period. Regression of the adenomas to varying degrees has occurred in six consecutive cases so treated. If regression does occur, it minimizes the trauma to the retained rectal segment incident to repeated excision and fulguration of the residual adenomas. This seems highly desirable in a markedly "unstable" mucosal epithelium, which is predisposed to tumor formation, and reduces the risk of stricture formation. It is even possible that repeated fulguration may have been a contributing factor in the development of cancer in some of the reported cases.

Summary

With the exception of those patients with adenocarcinoma of the rectum and those who, for a variety of reasons, cannot be relied upon to submit to periodic examination of the rectum, all patients with familial polyposis of the colon are best treated by colectomy and ileoproctostomy for the following reasons:

1. The risk of carcinoma in the retained rectal segment is not excessive in carefully followed patients, and its occurrence, with early recognition, does not preclude the possibility of cure.

2. Patients with total colectomy and ileoproctostomy lead completely normal lives without the social, psychological, and physical disability associated with a permanent abdominal ileostomy or the unsatisfactory fecal continence that accompanies other procedures.

3. Because this procedure does not cause disability, patients seek prompt attention for their disease. This is also a most important consideration in encouraging early examination in asymptomatic members in a family carrying the genetic trait. Of particular importance, in this regard, is the willingness of parents to present their children for earlier examination and diagnosis. One cannot underestimate the importance of this point in the selec-

tion of a surgical procedure and control of the disease in the general population.

4. Permanent abdominal ileostomy carries a 3 per cent mortality rate and ileoanal anastomosis or pull-through procedures are unsatisfactory in most reported series with a high morbidity rate.

5. Spontaneous regression of the adenomas in the retained rectal segment will occur in a significant number of patients following total colectomy and ileoproctostomy, and is influential in our selection of this surgical procedure.

The author wishes to express his gratitude to the staff of St. Marks Hospital, London, for making possible portions of this report.

References

1. Bacon, H. E.: Abdominoperineal proctosigmoidectomy with sphincter preservation. J. A. M. A., *160*:628, 1956.
2. Best, R. R.: Evaluation of ileoproctostomy to avoid ileostomy in various colon lesions. J. A. M. A. *150*:637, 1952.
3. Cole, J. W., and Holden, W. D.: Postcolectomy regression of adenomatous polyps of the rectum. Arch. Surg., *79*:385, 1959.
4. Cole, J. W., McKalen, A., and Powell, J.: The role of ileal contents in the spontaneous regression of rectal adenomas. Dis. Colon Rectum, *4*:413, 1961.
5. Cole, J. W., and Morson, B. C.: Unpublished data.
6. Dukes, C. E.: Cancer control in familial polyposis of the colon. Dis. Colon and Rectum, *1*:413, 1958.
7. Dunphy, J. E., Patterson, W. B., and Legg, M. A.: Etiologic factors in polyposis and carcinoma of the colon. Ann. Surg., *150*:488, 1959.
8. Hubbard, T. B., Jr.: Familial polyposis of the colon: the fate of the retained rectum after colectomy in children. Am. Surg., *23*:6, 1957.
9. Lockhart-Mummery, H. E., Duke, C. E., and Bussey, H. J. R.: The surgical treatment of familial polyposis of the colon. Brit. J. Surg., *43*:476, 1956.
10. Ravitch, M. M., and Sabiston, D. C.: Anal ileostomy with preservation of sphincter. A proposed operation in patients requiring total colectomy for benign tumors. Surg., Gynec. and Obst., *84*:1095, 1947.
11. Ravitch, M. M.: Total colectomy and abdominoperineal resection (pan-colectomy) in one stage. Ann. Surg., *144*:758, 1956.

Excision of the Rectum or its Mucosa in the Surgical Management of Polyposis

Mark M. Ravitch

Johns Hopkins University School of Medicine

The central factor involved in the choice of treatment for multiple polypoid adenomatosis of the colon is the inevitability of the development of cancer. Whatever may be the ultimate outcome of the present day polemic over the carcinogenic significance of sporadic polyps in the colon, there is essential agreement concerning the significance of polyps in patients with polyposis coli. All such patients will ultimately die of cancer of the colon, unless they succumb to some other cause first, or have all of the colonic mucosa removed. The youngest patients with cancer of the colon in association with this disease, whom we have treated, have been seventeen and eighteen years of age, but patients a decade or more younger are on record. Multiple simultaneous carcinomas are not uncommon, and the unfortunate fact is that bleeding, diarrhea, and tenesmus, which might otherwise signal the presence of a cancer, are precisely the symptoms of the pre-existing, underlying disease. In this day, when so much effort is devoted to prophylaxis and prevention of cancer, one would suppose that there would be little temptation to compromise in a condition that invariably leads to cancer, and for which an absolutely curative operation is available which is, at the same time, a certain prophylactic against cancer.

Excision vs. Preservation of Rectum

The operation of abdominal colectomy, with preservation of the rectum and an ileorectal anastomosis, is widely performed. This radical disregard of the malignant potentiality of the mucosa in the retained rectum is nevertheless supported by a number of arguments. Undeniably the patient retains normal defecatory apparatus, at the price, perhaps, of some modest change in bowel habit. The operation is generally performed after repeated endoscopic fulgurations have destroyed the polyps in the segment of rectum to be retained, and the subsequent plan entails lifelong observation of the patient, with periodic endoscopic examination and fulguration of recurrent polyps. The first such operation done successfully may well have been that of Lillienthal[4] some fifty years ago, and Lockhart-Mummery[5] and others have reported long-term survivals without occurrence of cancer in the retained rectal stump. On the other hand, a substantial number of patients have been reported in whom cancer has, soon or late, occurred in the retained rectal stump, often being discovered at a time when a curative operation was no longer possible.[3] The symptoms of the carcinoma, of course—bleeding, tenesmus, change of bowel habit, etc.—are precisely those of the underlying basic disease, and might not necessarily be alarming to the patient. Understandably there is less enthusiasm for publishing ultimate failures in such procedures than ultimate successes, and it may fairly be assumed that a larger proportion of the successes than of the failures have been reported. Difficulties in the follow-up of such patients are obvious. Either the patient or the physician may fail to maintain the regular re-examination schedule. Fulguration may be inadequate to destroy some of the polyps, so that carcinoma may actually develop between the periodic visits. The polyps may be so numerous, essentially carpeting the mucous surface, that destruction of all the polyps by fulguration cannot reasonably be achieved. Finally, the anastomosis may be sufficiently high, or the bowel so fixed and angled after operation, as to make it difficult or impossible to inspect with certainty every bit of the mucosal surface of the retained rectum.

When all is said and done, this is a genetically determined disease. The regenerated mucosa, no matter how often fulgurated, retains its genetic predisposition to form polyps, and these, in turn, retain their capacity for developing into cancer if inadequately treated, or left untreated. The risk seems a great one to take, and the potential price a heavy one to pay for preservation of the rectum.

The Patient Makes the Decision

In our own practice we present patients with two alternatives. Having mentioned the operation of preservation of the rectum, we advise the patient that this is not an alternative which we are prepared to discuss, since we are unwilling to allow them to take the mortal risk involved, and that if this is the operation they are determined to have, it will have to be performed by another surgeon. We explain that it is necessary to remove all of the mucosa of the colon and rectum.

Pancolectomy with Abdominal Ileostomy

The simplest procedure, the most definitive and most calculable in its results, is pancolectomy (total colectomy plus abdominoperineal resection of the rectum) in one stage, with an abdominal ileostomy. This involves a two- or three-week hospitalization, at the end of which time, to all intents and purposes the patient can expect to be well, to have reached a stable condition, and to be able to make his life plan without the expectation of interruption, once he has regained the strength lost by the preoperative manifestations of his disease, and by the operation itself. Abdominal ileostomy today, with the maturation of the ileostomy at the time of laparotomy (a maturation which we prefer to perform by the Brooke technique) and with the use of a wide variety of acceptable ileostomy devices, is not the incapacitating and unpleasant thing that it was twenty years ago, although it can still hardly be rated as a social asset. Nevertheless, whereas it was once a truism that a young woman with an ileostomy could never expect to marry, all of us have now seen numerous girls go to maturity and marriage despite an ileostomy.

Total Colectomy with Anal Ileostomy

The other alternative which we offer to patients is total colectomy with anal ileostomy,[1, 7-9] by the technique to be presently described. In this situation we are forced to explain that the mortal risk of operation, which is almost nil in the one stage pancolectomy with abdominal ileostomy, is somewhat higher, that the complication rate after operation is higher, (even in patients with ultimate first-rate outcome, there may be a period of months during which the patient must become accustomed to and overcome an increased frequency of stools), and finally, that there is the possibility of technical failure, which would require a second operation and establishment of an abdominal ileostomy. While most patients presented with this choice nevertheless opt for the anal ileostomy, an occasional one prefers the quick definitive procedure with the smallest likelihood of subsequent distress or danger.

The operation of anal ileostomy is based on the concept that in benign disease it is necessary only to remove the mucosa and submucosa and that the muscular coats of the rectum can be left behind. This allows the sphincters and the levatores, the effector mechanisms controlling continence, to be left intact, and, as well, allows the sensory portion of the reflex arc in the rectum to receive the impression of fullness and initiate the sequence of muscular contractions that prevent involuntary evacuation. We now have a 17-year experience with this operation, applied to operations for preserving the sphincter and the normal mode of defecation in patients requiring total colectomy in the presence of either polyposis or ulcerative colitis, in patients requiring excision of the rectum for villous adenoma, and in patients with destruction of the rectum from lymphopathia venerea. Obviously in the patients with ulcerative colitis and polyposis, it is the ileum that is brought down through the intact tube of rectal musculature, and in patients with villous adenoma and with lymphopathia venerea, it is the more proximal colon that is brought down. In one patient with lymphopathia, in fact, a loop of ileum was brought down and interposed between anus below and descending colon above. Furthermore, there has now been an experience of several years, chiefly in Brazil,[6] with the application of this same technique to resection of the rectum for the acquired type of aganglionic megacolon that is due to Chagas disease—Brazilian trypanosomiasis, and in Brazil,[11] and in Italy[12] and France,[2] the same technique was applied to the congenital form of true Hirschsprung's disease. From all these experiences it can be stated that the aim of the operation in respect to the production of continence can regularly be achieved if the bowel that is brought down is viable and heals without infection, which is ordinarily the case. If the proximal colon is brought down, there is ordinarily little or no period of adjustment, and when the wound is healed, the patient, in essence, is well, except insofar as any large operation on the rectum or left colon may lead, for a while, to irregularity of bowel habit and perhaps increased frequency of stools. When the ileum is brought down, continence is similarly perfectly secure. The difficulty here lies in the persistence of frequent evacuations of liquid stool. Our experience and the reports of others show considerable variation in the patterns ultimately achieved, and the speed with which they are achieved. We have had patients leave the hospital in three weeks, clean and continent, and having only three or four stools a day, and we have had other patients who eventually achieved completely successful results, but required six to nine months before achieving a satisfactory modus vivendi. At first the necessity for nocturnal evacuations is annoying, and at times these, being liquid, may escape in part before the patient awakes. All our patients have ultimately overcome the need for nocturnal evacuations, and the usual pattern is three to six evacuations a day. During the initial postoperative phases, when evacuations of watery ileal contents are frequent, there may be perineal burning and excoriation. This has not been a persistent problem. In patients with ulcerative colitis the operation has proved to be quite difficult to perform, failures have been frequent, and although we can claim two long-term successes more than 15 years later, which are very good, we doubt, because of the special nature of the inflammatory disease and the special personality problems of the patients, that the operation in general is justifiable in this condition. In patients with polyposis the success rate has been extremely high, and in fact, failures have occurred only when the bowel has been improperly or unsuccessfully mobilized, so that the end of the ileum brought down to the anus has not been viable.

Technique for Total Colectomy with Anal Ileostomy

The technique is described here in some detail because so often its principle appears to have been misunderstood, and it is common, in discussions of this general problem, to have the results from extremely low rectal anastomoses below the level of the levatores or from pull-through operations, after removal of the entire rectum, equated with results of the procedure presently under discussion.

From within the abdomen the right and left colons are freed from their peritoneal reflections, the gastrocolic omentum is divided, the mesenteric blood supply of the colon is divided, and the pelvic peritoneum incised. At this point one has a choice of beginning the submucosal dissection from above, or descending to the perineum and initiating it from below, or, in fact, employing a combination. In either case the submucosal section is best accomplished if saline solution with epinephrine is injected into the submucosal plane to allow for easier dissection and separation of the tissues, and to minimize bleeding from small vessels. If one begins above, the injection is administered just below the level of the peritoneal reflection; by blunt dissection the muscular coats are reflected and, traction being made on the mucosa and submucosa, dissection is carried down between these coats essentially to the anus.

The patient, from the first, is in the combined lithotomy-Trendelenburg position. In the anal portion of the operation one seizes the mucocutaneous junction with four Allis clamps, makes a circular incision at the mucocutaneous junction, and then, again, aided by injected saline solution, dissects the mucosa and submucosa from the rectum, ultimately, therefore, delivering the specimen, which consists of the full thickness of the entire colon down to the rectum, of which only the mucosa and submucosa are removed, leaving behind an intact tube of rectal musculature with its sphincteric and levator components and attachments. The terminal ileum is now divided, and with considerable care and thought, appropriate mesenteric vessels are divided, so that a sufficient length of viable ileum is secured to reach down through this muscular tube to the anus. We have preferred, in the past, to take sutures between the outer coats of the ileum and the muscular coats of the rectal tube, as well as to put silk sutures through and through the ileum and the skin. Soave,[12] in performing this operation for Hirschsprung's disease recommends that the pulled-through bowel be permitted to protrude for several centimeters and to heal in place without sutures, being then trimmed away 10 or 12 days later. This should be an entirely acceptable alternative. We have not employed a preliminary ileostomy or a simultaneous proximal decompressing ileostomy, although this has been recommended by some,[10] and may have some merit.

Summary

Polyposis coli is a potentially and inevitably fatal disease, all patients succumbing to cancer of the colon eventually. Under the circumstances, we feel that there is no justification for withholding a certainly prophylactic operation, and the choice lies between the relatively simple and direct and predictable operation of pancolectomy with abdominal ileostomy, or total colectomy with endoanal mucosal resection and anal ileostomy. While either is acceptable and can be recommended with propriety, we prefer the anal ileostomy.

References

1. Devine, J., and Webb, R.: Resection of rectal mucosa, colectomy, and anal ileostomy with normal continence. Surg., Gynec. and Obst., *92:*437, 1951.
2. Duhamel, B.: Personal communication.
3. Gupstill, P.: Familial polyposis of the colon. Surgery, *22:*286, 1947.
4. Lilienthal, H.: Hyperplastic colitis: Extirpation of the entire colon, the upper portion of the sigmoid flexure and four inches of the ileum. Am. Med., *1:*164, 1901.
5. Lockhart-Mummery P.: Diseases of the Colon and their Surgical Treatment. New York, W. Wood and Co., 1910.
6. Raia, A.: Megacolo adquirido-Tratamento cirúrgico. Proceedings of Anais do I Congresso Latino-Americano II Internacional e X Braxileiro de Protologia. p. 296–305, Sept. 1960.
7. Ravitch, M. M.: Anal ileostomy with sphincter preservation in patients requiring total colectomy for benign conditions. Surgery, *24:*170, 1948.
8. Ravitch, M. M., and Handelsman, J. C.: One stage resection of entire colon and rectum for ulcerative colitis and polypoid adenomatosis. Bull. Johns Hopkins Hosp. *88:*59, 1951.
9. Ravitch, M. M., and Sabiston, D. C., Jr.: A proposal for preservation of the sphincter with anal ileostomy in patients requiring total colectomy for benign lesions. Surg., Gynec. and Obst., *84:*1095, 1947.
10. Schneider, S.: Anal ileostomy: experiences with new three stage procedure. A.M.A. Arch. Surg., *70:*539, 1955.
11. Simonsen, O., Habr, A., and Gazal, P.: Rectossigmoidectomia endoanal con resseccas de mucosa rectal. Rev. Paulista med., *57:*116, 1960.
12. Soave, F.: Hirschsprung's disease: a new surgical technique. Arch. Dis. Childhood, *39:*116, 1964.

Idiopathic
Ulcerative Colitis

Introduction

As the term "idiopathic" implies, little has been learned about the etiology of ulcerative colitis; hence the treatment of this condition takes many a divergent course. With the advent of corticosteroid therapy there are some new controversial aspects of the medical management, while the type of surgical management seems to have become less controversial. In the surgical field, for instance, ileostomy alone is seldom done as the primary treatment, and the use of vagotomy has run its short-lived course. On the other hand, the improvement in surgical technique and the availability of better supportive therapy has led to almost universal acceptance of total colectomy as the surgical treatment most likely to succeed. There is some disagreement as to whether the rectum ought to be removed or preserved by ileoproctostomy and, furthermore, whether operations should be staged. Factors to be considered include the usual involvement of the entire colon and rectum with mucosal disease, the nature of the complications that require operation, and the acuteness (or chronicity) of the disease. The very ill patient may require the total removal of colon and rectum instead of lesser procedures, contrary to former considerations.

Better surgical techniques, including the meticulous fashioning of the ileostomy and its continuing care, have improved the results of surgical treatment so that patients are being referred for operation earlier than formerly; operations thus performed before the moribund stage is reached also have had a salutory effect on the overall results.

The following articles are presented for their controversial aspects regarding the surgical management of ulcerative colitis. Each describes views based on extensive surgical experience.

S. R. F.

Multistaged
Operations for Ulcerative Colitis

Robert Tidrick

University of Iowa College of Medicine

Introduction

In the early history of surgical treatment of ulcerative colitis, the multistaged operative approach was the rule, and three or even four stages were commonly employed. Staging gradually evolved into the present use of two operations. In the past decade the employment of single-stage proctocolectomy with ileostomy as the procedure of choice in patients requiring elective ablative therapy has had considerable support. It is believed in some circles that with the one-stage operation the mortality rate is lower and the period of hospitalization shorter than with the multistaged approach. In the opinion of this writer, this view has limited application.

As a measure of apparent inconsistency, the author favors single-stage proctocolectomy with ileostomy in most patients with familial polyposis. The usual patient with ulcerative colitis is a substandard risk and not in the same category as the average young patient requiring proctocolectomy in familial polyposis.

The University Hospitals have a constant population of patients with ulcerative colitis, averaging about 25 new case registrations each year. The substantial majority are registered as indigent or on a part-pay basis, because the disease has exhausted them economically as well as physically. A relatively high percentage of these patients have significant complications of the disease. Many of the operations are performed by members of the resident staff with the assistance of a senior staff member.

The complications of massive hemorrhage, acute perforation, and cancer comprise special categories that need individualization in management, and each will be commented upon briefly. The other complications, both systemic and local, have been present almost constantly in patients coming to elective operation in the University Hospitals. A majority, indeed today essentially all, of them have been exposed to corticosteroid hormone treatment. Some have obvious and advanced side effects. These patients, as a group, have altered response to blood loss, to some anesthetic agents and drugs, and to bacterial contamination, and demonstrate altered wound healing. The incidence of wound infection in these patients is exceptionally high.

Staged Approach and Operative Technique

Meticulous attention to operative technical details reduces a number of the troublesome complications that have long beset surgeon and patient alike. When wound complication does occur, transverse and oblique incisions have been associated with fewer instances of massive breakdown and evisceration than vertical incisions. The performance of meticulous ileostomy as a plastic procedure, with a predetermined site selected and identified by preoperative tattooing, has paid creditable dividends. We have employed a coned-out hole superior to the semicircular line and have closed the ileocolic gutter with a terminal mesenteric flap. For a number of years we have created a protruding rosebud stoma similar to that advocated by Brooke. By using rubber sheets, thereby avoiding small bowel serosal contact with sponges, cloth pads, and wound draping fabrics, we have reduced the incidence of postoperative ileus and, we believe, the late incidence of small intestinal adhesions and obstruction. The greater omentum is spared. The mesenteries are dissected sharply and with care to avoid crushing the mesenteric lymph nodes, since cultures of these nodes, in the past decade, have revealed significant pathogenic organisms in the majority of patients. Reperitonealization is done. Colectomy in the planned two-stage procedure is carried out to a convenient area in the sigmoid, the stump of which is brought out as a mucous fistula through a short muscle-splitting incision in the left lower abdominal quadrant. The patient's response is usually rapid, and as soon as ileostomy adjustment and wound healing are apparent the patient is ready for discharge from the hospital.

The second, or proctectomy, stage is generally done through a left lower abdominal quadrant transverse incision, with excision of the mucous fistula or dimple representing its previous site. The aim is to ablate rectum and remaining sigmoid with sharp dissection techniques, and with dissection as close to the rectal wall as possible. We usually spare the levatores ani and anal musculature and open the anus in the posterior midline to effect complete excision of the epithelium in the anal canal. The use of a pack in the rectum, as advocated by Hill, is helpful. Meticulous attention is directed to restoring the perineal floor, reperitonealizing the left pelvic gutter, and loosely closing the levator sling. These several measures contribute to reduction in the incidence of impotence, dyspareunia, painful, sensitive perineum, and urinary tract difficulties.

Categories for Individualization

One may be certain that there are indications for single-stage proctocolectomy with ileostomy, as well as indications for multiple-stage procedures,
even exceeding the conventional two stages. These varying conditions are
found principally in patients experiencing the gravest complications, namely
perforation, massive hemorrhage, and cancer.

It is our present policy to avoid extensive resection in the face of perforation. In instances of concealed leakage, usually in association with
fulminating ulcerative colitis with gross dilatation of the colon, we prefer
the use of double ileostomy with a decompression tube introduced through
the distal or defunctionalized ileal stoma. A recent review of our experience
with 13 patients with fulminating ulcerative colitis and colonic wall necrosis
outlines this technique. In instances of massive perforation, limited resection
or even exteriorization may be done in conjunction with ileostomy.[5]

In operations for massive hemorrhage, extensive resection may be required, including single-stage proctocolectomy, as the hemorrhage may
be diffuse and require this extensive procedure to effect control. The first
one-stage total proctocolectomy performed at the University Hospitals a
decade ago was done in such a situation. Two instances of inadequate resection in the face of massive bleeding were encountered in the past 15
years. In one, the resection had to be extended only five days after ileostomy and partial colectomy, certainly not a propitious time. However, in
another patient, a single-stage proctocolectomy with ileostomy was done
under such unfavorable circumstances as massive hemorrhage and demonstrated septicemia. He had been receiving large-scale corticosteroid therapy
for a year. He succumbed three weeks postoperatively from massive sepsis
and wound complications, including evisceration through the vertical midline wound which had been employed. The degree of involvement of the
sigmoid and rectal mucosa was significantly less prominent than that of the
proximal colon, and a less extensive operation could certainly not have
been any less disastrous.

Cancer of the colon complicating ulcerative colitis, as has been pointed
out by a number of authors, including some from our University Hospitals,
is often multifocal and occasionally spreads for long distances intramurally.
Under conditions of reasonable risk, therefore, one-stage proctocolectomy
with ileostomy is indicated as a curative approach in these patients.

Elective Procedures for Chronic Ulcerative Colitis

In a large number of patients, elective proctocolectomy is indicated
for treatment of the chronic disease. In our opinion the sum of two planned
operative procedures of reasonable scope affords less combined risk of
death and serious complication than does one, which, in average surgical
hands, would be a massive procedure. Since a large percentage of these

procedures are performed by surgical residents or by surgeons who only occasionally treat ulcerative colitis, the indication for planned staging appears even stronger. The argument that the disease continues apace, without significant amelioration, in the absence of total immediate ablation, is not borne out by careful examination of the records of our patients. There are only occasional exceptions: patients with active rheumatoid arthritis and those with ocular, oral, or cutaneous complications that may not show immediate salutary response. The usual patient presents a prompt favorable response after the initial stage of elective ileostomy and partial colectomy.

Mortality rates are difficult to assess as a means of determining whether proctocolectomy should be performed in one or in several stages. Of 114 patients subjected to proctocolectomy during a 12-year period, there were four deaths: two in patients requiring emergency operation for hemorrhage, one in a patient with ankylosing spondylitis who had elective ileostomy and partial colectomy, and one from unrelated causes. The mortality rate is obviously likely to be higher in those series having a considerable proportion of patients having massive hemorrhage or perforation.

An argument sometimes forwarded in favor of staging proctocolectomy is that of delaying the decision in relation to possible ileoproctostomy, especially in those instances where there is active disease in the rectal segment. We would not forward this as a significant point, but view the subject as still under consideration. We are subjecting a small group of patients with remaining rectal and sigmoid segments to a carefully observed program of local corticosteroid administration with frequent observation and biopsy. In only one of these has there been apparent complete remission of the remaining segment. In most of them, it has been disappointing, and it is our current impression that those applicable to subsequent ileoproctostomy constitute only a small percentage of the total.

Summary

In considering the total removal of the colon and rectum in patients with chronic ulcerative colitis, it is the view of this author that the sum of two carefully planned procedures, with provision for much attention to technical operative detail, provides less risk to life and to complications than a single procedure of greater scope, magnitude, and time. It is further stressed that individualization in both directions, that is for multistaged procedures and for single-stage proctocolectomy, is indicated in dealing with the three principal catastrophic complications of this disease.

References

1. Aylett, S.: Total colectomy and ileo-rectal anastomosis as a treatment of choice in ulcerative colitis. Acta chir. Belg., 58:597, 1959.

2. Bacon, H. E., and Nuquid, T. P.: An improved technic of colectomy for ulcerative colitis and disseminated adenomatosis. Dis. Colon Rectum, 4:159, 1961.
3. Brooke, B. N.: Ulcerative Colitis and Its Surgical Treatment. Edinburgh and London, E. & S. Livingstone Ltd., 1954, Chap. VI.
4. Hickey, R. C., and Tidrick, R. T.: Cancer in patients with chronic ulcerative colitis. Cancer, 11:35, 1958.
5. Hickey, R. C., Tidrick, R. T., and Layton, J. M.: Fulminating ulcerative colitis with colonic wall necrosis. Arch. Surg. 86:764, 1963.
6. Hill, L. D., Stone, C. S., and Pearson, C. C.: Surgical aspects of ulcerative colitis. A.M.A. Arch. Surg., 72:968, 1956.
7. Hill, L. D., Stone, C. S., and Baker, J. W.: One-stage abdominoproctocolectomy and ileostomy. A.M.A. Arch. Surg. 83:98, 1961.
8. Hoxworth, P. I., and Culberston, W. R.: Removal of the large bowel in one stage in selected cases of ulcerative colitis. A.M.A. Arch. Surg., 61:834, 1950.
9. Tidrick, R. T., and Hickey, R. C.: The catastrophic complications of ulcerative colitis: cancer, perforation and massive bleeding. J. Iowa M. Soc., 46:485, 1956.
10. Turnbull, R. B., Jr.: Management of the ileostomy. Am. J. Surg., 86:617, 1953.

One-Stage Colectomy, Proctectomy, and Ileostomy for Idiopathic Ulcerative Colitis

Karl E. Karlson *and* Clarence Dennis

State University of New York, Downstate Medical Center

Our observation of the natural history and results of treatment of idiopathic ulcerative colitis has led us to the conclusion that the optimal surgical therapy for the majority of patients coming to operation is colectomy, proctectomy, and ileostomy, performed at a single operative procedure.[1] It became apparent more than a decade ago that colectomy was the procedure of choice when operation was necessary. The mortality from ileostomy alone was many times that of colectomy, even in the sickest patients. It became further apparent that the usefulness of the rectum to the great majority of patients was so limited that resection of the rectum was advantageous. Therefore, this operation has been performed by choice in those patients who could tolerate colectomy and proctectomy during a single procedure.

Indications for Resection

In the acute stages of the disease, emergency surgical intervention is occasionally necessary because the disease is uncontrollable by nonoperative management. Hemorrhage, peritonitis, or generalized sepsis may be the major indications for operation. More frequently, however, the disease progresses to a subacute or chronic stage, and operation may be undertaken on an elective or semielective basis. Intractable colitis, together with arthritis, pyoderma, furunculosis, fistulas, or liver abnormalities, may be the indication. Chronic colitis is associated with a significant incidence of cirrhosis of the liver. The incidence of nonneoplastic complications in our experience is tabulated in Table 1.

The risk of carcinoma as a complication of chronic ulcerative colitis

Page 414

TABLE 1. NON-NEOPLASTIC COMPLICATIONS OF IDIOPATHIC ULCERATIVE COLITIS*

Perforation of colon		10 (3.7%)
Perianal abscess		8 (3.0%)
Fistula in ano		4 (1.5%)
Rectovaginal fistula		3 (1.1%)
Ileocolic fistula		2 (0.8%)
Massive hemorrhage		4 (1.5%)
Liver abnormalities		50 (18.7%)
Cirrhosis	12 (4.5%)	
Atrophy	2 (0.8%)	
Lesser abnormalities	14 (5.2%)	
Abnormal function tests	22 (8.2%)	
Arthritis†		19 (7.1%)
Thromboembolic disease		20 (7.5%)
Fatal pulmonary embolism	10 (3.7%)	
Pyoderma		9 (3.4%)
Cholelithiasis		6 (2.2%)
Nephrolithiasis		3 (1.1%)

* From Dennis, C., and Karlson, K. E.: Surgery, *32:*892, 1952.
† Ninety-two per cent having surgical therapy improved after operation.

is significant. The overall incidence of carcinoma associated with colitis in our series of patients was 7.4 per cent, with one patient developing two cancers.[2] This patient had a colectomy for a carcinoma of the ceum, at which time the rectum was left in situ. The patient persistently refused proctectomy and a rectal carcinoma subsequently developed. Proctectomy was then performed. Although others have recorded the development of carcinoma three to four years after the onset of colitis, 10 years has been the shortest duration of colitis before the development of carcinoma in our series. A review of those patients who were under observation on and subsequent to the tenth anniversary of their colitis showed that these patients were continually subject to a risk of carcinoma, which was 4 per cent per year. In those patients in whom the colon had been removed but the rectum left in situ, the risk of carcinoma was 1 per cent per year in the retained rectum.

Consideration of the risk of the development of carcinoma brings one to the conclusion that the annual risk of carcinoma in patients who have had colitis for more than a decade is greater than the operative risk for removal of the colon and rectum. Therefore, on the basis of operative versus cancer mortality alone in any single year, it would appear to be advantageous to resect the colon of any patient with longstanding chronic ulcerative colitis. Because patients with chronic colitis almost never recover from their disease, but continue to have abnormal mucosa, colectomy and proctectomy are recommended after the disease has been present for 3 to 4 years, unless more pressing indications dictate colectomy before this time.

Indications for Proctectomy

The only bowel that may be considered immune to the complications of colitis, including carcinoma, is that which is entirely normal. It is extremely rare to see a fully normal rectum in a patient with chronic ulcerative colitis. Therefore, the retention of a rectum in such a patient is associated with an inherent risk. As already stated, the risk of carcinoma in a rectum retained after colectomy, whether the fecal stream is deviated from the rectum or passes through the rectum, is 1 per cent per year per patient.

When one couples this risk of carcinoma with the generally unsatisfactory results obtained from ileoproctostomy, most of our patients in retrospect would prefer to have had the rectum excised. The morbidity and mortality of ileoproctostomy are definitely greater than those of proctectomy and ileostomy. Of 41 cases followed after completion of ileoproctostomy, five died as a result of complications of their disease. There was one late (2 months) death after perforation at the suture line and pelvic peritonitis, three deaths from carcinoma of the rectum, and one death associated with severe recurrent proctitis. One additional patient survived after ileostomy was performed for severe proctitis. Further, the anticipation of being socially comfortable with ileoproctostomy is not good since, in our experience, less than half the patients have 5 or fewer stools per day after ileoproctostomy.

One of the significant complications of colitis, pulmonary embolism, appeared to be associated with the retention of diseased rectum. Excision of the rectum reduces considerably the incidence of pulmonary embolism.

Proctectomy may be performed in these patients when there is no evidence of carcinoma without risk of sexual dysfunction postoperatively. In the absence of carcinoma, the dissection of the rectum may be very close to the rectal wall.

As far as operative technique is concerned, the lumen is carefully irrigated with an antiseptic solution before performing perineal excision of the rectum. Dissection may then be greatly facilitated by inserting a finger into the rectum as a guide to the rectal wall. The nervous pathways essential to sexual function are then left undisturbed. In our series of over 100 proctectomies for colitis, sexual function has been retained in all. When proctectomy is necessary after the development of carcinoma, wide excision of the ischiorectal fat and levator ani muscles is indicated. It is after this type of procedure that sexual incapacity commonly occurs.

In those patients in whom elective colectomy is to be performed, proctectomy may be added to the initial procedure without increased mortality or morbidity. We have found that even in those cases in which operation is done for fulminating colitis on an emergency basis, it has frequently been possible to continue the operation to include proctectomy. Recovery occurs sooner if all of the diseased bowel is removed than if a diseased rectum or rectosigmoid is retained.

If at any time during operation it becomes apparent that it is wise to terminate the procedure with the resection of the colon and performance of the ileostomy, the rectosigmoid may be left in situ. In this event, the proximal end of the terminal bowel may be either brought out as a mucous fistula to the anterior abdominal wall or inverted with suture closure. In our experience, suture closure has been without complication, but mucous fistula has been associated with a high incidence of severe wound infections. The terminal colon and rectum may then be removed at a second procedure, which has been associated with no mortality in our hands.

An occasional patient will refuse to have proctectomy despite the high morbidity and despite the definite risk of malignant change in the rectum. Such a patient must undergo proctoscopic examination regularly at intervals of 3 or 4 months, and biopsy must be obtained from any suspicious area. Carcinoma may develop in a bowel afflicted with colitis in the absence of any symptom or abnormality of bowel habits.

Summary

Colectomy is recommended for the treatment of all patients with chronic idiopathic ulcerative colitis who have had the disease for more than 3 or 4 years. After the disease has reached this stage, progression with recurrent episodes of hemorrhage and fibrosis mask the early symptoms and signs of developing carcinoma. After 10 years of colitis, the incidence of carcinoma is such that it entails a risk in each year of the patient's life greater than that of colectomy. Because ileoproctostomy provides generally unsatisfactory bowel function in the face of higher mortality and morbidity, and because the risk of carcinoma development persists, proctectomy is recommended at the time of colectomy in the absence of a completely normal rectum. The operative mortality appears to be no higher when proctectomy is added to the colectomy in those patients who will tolerate the additional procedure, and the morbidity postoperatively is very much lower.

References

1. Dennis, C., and Karlson, K. E.: Surgical measures as supplements to the management of idiopathic ulcerative colitis; cancer, cirrhosis, and arthritis as frequent complications. Surgery, 32:892, 1952.
2. Dennis, C., and Karlson, K. E., Cancer risk in ulcerative colitis; formidability per patient-year of late disease. Surgery, 50:568, 1961.

Ileoproctostomy in Ulcerative Colitis

Ward O. Griffen, Jr., Richard C. Lillehei, *and* O. H. Wangensteen

University of Minnesota School of Medical Sciences

Outside of the continuing debate of medical versus surgical therapy for chronic ulcerative colitis, the most controversial issue is whether the anal sphincter can be preserved in these cases. The enthusiasm for less direct procedures such as ileostomy, appendicostomy, and vagotomy has waned. Total colectomy and proctectomy with ileostomy is a discouraging and at times unnecessary handicap to place on these patients, especially if some procedure acceptable to both patient and surgeon will suffice. The question then is: Must the rectum be sacrificed in all cases of chronic ulcerative colitis treated surgically?

Results of Treatment

In 1943, a one-stage colectomy with ileoproctostomy was advocated as a satisfactory method of removing the major portion of the diseased bowel for ulcerative colitis while preserving the anal sphincters.[5] In 1948 a group of 13 patients so treated was reported.[6] Since that time, 53 patients have undergone such a procedure in this institution.[3] All the patients had chronic ulcerative colitis diagnosed by history and verified by x-ray studies, proctosigmoidoscopic examinations, and gross and histological examination of the excised surgical specimen. A few patients had only segmental involvement of the colon. A long history of bloody diarrhea with remissions and exacerbations was usual; 26 of the patients had undergone previous operative treatment directed at the illness.

At operation, total colectomy was performed. Restoration of intestinal continuity was accomplished by primary ileoproctostomy (46 patients), cecoproctostomy (1 patient), and ileal pull-through (5 patients). In one patient only, a left hemicolectomy was performed because the disease was segmental in nature. A diverting ileostomy was made at the time of colorectal resection in only one patient.

Thirteen patients had complicated postoperative courses; four required ileostomy in the immediate postoperative period for relief of persistent diarrhea or obstructive symptoms. Two of these have undergone subsequent closure of the ileostomy. Two postoperative deaths occurred, one following a decompressive ileostomy on the second postoperative day, the other as the result of a subdural hematoma secondary to an unsuspected congenital cerebral vascular lesion.

Excluding the two postoperative deaths, 51 patients have been followed in this clinic. Thirteen patients have died since dismissal from the hospital. One patient who had had an ileal pull-through died after an operative reversal of a segment of ileum was done in an attempt to control diarrhea. Two patients developed carcinoma in the retained rectum and eventually died as a result of the malignancy. Two other patients had carcinoma of the colon in addition to chronic ulcerative colitis at the time of the original operation; both died of recurrent cancer. Three patients died as a result of recurrent ulcerative colitis and its complications. The remaining five patients died of causes unrelated to the original disease.

Of the 38 patients available for recent follow-up studies, 30 patients have been seen in the outpatient department within the last two years. The other 8 patients provided pertinent data by answers to questionnaires and letters. Evaluation of the results as good, fair, or poor has been based on weight gain, number of stools per day, continuation or recurrence of associated lesions, and ability to hold a job or carry on a former occupation. The patients' subjective feelings about their condition also were considered in the evaluation.

All but eight patients gained weight postoperatively. Twenty-five of the patients were considered to have obtained a good result (no more than four stools per day, weight gain, and working at a full-time job). Nine of the patients were classified in the fair result group (five to ten stools per day, weight gain, and still working, but not as vigorously as before). Seventeen patients were considered to have a poor result (more than 10 stools per day, weight gain poor, further operation needed, or recurrence of disease). Among the 17 patients in this group are the 2 who developed carcinoma in the residual rectum as well as the 2 in whom coincidental malignancy was present in the original specimen. Three patients required proctectomy and permanent ileostomy. The other patients have had up to 25 bowel movements per day.

All five patients who had an ileal pull-through procedure were classified in the poor result group. All of these had less than 10 cm. of ileum excised, but difficulty with the anal ileostomy led to the establishment of a permanent abdominal ileostomy in four patients. The other patient died following a second procedure as recounted previously. Of the eight patients who were regarded as having fair results, one required further surgical treatment, a vagotomy, which apparently has served to allay the symptoms. The other patients in this group, although maintaining a relatively normal life, still have five to ten stools per day.

Analysis of Results

Careful analysis of the cases brings to light the factors that are likely to lead to a good result from ileorectal anastomosis in patients with chronic ulcerative colitis. The first of these factors concerns the selection of patients. Sixteen (64 per cent) of the 25 patients in the good result group had either no involvement or slight involvement of the rectum at the time of the ileoproctostomy. In contrast, 67 per cent of the poor result group had moderate or severe rectal disease when operated upon. Thus it is evident that when an ileoproctostomy is contemplated, the patient should have, at most, minimal disease in the rectum. Although severe rectal disease has been observed to improve following ileorectal anastomosis, there are risks in effecting an ileorectal anastomosis under these conditions.

The other two factors insuring a good result are concerned with the technique of the procedure. Since 60 per cent of the patients in the good result group had only 10 cm. or less of ileum removed, it would seem that resection of as small an amount of ileum as possible, is important. Unless the ileum exhibits evidence of disease, there is no need to excise more than a centimeter or two in making the anastomosis. Secondly, the level of anastomosis appears to play a significant role in the outcome. In 64 per cent of the good result group ileorectal anastomosis was performed at 10 cm. or less from the anus. This facet of a successful outcome also is stressed by Aylett, who maintains that lesions of chronic ulcerative colitis are least common in the rectal ampulla and most common at the rectosigmoid level, and he therefore urges that the anastomosis be made as low as possible.[1] This concept seems to be valid in view of the results in our own cases. The use of a diverting ileostomy proximal to the anastomosis does not seem to be essential to the success of the procedure.

It must be stressed that patients with chronic ulcerative colitis treated by ileoproctostomy be kept under constant surveillance. Two patients in this series developed carcinoma in the remaining rectum, a complication that has been observed by others.[3] Neither of these patients had reported to the outpatient clinic regularly. Moreover, it has been pointed out that rectal carcinoma developing in the course of ulcerative colitis can occur during a quiescent period when the patient is asymptomatic and the bowel mucosa has no evidence of colitis.[2] Therefore, regular proctoscopy must be performed regardless of the patient's symptoms. Inability to maintain adequate follow-up has invited failure of the procedure.

Another point of discussion is one recently raised by Rosenquist.[4] If ileorectal anastomosis can be used moderately successfully in these cases, would not earlier operation give better results? The evidence is not yet certain that early cases have less rectal involvement. Should this be the case, early operative intervention would require close cooperation between internists and surgeons.

Advantage of Ileoproctostomy

The distinct advantage of an ileoproctostomy is that it does afford the patient a chance to lead a relatively normal life in many instances. Perusal of the literature regarding surgical therapy for ulcerative colitis indicates that more than 50 per cent of the reported cases of ileorectal anastomosis have returned to a useful, uncomplicated life. If the procedure fails, further operation can be performed. Colectomy and proctectomy with permanent ileostomy as the initial surgical endeavor against this disease represents a policy from which there is no return.

Summary and Conclusions

Ileoproctostomy can be done safely on selected patients with chronic ulcerative colitis. Patients without rectal disease or with minimal rectal involvement are the best candidates for this procedure. Resection of only a few centimeters of ileum and anastomosis between the ileum and the rectum at 10 cm. or less from the anus insure the best result. Regular follow-up with frequent proctoscopic examinations is essential. Patients with advanced disease of the rectum are not candidates for an ileorectal anastomosis.

References

1. Aylett, S.: Ulcerative colitis treated by total colectomy and ileorectal anastomosis. A ten year review. Proc. Roy. Soc. Med., 56:183, 1963.
2. Dawson, I. M. P., and Pryse-Davis, J.: The development of carcinoma of the large intestine in ulcerative colitis. Brit. J. Surg., 47:113, 1959.
3. Griffen, W. O., Jr., Lillehei, R. C., and Wangensteen, O. H.: Ileoproctostomy in ulcerative colitis: long-term follow-up, extending in early Cases to more than 20 years. Surgery, 53:705, 1963.
4. Rosenquist, H.: Ulcerative colitis. The aims of surgery. Acta. chir. scandinav. 125:478, 1963.
5. Wangensteen, O. H.: Primary resection (closed anastomosis) of the colon and rectosigmoid: including description of abdominoanal methods for restoration of continuity accompanying excision of carcinoma of the rectal ampulla. Surgery, 14:403, 1943.
6. Wangensteen, O. H., and Toon, R. W.: Primary resection of the colon and rectum with particular reference to cancer and ulcerative colitis. Am. J. Surg., 75:384, 1948.

Congenital

Aganglionic

Megacolon

(Hirschsprung's Disease)

Introduction

Every patient with Hirschsprung's disease owes a debt of gratitude to Swenson for his contribution (1948) in calling our attention to the aganglionic concept in the pathogenesis of congenital megacolon. The surgical management popularized by him has saved many lives and has tended to clarify the previously muddled thinking about this condition. His reported results of his personal experience (Ann. Surg., *146*:706, 1957) are very good, and hard to match; indeed, other surgeons apparently are not as successful. He has, as will be noted in the following presentation, described a modification of his original technique to include partial anal sphincterectomy for the purpose of eliminating one of the complications, occasional "enterocolitis." Other surgeons also have noted this and other complications which, as is so often the case, has led to other surgical procedures and even modifications of them. The second presentation describes modifications of the Duhamel procedure as the surgical treatment of choice. In the third presentation in this chapter, State calls our attention to the radiologic evaluation of the functional capacity of the rectum and entire colon, which has led him to carry out "physiologic" segmental colon resection including the rectosigmoid. His excellent follow-up and careful study of his cases over many years (since 1948) are worthy of thoughtful consideration.

Since all surgical procedures in the management of this condition require definite assessment of the presence or absence of ganglion cells in Auerbach's plexus, by either permanent or frozen section, histologic confirmation by competent pathologists is very important. The demonstration of the histologic picture, including the increase in nerve fibers in the aganglionic area, can be improved markedly by sections prepared histo-chemically for enzyme activity. Histochemical analyses on cryostat-cut sections, in a laboratory prepared to do this, can yield unequivocal deter-minations in the same period of time required for ordinary histologic examination by frozen section.

S. R. F.

Prevention of Enterocolitis following Segmental Resection for Congenital Megacolon

Orvar Swenson

Northwestern University School of Medicine

It is now 18 years since we first proposed resection of the aganglionic segment of colon in the treatment of Hirschsprung's disease.[1] We have had opportunity to observe some patients almost two decades after resection. In examining our follow-up records, we are impressed with the uniformly good results. Patients who are now fifteen years and more from operation are perfectly normal individuals. Several have passed examinations for service in the Army, Air Force, and Navy. In fact, our first patient to undergo resection 18 years ago is in the Navy at present and is entirely normal.

In view of these excellent long-term results, we have been loath to change our technique of operation. There has been one problem, however, in very young patients and in patients in whom colostomy or resection has been performed during the neonatal period. We refer to the presence of rather severe intermittent enterocolitis, which has been a troublesome complication. Although not all patients have suffered episodes of enterocolitis postoperatively, a number have had this trying experience. The treatment for enterocolitis has been tedious, requiring irrigation with a large rectal tube to decompress the colon. The interesting thing about patients who develop enteritis, either pre- or postoperatively, is that the whole intestinal tract becomes paralytic, there is massive distention, and the bowel becomes enormous in size. The absorption of fluids is reduced virtually to nothing. At this point, one must insert a very large rectal tube to drain the colon, irrigating the tube frequently to dislodge any particle that might block the lumen, permitting a free flow of intestinal gases and fluids so that decompression is accomplished. Usually two or three days of careful treatment of this type is sufficient. In some patients in whom the condition is not recognized and has been permitted to become chronic, treatment is more prolonged. Such situations may necessitate a prolonged series of irrigations.

Three years ago, we postulated that patients who developed severe enterocolitis were in need of a more extensive resection. On examination of such patients, we had found a very firm, long anal canal with a tight internal sphincter. We began to do a partial sphincterectomy as part of the procedure for resection of the aganglionic segment, simply cutting the distal segment of bowel obliquely across, so that anteriorly about 2 cm. of mucosa remained above the dentate line and 1 cm. or less remained posteriorly. By angulating the cut we resected about half of the internal sphincter. We have operated now on 30 patients with this technique, and although some of these have had diarrhea just as any normal child would, they have not become distended or required irrigation. This is the only change in technique that we have undertaken, and we believe that the troublesome postoperative complication of enterocolitis can be virtually eliminated by this more radical resection.

It is interesting that the so-called Duhamel operation is being discarded by a considerable number of people. Grob, in Switzerland, has had much experience with this procedure, and because of poor results he has now given it up in favor of resection with anastomosis. This is not surprising, in view of the fact that the Duhamel operation violates the basic principles of treatment of Hirschsprung's disease by leaving a large aganglionic segment of colon in place.

Reference

1. Swenson, O.: Hirschsprung's disease in older infants—resection of aganglionic segment. *In* Pediatric Surgery. 2nd Ed. New York, Appleton-Century-Crofts, 1962, pp. 415–430.

Rationale for Segmental Colon Resection in the Treatment of Congenital Megacolon (Hirschsprung's Disease)*

David State

Albert Einstein College of Medicine

The macroscopic and microscopic pathologic changes in the large bowel and rectum in Hirschsprung's disease have been defined,[1] but alterations in function of the involved bowel have not been so clearly identified. Physiologic studies of the colon and rectum have yielded conflicting results. Whether the rectum and narrowed rectosigmoid segment are the primary sites of difficulty, with the distention and dilatation of the proximal colon a secondary manifestation, or whether the disease process involves the left side of the colon and spares the rectum and right half of the large bowel has not been resolved.

From a practical point of view, probably the best means of assessing the function of the bowel in congenital megacolon is by roentgenographic studies. If these studies are carried out with the intent of evaluating functional capacity of the rectum and entire colon, instead of merely defining the narrow rectosigmoid area for diagnostic purposes, the following important findings, which are usually overlooked, become apparent (Fig. 1):

1. The rectum appears normal in caliber, distensibility and contractility.

2. Proximal to the narrowed rectosigmoid, the left side of the colon, i.e., sigmoid, descending, and variable extents of the left side of the transverse colon, is markedly dilated and shows little if any evidence of peristalsis or haustrations.

3. The right side of the colon, i.e., cecum, ascending colon, and the right side of the transverse colon, presents good peristaltic activity and haustral markings.

* This work was supported in part by the National Institute of Health Training Grant No. 2A 5200.

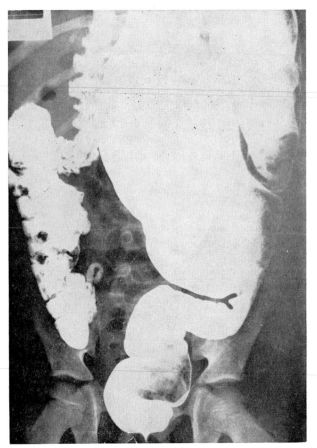

Fig. 1. Roentgenogram after a barium enema in a nine year old boy with congenital megacolon, showing normal caliber of the rectum; the narrowed rectosigmoid region; marked dilatation and absence of haustral markings of the left side of the colon; normal diameter and haustral pattern of the right side of the colon. The transition area is somewhere in the mid-transverse colon.

The rationale for segmental colon resection rests with the removal of those segments of the bowel that do not function normally and retention of those that do. In a general way, this means the removal of the left side of the colon from just *distal* to the rectosigmoid to the right half of the transverse colon or the ascending colon. The rectum is retained, and to it the residual proximal colon is anastomosed to establish bowel continuity. Since the success and acceptance of the operative procedure depend on a clear understanding of the extent of resection, it will be defined more specifically.

Extent of Resection (Fig. 2)

The *proximal extent* of resection is determined both by roentgenographic studies and by direct inspection at laparotomy. As described above, the differences between the right and left sides of the colon are easily ascertained roentgenographically. At surgery, the difference between normal and abnormal colon can also be easily seen, for in the former, the bowel wall is normal in thickness and the longitudinal muscular coat is in bands producing haustrations. In contrast, the abnormal bowel has a markedly thickened wall, and the outer muscle coat completely surrounds the bowel, so that the haustral pattern is absent. In the majority of patients the preferred level of proximal transection is either just distal or proximal to the hepatic flexure.

The *distal extent* of resection is through the upper part of the normal rectum immediately distal to the rectosigmoid junction. Dissection about the residual part of the rectum is kept to a minimum to prevent possible injury to the nervi erigentes. In actual measurement, depending on the age and size of the patient, the length of rectum remaining has varied from 6 to 10 cm. from the anal skin.

The anastomosis of residual colon to rectum was originally carried out by the closed technique over clamps, but more recently the anastomosis has been of the open variety, utilizing two rows of interrupted fine nonabsorbable sutures (Fig. 3).

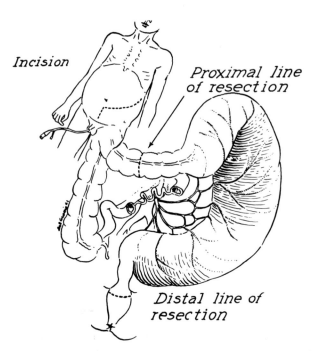

Fig. 2. Diagram showing the extent of resection just below the rectosigmoid distally and in the normal appearing colon proximally.

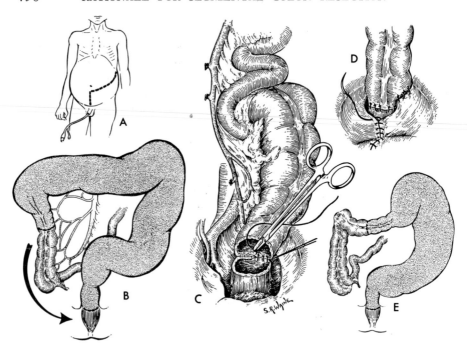

Fig. 3. *A,* Incision—an extensive hockey stick incision is employed. Note inlying urethral catheter. It is essential that the urinary bladder be decompressed.

B, The extent of resection is either proximal or (*E*) distal to the hepatic flexure.

C, The anastomosis is carried out in a two layer open technique (*C*) with care taken to reperitonealize the area of anastomosis (*D*).

Results

It can be properly argued that good immediate postoperative results in Hirschsprung's disease do not mean a great deal, for recurrent difficulties may not appear for 5 to 10 years after surgery. With this in mind, the first 18 patients treated by segmental colon resection were re-examined 10 to 14 years after operation, and it was found that the initial good results had been maintained throughout the years.

TABLE 1.   RESULTS OF SURGERY*

Year of Operation	*No. of Cases*	*Laxatives, Enemas, Abdominal Distention*			*Died*	*Fecal Incontinence*	*Daily Bowel Movements*		
		None	*Infrequently*	*Frequently*			1	2	3
1948–1951	18†	0	0	0	0	0	2	14	2

* From State, D.: Am. J. Surg., *105*:93, 1963.

† One patient needed enemas occasionally after operation, but for years (5) prior to this review had not needed any.

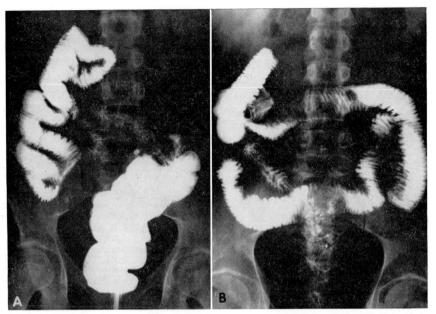

Fig. 4. Roentgenograms of colon of a 32 year old patient (R.F.) taken 12 years after colon resection and anastomosis between ascending colon and rectum. *A*, Residual colon distended with barium. *B*, Postevacuation film demonstrating the ability of the colon to empty.

Recent roentgenograms on 12 patients show moderate dilatation of the residual colon, but in all patients good peristaltic activity and evacuation of the colon was demonstrated (Fig. 4).

Other surgeons have reported large series of cases treated with segmental colon resection with good results. Hecker reports 40 patients on whom anterior resections were performed with no deaths and only one bad result,[3] while Rehbein and Nicolai report on 97 cases with good to excellent results in 81, and fair results in 9.[4] The latter group of patients were believed to have achalasia of the anal sphincter, and some responded to repeated sphincter dilatation or sphincterotomy.

Comments and Summary

The theory that the basic defect of congenital megacolon rests entirely in the aganglionic rectum and narrowed rectosigmoid area, and as a result functional obstruction and secondary dilatation of the proximal colon occur, cannot be accepted without some question for the following reasons:

1. The absence of ganglion cells is encountered to a variable extent in the dilated portions of colon as well as in the rectum and narrowed rectosigmoid area.

2. The rectum, as visualized by roentgenograms, appears to be normal in size, shape, distensibility and contractibility.

3. If the changes in the bowel proximal to the "narrowed" area were secondary to obstruction, one would expect the cecum, because it has the largest diameter of any portion of the colon, to have the maximum dilatation. Certainly this is true in other instances of colonic obstruction of an incomplete and chronic character (e.g., carcinoma, diverticulitis, and stenosis). In congenital megacolon, however, the maximum dilatation occurs in the sigmoid area rather than the cecum.

4. Roentgenographically, peristaltic activity is readily seen in the right side of the colon, but the dilated left side shows little or no peristaltic activity or contraction.

These observations would seem to indicate that in a congenital megacolon there is some unexplained defect in innervation of the entire left side of the colon, whereas the right side of the large bowel retains a normal nerve supply. In support of this theory, anatomically at least, we know the parasympathetic innervation of the two sides of the colon to be different; i.e., the vagus supplies the right side of the colon, whereas the left side is supplied by the pelvic parasympathetic outflow. The studies of Kamijo and co-workers also suggest that although the involved bowel is aganglionic, ganglion cells are present but located more centrally than normally.[5]

It must be emphasized that the operative procedure described is *not* merely a segmental sigmoid colon resection. The removal of the dilated sigmoid alone has yielded unsatisfactory results. It must be clearly understood that the extent of resection is based on physiologic studies and entails the removal of the narrowed rectosigmoid and portions of the inactive colon, proximally to the right side of the transverse colon or ascending colon, where good peristaltic activity can be seen by roentgenogram. In the majority of patients, the proximal line of resection has been immediately proximal or distal to the hepatic flexure, and the distal line of resection has left a rectal segment 6 to 10 cm. in length.

The possible advantages of this procedure over "pull-through" techniques are:

1. Resection and anastomosis of the colon and rectum are commonly performed operative procedures. Because of familiarity with the technique, surgeons can be expected to carry out the recommended surgical procedure for segmental megacolon with a low morbidity and mortality.

2. There is a possibility that the nervi erigentes may be damaged in the pull-through technique. Since Hirschsprung's Disease is seen predominantly in males, this possibility must be given serious consideration.

3. Since virtually the entire rectum as well as the anus are left undisturbed, the patient can be assured full fecal continence postoperatively.

4. A final evaluation of "physiologic" segmental colon resection (as is true for other procedures) must await several more decades. The initial results, over a 10- to 14-year period, however, have been most encouraging,

and have offered dramatic and gratifying rewards to the patient, parents, and surgeon.

References

1. Robertson, H. E., and Kernohan, J. W.: The myenteric plexus in congenital megacolon. Proc. Staff Meet. Mayo Clin., *13*:123, 1938.
2. State, D.: Segmental colon resection in the treatment of congenital megacolon (Hirschsprung's disease). Am. J. Surg., *105*:93, 1963.
3. Hecker, W. C.: Diagnosis and therapy of megacolon. Med. Welt., *NR33*:1621, 1963.
4. Rehbein, F., and Nicolai, I.: Surgery in Hirschsprung's disease. Deutsche med. Wchnschr., *88*:1595, 1963.
5. Kamijo, K., Hiatt, R. B., and Koelle, G. B.: Congenital megacolon. A comparison of the spastic and hypertrophied segments with respect to cholinesterase activities and sensitivities to acetylcholine, DFP and the barium ion. Gastroenterology, *24*:173, 1953.

Preservation of the

Rectum (Modified Duhamel

Operation) in Hirschsprung's Disease

Lester W. Martin

University of Cincinnati College of Medicine

The modern concept of the surgical management of Hirschsprung's disease first described by Swenson[21] in 1948 constitutes one of the major advances in abdominal surgery of our present generation. Not only has his operation saved countless lives, but his teaching and interest in the subject have stimulated others in the recognition and diagnosis of the disease in medical centers throughout the world. The condition formerly regarded as more or less a medical curiosity generally leading to death is now accepted as a condition that is curable through operation, after which there is a nearly normal life expectancy.

The operation described by Swenson consists of removal of the aganglionic segment of rectum and distal colon, and re-establishment of intestinal continuity by means of a primary end-to-end anastomosis just inside the anus. The operation, though lifesaving, is difficult to perform, and is followed by a discouragingly high rate of complications incident to removal of the rectum.

Duhamel,[4] in 1960, described a procedure that left the rectum in place, excluding it by establishing an oblique, end-to-side anastomosis at the skin level. Grob,[6, 7] concerned that incontinence might result, advised modifying Duhamel's operation by establishing the anastomosis at the level of the levator ani muscles.

The operation we have employed consists of a side-to-side anastomosis between the ganglion-containing colon and the entire aganglionic rectum from the level of the pelvic peritoneum to the levator muscles.[16]

Experience with Swenson's Operation

Prior to the adoption of this operation in the routine management

Page 434

of Hirschsprung's disease, fifteen consecutive patients were treated by the conventional method of resection of the rectum and aganglionic colon, and primary anastomosis just inside the anus. There were no deaths, but complications of a significant nature occurred in ten of the fifteen patients (66.6 per cent), and consisted of three instances of postoperative enterocolitis, one anastomotic stricture, and six instances of fecal soiling of the underclothing between bowel movements. The soiling persisted for six months in three children, and longer in the other three.

The literature was reviewed in order to evaluate the experience of others with the Swenson operation. A total of 625 cases were collected, including 200 patients reported by Swenson.[3, 5, 8–13, 20, 22, 23] In the 625 patients, there were 52 deaths, a mortality rate of 8 per cent (Table 1), and 274 major complications (Table 2). The exact complication rate is difficult to determine since some patients suffered more than one complication, but it appears to be between 30 and 35 per cent.

The leading cause of death was sepsis due to leakage from the anastomosis. Several deaths resulted when the operation was attempted on small infants. Most of the late deaths were due to rapid fulminating enterocolitis; and some resulted from strangulating bowel obstruction, which had been neglected because it was mistaken for functional distention and

TABLE 1.   CAUSE OF DEATH FOLLOWING "SWENSON" OPERATION
(52 DEATHS IN 625 PATIENTS)

Cause of Death	Number
Enterocolitis	16
Peritonitis	10
Intestinal obstruction	8
Shock	2
Aspiration pneumonia	2
Necrosis of proximal bowel	6
Cardiac arrest	1
Tracheobronchitis	1
Adrenal hemorrhage	1
Other causes	5
Total	52

TABLE 2.   COMPILATION OF NONFATAL COMPLICATIONS FOLLOWING
625 "SWENSON" OPERATIONS (12 AUTHORS)

Complication	Number	Per Cent
Anastomotic leak	38	6
Stricture	43	7
Constipation	56	9
Enterocolitis	21	3.5
Incontinence	71	11.3
Intestinal obstruction	19	3
Other	26	4.2
Total	274	30 to 35

thought to represent a recurrence of the symptoms of Hirschsprung's disease.

Of the 43 strictures that developed, it is interesting that several occurred even in the presence of a proximal diverting colostomy. The occasional one required further surgical operation.

Of the 38 instances of anastomotic leak, six died, one was treated with a permanent colostomy, 16 healed following the establishment of a proximal temporary diverting colostomy, and the remainder healed spontaneously.

Constipation was reported postoperatively as a complication in 56 patients. This complication was difficult to evaluate on the basis of the material presented in the various reported series, since it varied from mild irregularity to recurrent impactions. Wyllie[23] reported nine patients in whom constipation developed after one year of normal bowel movements.

Enterocolitis occurring following surgery was also difficult to assess because of varied terminology as well as wide variations in the degree of severity of the complication. It has been reported as colitis, enterocolitis, diarrhea, unexplained abdominal distention, etc. We were able to find 21 reported instances, although some authors refer to its management, but do not list it as a complication. In another reported series not included in this review, Bill and Chapman[2] reported enterocolitis in 24 of 48 patients, 8 of whom died. This complication was noted in some instances only as a periodic diarrhea associated with abdominal distention. Stool cultures in most instances were not abnormal, and the etiology of the complication has continued to be poorly understood. Swenson has recommended sphincterotomy as the preferred treatment.

Incontinence was reported as a complication in 71 instances. It was sometimes associated with either constipation or diarrhea. Some children were cured of the symptoms of Hirschsprung's disease; they had one to two normal bowel movements daily, but consistently soiled their underclothing between bowel movements. This suggested that the complication may in some way be related to the fact that the rectum is no longer present to serve as a temporary storage area, and the continued peristalsis of the colon periodically carries a small bit of stool by the unwary sphincter. One of the advantages of the operation we now employ has been the preservation of the storage function of the rectum.

Intestinal obstruction was reported as a complication in 19 patients. This somewhat higher incidence than one would anticipate from the usual laparotomy has been attributed to the length of the operative procedure, drying of the intestinal surface, extensive dissection and mobilization of the colon, and failure to reperitonealize the peritoneal floor.

In the male patients, impotence or disturbance of the ejaculatory mechanism as a result of the pelvic dissection has been discussed as a possible objection to proctectomy. The incidence of this complication is impossible to evaluate at this time because of the long follow-up required. If it does prove to occur at all, the legal implications alone could prove to be a strong deterrent against removal of the rectum from a child for a histologically benign disease.

Technique of the Modified Duhamel Operation

The operation we now employ[15, 16] is performed with the patient in the lithotomy position. The abdomen is opened through a generous left, paramedian incision, and the rectus muscle is retracted laterally. The rectum is divided just above the peritoneal floor, and the distal end closed with two layers of interrupted silk. The remaining aganglionic colon is then resected, the extent of the resection being determined by biopsy and microscopic examination using the "frozen section" technique (Fig. 1). Following removal of the aganglionic segment, the proximal end of the colon is closed with either a row of inverting Lembert sutures or a simple inverting

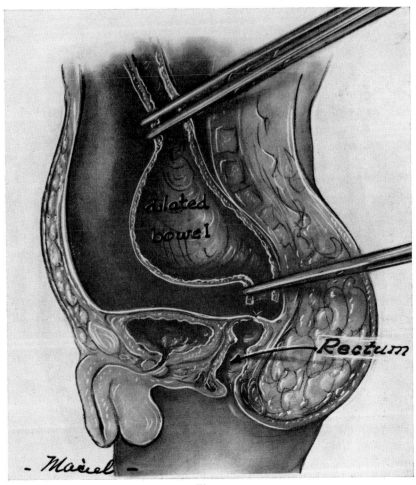

Fig. 1

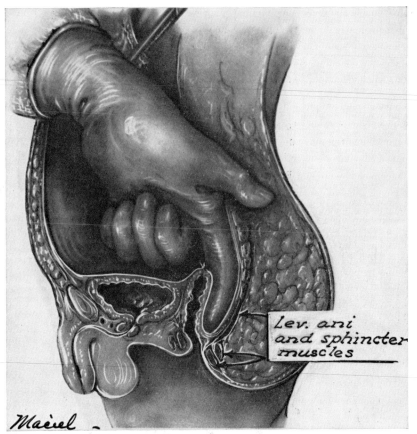

Lev. ani and sphincter muscles

Maciel

Fig. 2

purse-string suture. The ends of the sutures are kept long so that they may be grasped with a clamp which is subsequently inserted from below. The presacral space is opened next and the dissection carried downward directly in the midline posterior to the rectum; the finger is used for dissection until the level of the pelvic diaphragm has been reached (Fig. 2). The surgeon then moves to the perineal portion of the operation while the assistant remains at the laparotomy field. The anus is gently dilated and the rectum is thoroughly irrigated with saline solution, then with a mild antiseptic. During the irrigation, the assistant observes the closed end of the rectal stump and is prepared to reinforce any area of fluid leak. Sterile drapes are then applied to the perineal area. The assistant then places a long, curved hemostat into the presacral space from above, down to the levator muscles, and then separates the jaws of the hemostat as the tip contacts the posterior wall of the rectum. With his other hand, the assistant then applies mild upward traction on the rectal stump. From below, the surgeon then palpates the tip of the opened hemostat through the intact posterior wall of the rectum and makes a stab wound, between the hemostat tips, through the posterior wall of the rectum and into the presacral space (Fig. 3). The stab wound is then enlarged transversely 180 degrees. A curved clamp is then inserted through the stab wound, into the presacral space, and up into the abdomen. The end of the purse-string suture closing the proximal colon is then grasped, and the closed end of the colon withdrawn into the pelvis behind the rectum and through the stab wound in the posterior wall of the rectum. The position of the colon is arranged from above, by the assistant, so that the mesenteric border faces away from the rectum; otherwise its blood supply could be compromised when the long spur-crushing clamp is subsequently applied. Several fine, catgut sutures are then placed around the circumference of the stab wound, anchoring the wall of the rectum to the seromuscular layer of the end of the colon (Fig. 4).

The end of the colon may be opened immediately if the child has a proximal diverting colostomy already established. The purse-string suture in the end of the colon is simply removed and a spur-crushing clamp applied immediately (Fig. 5). One prong is inserted into the rectum and the other into the colon. The clamp should be of sufficient length to reach the apex of the rectal stump. Its position is confirmed by the assistant from above. We have found the *Gross' spur-crushing clamp* (Codman and Shurtleff) ideal for this maneuver, as the entire clamp lies within the

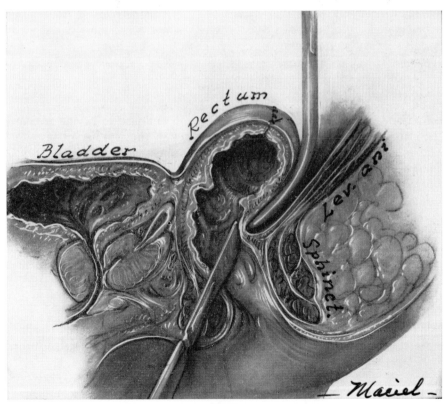

Fig. 3

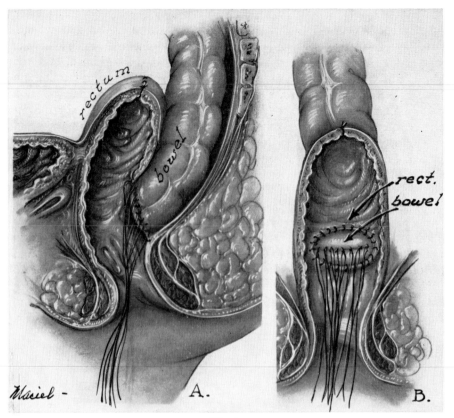

Fig. 4

rectum and, therefore, does not interfere with ambulation of the patient. The clamp is tightened daily. It will cut through the septum by pressure necrosis and pass with a bowel movement within three to five days time.

If the child does not have a proximal diverting colostomy, it has been our practice to defer application of the spur-crushing clamp for 24 to 48 hours. The perineal portion of the operation is discontinued after the wall of the colon has been sutured to the circumference of the stab wound in the posterior wall. The purse-string suture closing the end of the colon is left in place with the end of the suture protruding through the anus. After 24 to 48 hours, a brief general anesthetic is employed, and with the patient in the lithotomy position, the purse-string suture is removed. An Allis clamp is applied to either side of the midline of the septum for traction, and then the spur-crushing clamp applied. It is our feeling that the 24- to 48-hour delay allows the suture line to seal and prevents possible fecal contamination of the presacral space, which would occur if the colon were opened at the time of the initial operation.

The result of this operation is a long, side-to-side anastomosis between the ganglion-containing colon and the aganglionic rectum. The resultant

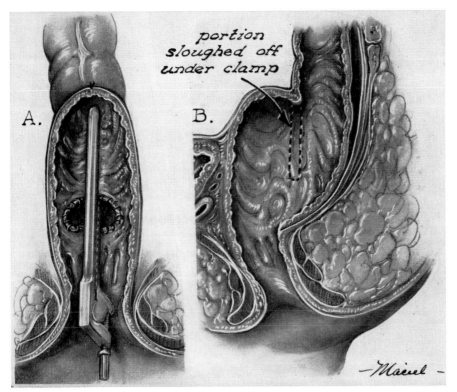

portion sloughed off under clamp

A.

B.

—Maèrel —

Fig. 5

rectal reservoir then is twice normal circumference and contains ganglion cells in the wall of half its circumference.

An alternate method for constructing the anastomosis has been described (Fig. 6) which provides an immediate anastomosis and avoids the spur-crushing clamp.[18] We have not employed this method because of the fear that the anastomosis would not extend to the apex of the rectum, thus leaving an undesirable, blind rectal pouch.

Results

In our series of 13 patients, we have had one complication, pelvic cellulitis, which we believe resulted from retraction of the rectum at the time of abdominal closure of the peritoneal floor. The patient's recovery, however, was uneventful. In the other 12 children, there were no complications.

In two of our patients with aganglionosis of the entire colon, no bowel was resected. The ileum, after being transected at the lowest level where ganglion cells were encountered, was brought down behind the rectum for a side-to-side anastomosis with the rectum. In one instance, the side-

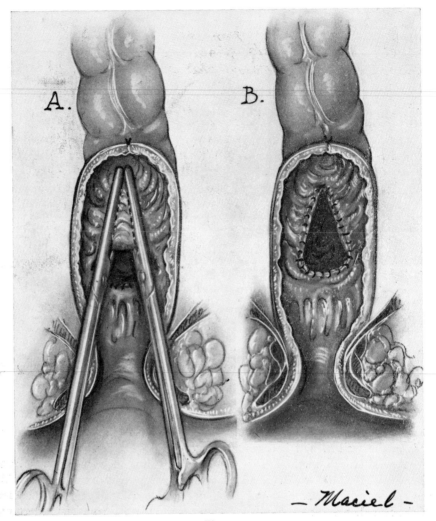

Fig. 6

to-side anastomosis was continued up to the level of the splenic flexure at laparotomy. An excellent result was obtained, and the child continues to do well three years later.

An attempt has been made to evaluate the complication rate of the operation in other medical centers.[1, 4, 7, 14, 16–19] Reports of 178 cases treated with the Duhamel type operation have been found, and no serious complications have been described. Several of the authors alluded to patients who required further division of the rectal septum. One author mentioned two patients in whom resection of the blind rectal pouch resulting from the alternate method, shown in Figure 6, became necessary.

If this operation is employed for a patient who has had a previous Swenson operation, special care must be exercised to preserve adequate blood supply from above to the rectal stump. One case has been reported in the literature in which this point had not been appreciated and, consequently, necrosis of the rectum was the result.

We have not encountered postoperative enterocolitis in any of our patients, and we have not found this complication reported in the literature following the Duhamel operation. Since we are not aware of its etiology, however, we cannot say that it could not occur. Incontinence of stool and soiling between bowel movements following the operation that we have described have been encountered only when the colorectal septum has not been divided high enough. It may be corrected by re-application of the clamp and crushing the spur up to the apex of the rectal stump. Impotence or disturbance of the ejaculatory mechanism would not be expected following this operation, since a minimum of pelvic dissection is performed and the rectum is left in place.

It is probably best to defer definitive surgery until the child is approximately one year of age.

Summary

Early experience with our modification of the Duhamel operation indicates that it is an effective surgical treatment for Hirschsprung's disease. In our 13 patients operated on by this method over the past three years, only one postoperative complication has been encountered. This consisted of pelvic cellulitis followed by recovery. Moreover, in a review of 178 reported cases of patients treated by the Duhamel type operation, we have been impressed by the almost complete absence of complications in comparison with the reported high complication rate following the Swenson operation.

It is noteworthy that the type of operation we have described allows the rectum to remain in place and to maintain its function as a reservoir. Complications resulting from its removal are avoided. The operation has been especially successful for two children with aganglionosis of the entire colon.

Our limited experience over the past three years indicates that this procedure has advantages that recommend its use for the management of patients with Hirschsprung's disease.

References

1. Beardmore, H.: Unpublished data.
2. Bill, A. H., Jr., and Chapman, N. D.: The entero-colitis of Hirschsprung's disease: its natural history and treatment. Am. J. Surg., 103:70, 1962.
3. Clausen, E. G., and Davies, O. G.: Early and late complications of the Swenson pull-through operation for Hirschsprung's disease. Am. J. Surg., 106:372, 1963.

4. Duhamel, B.: A new operation for the treatment of Hirschsprung's disease. Arch. Dis. Child., *35*:38, 1960.
5. Ehrenpreis, T.: Long-term results of rectosigmoidectomy for Hirschsprung's disease with a note on Duhamel's operation. Surgery, *49*:701, 1961.
6. Grob, M.: Intestinal obstruction in the newborn infant. Arch. Dis. Child., *37*:167, 1962.
7. Grob, M., Genton, N., and Vontobel, V.: Experience with surgery of congenital megacolon and suggestion of a new surgical technique. Zentralbe Chir., *44*:1781, 1959.
8. Hallenbeck, G. A., Brown, P. M., Waugh, J. M., and Stickler, G. B.: Surgical treatment of Hirschsprung's disease: a review of 40 cases. Arch. Surg., *83*:928, 1961.
9. Hays, D. M., and Norris, J. W.: Congenital aganglionic megacolon. California Med., *84*:403, 1956.
10. Hiatt, R. B.: A further description of the pathologic physiology of congenital megacolon and the results of surgical treatment. Pediatrics, *21*:825, 1958.
11. Kostia, J.: Results of surgical treatment in Hirschsprung's disease. Arch. Dis. Child., *37*:167, 1962.
12. Langer, B., and Thompson, S.: Hirschsprung's disease: nine years' experience at the hospital for sick children in Toronto, Canada. Surgery, *2*:123, 1959.
13. Lee, C. M., Jr.: Experience with the extended postoperative care of congenital megacolon. Am. Surgeon, *32*:705, 1956.
14. Louw, J. H.: The Duhamel operation for Hirschsprung's disease. South African M. J., *35*:1033, 1961.
15. Martin, L. W.: Preservation of the rectum in Hirschsprung's disease. Am. J. Surg., *106*:29, 1963.
16. Martin, L. W., and Altemeier, W. A.: Clinical experience with a new operation (modified Duhamel procedure) for Hirschsprung's disease. Ann. Surg., *156*:678, 1962.
17. Menghetti, L.: Considerations of the Duhamel operation for treatment of aganglionic megacolon and of other surgical diseases of the recto-sigmoid. Acta chir. Ital., *16*:107, 1960.
18. Sieber, W. K., and Kiesewetter, W. B.: Duhamel's operation for Hirschsprung's disease. Arch. Surg., *87*:111, 1963.
19. Snyder, W.: Personal communication.
20. Swenson, O.: Follow-up on 200 patients treated for Hirschsprung's disease during a ten year period. Ann. Surg., *146*:706, 1957.
21. Swenson, O., and Bill, A. H.: Resection of rectum and recto-sigmoid with preservation of the sphincter for benign spastic lesions producing megacolon. Surgery, *24*:212, 1948.
22. Swenson, O., and Fisher, J. H.: Resection of the colon for Hirschsprung's disease. S. Clin. North America, *36*:821, 1956.
23. Wyllie, G. G.: Treatment of Hirschsprung's disease by Swenson's operation. Lancet, *1*:850, 1957.

Villous Adenoma

of the

Rectum and Colon

Introduction

Villous adenomas of the colon and rectum lead to controversial view-points of management because of the difficulty in determining whether the lesion is benign or malignant. The villous lesion, said to have a greater potential of malignancy than the ordinary adenomatous polyp, is usually so large and bulky, with its soft fronds of tissue, that it is not only difficult to palpate, but even more elusive when one attempts to obtain representative biopsy specimens. They are usually located in the rectum or distal colon, but may also be found in the right colon. There have been instances (not reported) when a cecal villous adenoma could not be palpated or detected at laparotomy. The diagnosis can be enhanced by the clinical observation of a history of watery diarrhea and evidence of hypokalemia by serum values and electrocardiographic studies. Proctosigmoidoscopic and barium enema studies usually reveal the lesion, but many biopsies often fail to determine the presence or absence of malignancy. The latter circumstance, together with the usual large size of the lesion, may preclude local excision as the treatment of choice; yet if the lesion proves to be benign, a local excision, particularly for the smaller lesions, obviously would have been better for the patient.

Whether local excisions or more extensive resections should be carried out for villous adenoma is discussed in the two following presentations.

S. R. F.

Segmental Resection for Villous Lesions of the Colon and Rectum

Oliver H. Beahrs *and* Robert M. Appleman

Mayo Clinic and Mayo Foundation

Incidence and Diagnosis

If a particular type of tumor is obviously either malignant or benign, there usually is little controversy as to the extent of surgical treatment that is necessary for its management. On the other hand, if a type of tumor shows benign characteristics in one patient and malignant characteristics in another, considerable discussion ensues regarding the philosophy of treatment. Certainly villous tumor of the colon is one of the latter.

When a lesion such as a villous tumor is known to be associated with a significant incidence of malignant change, there should be no question that the surgical approach usually should be radical rather than conservative. This is especially true if the experience of a surgeon or of a surgical group has demonstrated that the more extensive operation can be accomplished safely and with an acceptable mortality rate (about 3 per cent), with a high incidence of cure, and without significant morbidity, cosmetic deformity, or functional disability to the patient.

Rokitansky first reported on villous tumors as malignant new growths in 1846.[1] Quain, a few years later, in discussing these tumors, considered them not to be cancerous.[2] Since that time, especially in the past several decades, sufficient information has accumulated to indicate that the incidence of malignancy in these tumors ranges from 20 to 40 per cent. Welch and Dockerty,[3] in reviewing 1216 surgical specimens of cancer of the colon, which were obtained during a 2-year period, found that 82 could correctly be called villous tumors. Forty per cent of these lesions were associated with nodal metastasis. Harp and associates,[4] in a search for villous lesions, reviewed 1379 adenomatous tumors removed during a 7-year period and found 76 that could be considered to be benign villous adenomas, but in the same survey found 21 villous tumors that could frankly be considered to be cancers. It has been amply demonstrated, unfortunately, that any one villous tumor might show histologically completely benign tissue on its surface or periphery, but show invasive cancer in its central or deeper part. For this reason, when a villous tumor is accessible to biopsy on proctoscopy, it is essential that multiple specimens be removed for study. Even then, the true character of the tumor may not be uncovered. In 12 of 51 cases studied by Welch, the biopsy specimens were considered benign, but examination of surgical specimens revealed invasive cancer. Wheat and Ackerman,[5] in a study of 49 biopsy specimens from 35 patients, stated that the significant pathologic changes were missed in 26 per cent of the patients. Inspection or palpation of the lesion, when it can be seen or felt, likewise is of little aid in determining the nature of the tumor. The lesion is frequently bulky and appears to be entirely benign. Often the lesion is so soft and "silky" that it is difficult to feel, but under its surface cancer is present. Size of the tumor alone does not support benignancy or malignancy. Symptoms are about the same and occur as often for patients with benign lesions as for those with malignant tumors.

Second lesions can exist in the presence of a villous tumor; these may be polyps or other cancers. Additional lesions were found in 22 of 82 cases studied by Welch. Twenty-two per cent of cases reviewed by Harp had polyps, while Wheat and Ackerman reported an incidence of 16 per cent in their cases, and Bacon and associates 10.7 per cent in theirs.[6] These incidences are higher than the incidence of 8 per cent usually given for the general population.

Indications for Resection

Because villous tumors are malignant in a significant number of cases and because the presence of malignancy cannot always be determined without study of the entire specimen, it seems reasonable not only that surgical removal always should be adequate, but also that it should provide a wide margin of normal tissue in case cancer is found to be present. Transcolonic polypectomy and local removal of these tumors via the anus should be done only when the tumor is small enough to afford an adequate circumference of normal mucosa. The use of fulguration to destroy the tumor is to be condemned, as zones of malignant infiltration, requiring more radical surgical intervention, may be missed.

For any villous tumor of the rectosigmoid colon and any part of the colon above this level, unless the tumor is very small and pedunculated, the minimal operation should be segmental resection of the involved segment of bowel. If, on gross inspection of the tumor, cancer is suspected, the resection should be the same as for any cancer of that segment of the bowel, including removal of the tissues containing the regional lymphatics.

For villous tumors of the upper third of the rectum, a low anterior resection had best be used, unless the lesion is small, involves only the mucosa, and can be completely excised through the proctoscope. A low anterior resection will be suitable for most of these lesions, since the bowel distal to the lesion can be transected safely immediately below the tumor, while for the usual adenocarcinoma the area of resection should be 3 to 5 cm. below it.

When the tumor is in the middle third of the rectum, a low anterior resection can frequently be done by transecting the bowel at the levator ani muscles or just above them. If an anastomosis cannot be accomplished, then a pull-through operation can be considered.

Lesions that are in the lower third of the rectum will almost always require a combined abdominoperineal resection, and this procedure is justified for tumors other than those that are highly selected and that possibly could be treated by conservative measures, such as local excision or fulguration after adequate biopsy, in order to preserve anal function. Cases in which the tumor is treated by local excision must be followed carefully; then, if the tumor should recur, the more radical operation must be seriously considered. In the series of cases reported by Harp, only six of 59 patients required the Miles operation.

In accepting the more aggressive approach in the management of villous tumors of the colon, patients with lesions that prove to be malignant (20 to 40 per cent) can anticipate a 5-year survival rate of more than 50 per cent (54 per cent, Welch and Dockerty), while those who have benign tumors will not very often be overtreated and will not have been exposed to undue risk.

References

1. Rokitansky, C.: A Manual of Pathological Anatomy. (Translated by W. E. Swaine.) London, The Sydenham Society, 1854, vol. 1, pp. 290–292.
2. Quain, R.: The Diseases of the Rectum. Ed. 2, London, Walton and Maberly, 1855, pp. 295–298.
3. Welch, J. S., and Dockerty, M. B.: Villous carcinoma of the colon. Dis. Colon & Rectum, 1:251, 1958.
4. Harp, R. A., Waugh, J. M., and Dockerty, M. B.: Noninfiltrating villous colonic tumors: partial review of literature and report of 63 cases. Dis. Colon & Rectum., 5:121, 1962.
5. Wheat, M. W., Jr., and Ackerman, L. V.: Villous adenomas of the large intestine: clinicopathologic evaluation of 50 cases of villous adenomas with emphasis on treatment. Ann. Surg., 147:476, 1958.
6. Bacon, H. E., Lowell, E. J., Jr., and Trimpi, H. D.: Villous papillomas of the colon and rectum: A study of twenty-eight cases with end results of treatment over a five-year period. Surgery, 35:77, 1954.

Local Excision of
Villous Adenoma of the Rectum

Sidney E. Ziffren

University of Iowa College of Medicine

Villous adenoma or papillary adenoma of the rectum has been labeled a dangerous lesion, and radical excision is commonly advised as its treatment. Primarily this has resulted because the villous tumor is commonly considered in conjunction with adenomatous polyp when polyps are discussed. In contrast to the adenomatous polyp, there is no question that the incidence of cancer is much higher in villous adenomas.[5] However, what is apparently not realized is that a majority of villous adenomas never have and most likely never will develop cancer. Once a pathologist says cancer is present, the surgeon too often, without giving thought to the appearance of the lesion under the microscope or what effect such an operation will have on the aged patient harboring the lesion, proceeds to do a radical resection. Often this is an abdominal perineal resection, which may result in great morbidity or even a mortality. In fact, had the surgeon himself taken the time to study the lesion under the microscope, he would have realized that its malignant potential was extremely low and that a far lesser procedure for cure would have sufficed. What he has failed to realize is this: Even if a cancer focus is present, if the muscularis mucosae has not been penetrated, the probability of cancer recurrence after local excision is quite unlikely.

Reasons for Local Excision

This discussion has nothing to do with lesions that on biopsy prove to be invasive cancer. Whenever the statistics for local excision of villous adenoma are examined, it is important to separate those cases in which invasive carcinoma is present and those in which it is not. The term "invasive" refers to carcinoma that has penetrated through the muscularis mucosae. In the statistics of villous adenoma without invasive cancer, in

Page 450

practically every instance no recurrence of cancer is noted after a local excision.[2, 4–7, 9, 11–14] Occasional recurrences have been noted, probably owing to inadequate excision. In rarer instances recurrence may be due to a field change in the epithelium with development of a new lesion.[12] But when recurrences do occur, they are benign recurrences, that is, having the same character as the lesion previously removed.

These lesions almost invariably occur in the older age group of patients. The average age statistically varies from 60 to 65 years. When first noted the lesion may appear massive, mimicking cancer on gross examination. This may frighten the surgeon into injudicious action. If multiple biopsies are taken, they are reported as typical of villous adenoma or papillary adenoma or papilloma, as others prefer to call them. In a few instances a biopsy may show a focal area interpreted as carcinoma, yet if it does not invade through the muscularis mucosae it should not frighten the surgeon. But the word, carcinoma, does. On other occasions the surgeon cannot believe that such a large lesion, which appears grossly like carcinoma and is sessile and not on a stalk, is not cancer, and he proceeds to do a radical resection. This can properly be termed as operating out of fear and not out of reason. Usually ulceration or fixation indicate that biopsy will show malignancy. But induration often does not mean malignancy. It may only signify inflammatory reaction within the lesion itself. Since the vast majority of these patients are in the older age group, a radical operation, an abdominal perineal resection, carries a much higher operative mortality rate than does a local excision. In addition, such an operation means a much longer period of morbidity and a permanent colostomy. If the patient returns after a local excision and shows recurrence, and biopsy shows the same type of lesion, a repeat local excision is indicated, because almost invariably the lesion is still benign. In my own experience, I have never seen a benign lesion change into a malignant one. In our small series of lesions that were diagnosed as invasive carcinoma, but in which the patient was deemed too poor a risk for a radical operation, two-thirds of the cases have not recurred after local excision. This, too, would seem to indicate that such lesions are of low-grade malignancy. I cannot support a radical operation, which jeopardizes a patient's life and destroys the anal sphincter, when a simple excision will suffice.

Similarity to Papillary Tumors of Bladder

A remarkable similarity exists in the gross and low-power microscopic appearance of villous adenoma and papillary tumors of the urinary bladder. For many years, the urologists have treated these tumors in the bladder by conservative means. If such a lesion shows no more invasion than halfway through the muscularis of the bladder, it is assumed it can be treated by local excision and fulguration. The results have been excellent.[8] Recurrences are treated in the same fashion. In the bladder the muscularis is much thicker than in the rectum. It is also true that the type of carcinoma that may develop in the bladder is a transitional cell type, in contrast to adenocarcinoma that may occur in the rectum. But the fact remains that both lesions are grossly similar in appearance and both arise from epithelium. Probably we have something to learn from the urologists in dealing with such lesions.

Technique of Management

When such a lesion is encountered the surgeon should take multiple biopsies from the periphery, the center, and especially any area that is indurated, ulcerated, or fixed. If none of the biopsies show invasive carcinoma, he should plan to do the operation most suitable to the size and location of the lesion. The tumor should be excised with a margin of normal mucosa of about 1 cm., and preferably in toto. The lesion can be excised through the anus by either dilating the sphincter or cutting the sphincter in the midline posteriorly.[3] After removing the lesion the mucosa is reapproximated. If the tumor is in the mid-rectum (4 to 7 cm. from the anorectal line), a posterior approach, excising the coccyx, can also be utilized.[10] After excision of the lesion the bowel is reapproximated. A pull-through operation, as advocated by Black,[1] can also be done; however, this is a much more extensive operative procedure. Above the peritoneal reflection a simple local excision or sleeve resection is adequate. For local recurrence we have, on occasion, used fulguration following biopsy. We do not advocate the use of irradiation therapy.

Conclusion

Most villous adenomas of the rectum are benign. In the absence of invasive cancer, local excision of the lesion is advocated, with the likelihood of successful eradication of the tumor and preservation of the anal sphincter.

References

1. Black, B. M.: Combined abdominoendorectal resection. Technical aspects and indications. A.M.A. Arch. Surg., 65:406, 1952.
2. Boling, E., and Finch, H.: Villous tumors of the colon and rectum. Am. Surg., 29:413, 1963.
3. David, V. C.: The management of polyps occurring in the rectum and colon. Surgery, 14:387, 1943.
4. Enterline, H. T., Evans, J. W., Mercado-Lugo, R., Miller, L., and Fitts, W. T., Jr.: Malignant potential of adenomas of colon and rectum. J.A.M.A., 179:322, 1962.
5. Grinnell, R. S., and Lane, N.: Benign and malignant adenomatous polyps and papillary

adenomas of the colon and rectum. An analysis of 1856 tumors in 1335 patients. Int. Abst. Surg., *106*:519, 1958.

6. Hanley, P. H., Hines, M. O., Ray, J. E., McPherson, F., and Hibbert, W. A.: Villous tumors: experience with 163 patients. South. M. J., *55*:233, 1962.

7. Harp, R. A., Waugh, J. M., and Dockerty, M. B.: Noninfiltrating villous colonic tumors. Partial review of literature and report of 63 cases. Dis. Colon and Rectum, *5*:121, 1962.

8. Jewett, H. J.: Tumors of the Bladder. *In* Campbell, M. F. (Ed.): Urology. Vol. II. Philadelphia, W. B. Saunders Co., 1963.

9. Liechty, R. D., and Raterman, L.: Villous adenoma, a surgical dilemma. A.M.A. Arch. Surg., *87*:107, 1963.

10. Lockhart-Mummery, J. P.: Diseases of the Rectum and Colon and Their Surgical Treatment. 2nd ed. Baltimore, W. Wood & Co., 1934.

11. Rhoads, J. E., Moderator: Panel Discussion: 1. Adenomas of Large Intestine and Their Malignant Potential. Am. J. Surg., *101*:91, 1961.

12. Sunderland, D. A., and Binkley, G. E.: Papillary adenomas of the large intestine. A clinical and morphological study of forty-eight cases. Cancer, *1*:184, 1948.

13. Turell, R.: Diseases of the Colon and Rectum. Vol. I. Philadelphia, W. B. Saunders Co., 1959.

14. Wheat, M. W., Jr., and Ackerman, L. V.: Villous adenomas of the large intestine. Clincopathologic evaluation of 50 cases of villous adenomas with emphasis on treatment. Ann. Surg., *147*:476, 1958.

Repair

of Inguinal

Hernia in the Adult

Introduction

One of the many controversies regarding the repair of inguinal hernias has not been discussed in Current Surgical Management. The exception, included in Volume I, presented the inguinal versus the combined inguinal-abdominal approach for the repair of sliding indirect inguinal hernias. Once again, we are incorporating alternative viewpoints on the approach to the repair of groin hernias, i.e., conventional inguinal versus the preperitoneal. Having reviewed the manuscripts supporting each of these concepts, it is at once apparent that the editorial comments of one of us (JHM) concerning the approach to groin hernias are still valid, "a clear appreciation of the complex anatomic distortions makes the operation simple—conversely, a foggy notion of the fundamental changes (anatomy) makes the operation difficult." Each author reviews his concept of the important anatomical structures of the groin, and both agree to the important role of the transversalis fascia. The advantages and disadvantages of the anterior and posterior approach are well presented, and two different repairs using the fascial tissues available are described.

The third contributor introduces still another viewpoint, namely, the use of a subfascial prosthetic mesh to close the defect when faced with a direct inguinal hernia. The technique employed is well illustrated in the accompanying diagrammatic drawings.

E. H. E.

Conventional Inguinal Approach in Herniorrhaphy

Robert S. Monk

Marquette University School of Medicine

General Comment

Since the beginning of hernia surgery the literature has been replete with suggested techniques for solving the problem of postoperative hernia recurrence. During this 100 year period few surgical problems have attracted more attention in the medical literature of the world. Thirty years ago 25 to 40 per cent of direct hernia repairs resulted in recurrence, but recently we have seen the reported incidence of recurrence reduced to approximately 2 per cent.

The achievement of this reduction in recurrence rate can be directly attributed to the tendency of surgeons to direct attention from the more superficial layers to the deeper lying transversus stratum in the repair of hernia. The anatomical artifacts and inaccuracies perpetuated in textbooks for many years have been made obsolete by the more recent clear and accurate descriptions of this fascial continuity. The publications of laboratory dissections by Anson and McVay are classics, and have served as the anatomical basis upon which the principles advanced by Dr. McVay are founded. Today there is general agreement that the most important layer to be considered in hernia repair is the transversalis fascia and its aponeurosis.

Whenever there is an inguinal or femoral hernia there must be a derangement in the anatomy of the transversus lamella. Similarly, if there is no abnormality of the transversalis fascia there is no hernia, except in the small indirect hernia of an infant. Then, indeed, this layer becomes the essence of our consideration of hernia repair. The ability of the surgeon to accurately identify the specific derangement, and his skill in the restoration of this fascial continuity to normal are, above all else, the most important factors in reducing hernia recurrence to a minimum. This basic concept is considerably more important than the method by which it is accomplished.

Brief Comment on Anatomy

The ability of a surgeon to reconstruct the transversus stratum to normal presupposes a knowledge of anatomy. The transversalis fascia is that portion of the endoabdominal fascia lying immediately beneath the transversus abdominis muscle and the first membranous layer superficial to the extraperitoneal fat. The muscle bundles of the transversus abdominis muscle are not present as low as the inguinofemoral level, but many of their terminating tendinous fibers arch and descend with the transversalis fascia to insert onto the superior pubic ramus. This attachment to Cooper's ligament extends from the pubic tubercle lateralward to the femoral vein, where it is reflected anteriorly, becoming an integral part of the anterior femoral sheath. The most lateral attachment of the transversalis fascia onto Cooper's ligament creates the normal medial border of the femoral ring. This must be reconstructed in femoral hernia repair. In a direct hernia, after the attenuated portion of the transversalis fascia is excised, there is approximately 1 cm. of transversalis fascia inferiorly, with a varying degree of integrity and a normal insertion on Cooper's ligament. This remaining tissue contains the so-called "iliopubic tract," as described by Nyhus. Because this is frequently thin and weak, McVay has recommended attachment of the incised upper edge of transversus to Cooper's ligament. Without excising the attenuated fascia, Nyhus, in his preperitoneal approach, sutures the upper border of the direct defect to its lower border, the latter being the 1 cm. of tissue anterior to Cooper's ligament.

The variable nature of the descending aponeurotic fibers within the transversalis fascia has, in the past, led investigators to describe specific ligaments within this stratum. A lateral thickening was called the "interfoveolar ligament," and a medial one was referred to as the ligament of "Henle." It seems appropriate to express some concern about the current descriptions of Nyhus. The diagrammatic representation of the "iliopubic tract" seems misleading, for this suggests a consistent thickening of this layer two or three times the density of the transversalis fascia above and below it. This is mentioned because in our hands, wide biopsies of this layer down to Cooper's ligament have not revealed its existence in the majority of the patients, as determined by either measurement or transillumination. This is not to discredit the importance of the transversus lamella, but to call attention to the variability of existing aponeurotic fibers in both number and quality and to resist erroneous impressions, which are confusing to both students and surgeons. The work of Nyhus has been excellent, and his fine publications along with the teachings of McVay should reaffirm the importance of the transversus aponeurosis in hernia repair. Though they approach the problem differently, in effect their repairs are similar, as each reconstitutes the transversalis fascial continuity to normal.

Disadvantages of Preperitoneal Approach

With the supposition that those surgeons using the conventional inguinal approach do so to diagnose and correct the pathology of the transversus stratum, it would appear that today we are sufficiently sophisticated in this matter to pursue the question of surgical approach.

One characteristic of the well trained surgeon is his competency in all methods of managing a given problem. Rarely is one technique suitable in all variations of a surgical problem, and the treatment of hernias is no exception. In other words, for the primary hernias we prefer the anterior approach. However, in the case of a patient with a direct recurrence following his third herniorrhaphy, a preperitoneal approach may be preferable. Traversing a densely scarred inguinal canal is hazardous, especially when the type of former repair is unknown. This type of patient and one with an incarcerated femoral hernia may be the two strongest indications for the preperitoneal approach. But a word of warning should be issued. All is not as it appears in an artist's diagrammatic illustration. Surgeons familiar with the anterior approach will find considerable uneasiness and uncertainty in anatomical orientation. This has been the experience of mature surgeons well versed in anatomy. Because of the obscurity of this anatomy, as exposed from the posterior aspect, a significant rise in recurrence rate would be anticipated should all surgeons adopt this as a routine approach in hernia repair.

Advantages of the Conventional Inguinal Approach

In general the inguinal approach is a more direct attack, permitting better exposure by less vigorous retraction, and does not require extensive development of a fascial space unnecessarily. When the spermatic cord is elevated and the extraperitoneal fat is encountered, either by dissecting high on the neck of an indirect sac or by excising the attenuated transversalis fascia in a direct hernia, one has at that moment a truly "preperitoneal" approach. One can at this point accomplish any repair that is possible, using the proposed preperitoneal exposure. One has the advantage of dissecting an indirect sac from the cord and the distinct advantage of removing extraneous fat and areolar tissue. This permits a careful closure of the abdominal ring that is small enough to resist recurrence without producing swelling of the testis. The technique of abdominal ring closure is of foremost importance. The opportunity to reduce the bulk of the cord, carefully approximate transversalis fascia, both medial and lateral to the ring, along with the opportunity to appraise the arterial pulsations and possible venous distention, all constitute strong support of the anterior approach.

The constricting mechanism of an incarcerated indirect hernia is occasionally the subcutaneous inguinal ring. This is easily relieved during the routine anterior inguinal approach, whereas with the preperitoneal approach an additional plane of dissection is required.

It would seem that for the same reason that the preperitoneal approach is not recommended for infant hernia repair, it is not to be recommended for the primary repair of indirect hernias in adults. It is simply more surgery than is necessary to effect a cure.

It is important to repair a direct hernia with tissue that has not been stretched and weakened. To evaluate the strength and composition of the upper edge of a direct hernia it is helpful to visualize this from both surfaces and to note its transparency. After excision of the attenuated portion, and with the extraperitoneal fat retracted, Cooper's ligament or the lower-most attachment of transversalis fascia may be used to attach the free upper edge. To permit the approximation of this strong superior edge of the transversus aponeurosis without tension on the line of closure, a relaxing incision, if needed, may be accomplished by vertically incising the anterior rectus sheath near the midline, with the aponeurosis of the external oblique retracted medially. Though it is not being used by Nyhus and Harkins in their approach, we believe the relaxing incision is important in surgery of direct and large indirect hernias.

The conventional inguinal approach for either type of groin hernia permits the diagnosis of another coexisting hernia as effectively as the preperitoneal exposure.

The proponents of each method of repair report similar recurrence rates. Therefore, the approach, per se, is not a major factor in influencing recurrence rates. Propitiously, a postoperative incisional hernia following preperitoneal herniorrhaphy does not affect the statistics because the incision is not inguinal. However, should this complication occur with a coexisting inguinal recurrence, a syndrome for which the preperitoneal approach is indicated has been created.

Summary

1. Identification of the specific defects within the transversalis fascia and restoration of this fascial continuity to normal is fundamental in every herniorrhaphy, and can be accomplished by either the preperitoneal or the conventional inguinal approach.

2. The exposure of the transversalis fascia from the posterior view is difficult, and details of anatomy are obscure. Experienced surgeons have difficulty remaining anatomically oriented.

3. The preperitoneal approach is applicable in recurrent direct and incarcerated femoral hernias.

4. The conventional inguinal approach is recommended for use in the primary repair of inguinal and uncomplicated femoral hernias.

References

1. Anson, B. J., Morgan, E. H., and McVay, C. B.: Surgical anatomy of the inguinal region based upon a study of 500 body halves. Surg., Gynec. and Obst., *111:*707, 1960.
2. McVay, C. B., and Anson, B. J.: Aponeurotic and fascial continuities in the abdomen, pelvis and thigh. Anat. Rec., *76:*213, 1940.
3. Nyhus, L. M.: An anatomic reappraisal of the posterior inguinal wall. S. Clin. North America, *44:*1305, 1964.
4. Nyhus, L. M., Condon, R. E., and Harkins, H. N.: Clinical experiences with preperitoneal hernial repair for all types of hernia of the groin. Am. J. Surg., *100:*234, 1960.

Preperitoneal Approach in the Repair of Inguinal Hernia in Adults

Lloyd M. Nyhus

University of Washington School of Medicine

Introduction

The subject of groin hernia is of interest to all. Standard methods of repair, while not completely in accord, have become fairly well crystallized during the past 25 years. An alternative viewpoint has evolved in the past few years concerning the operative approach and method of repair of the hernial defect, *the preperitoneal approach and the iliopubic tract repair.* To indicate that the preperitoneal approach and repair is the only method whereby groin hernias can be properly treated would be ludicrous. However, under certain conditions there seem to be definite advantages to this technique as compared with more standard modalities of treatment. If clinical experience with the technique demonstrates a low hernial recurrence rate, the surgeon will eagerly add the operation to his armamentarium for selected patients.

The early history of this posterior approach dates back to the late nineteenth century and the reports of Annandale (1876), Tait (1883), and Ward (1886). The concept of the preperitoneal or extraperitoneal approach to the posterior inguinal wall is usually credited to Cheatle (1920) and Henry (1936). These latter authors suggested that this approach might facilitate the technical handling of inguinal and femoral hernias. However, except for a very few exceptions, the approach was used only for femoral hernias. There was little use of the approach for direct hernias.

We were perplexed over the failure of this method to flourish. In 1955 we began a clinical investigation in a deliberate attempt to explore the potential of the approach and to secure a large clinical group in which a long-term follow-up could be accomplished and reported upon. During the ensuing few years, our technique for the repair of indirect and direct inguinal and femoral hernias evolved.[11-14]

Anatomic Considerations

The entire peritoneal cavity is encompassed by a fascial layer known as endoabdominal fascia. This fascial layer has many names, which are derived from adjacent muscular, aponeurotic, and vascular structures. Thus, in the region of the diaphragm it is called diaphragmatic fascia; in the region of the esophagogastric junction it is called the phrenoesophageal ligament; and in the region of the transversus abdominis muscle it is known as the transversalis fascia. Groin hernias result because of disruptions or relaxations in the endoabdominal fascial layer, and specifically in that portion known as transversalis fascia. In the repair of groin hernias, the essential task is the repair and restoration of the transversalis fascia lamina. Fortunately, there are thickenings (transversalis fascia analogues) within this layer of the posterior inguinal wall, which are present in most, if not in all, patients with groin hernias, and these thickenings are of use in the repair. Included among these important structures are: (1) iliopubic tract; (2) crura of the internal ring; and (3) arch of aponeurosis transversus abdominis.

Iliopubic Tract

This anatomic structure was first described by Alexander Thomson in 1836. Thomson recognized this important thickening in the posterior inguinal wall as an entity distinctly separate from the inguinal ligament. He wrote, "There is not one single fiber coming from the external oblique muscle. . . . We always find behind the tendinous portion of the external oblique, which forms Poupart's ligament, a strong aponeurotic bandelette, which has been, but wrongly, confused with the tendon itself."

The importance of the transversalis fascia and the internal abdominal ring in the repair of groin hernias has been recognized by many authors. The role of the iliopubic tract in these matters, however, has been obscured.

Clark and Hashimoto, in 1946,[3] focused attention on the iliopubic tract in the modern era of hernial repair. These authors demonstrated the iliopubic tract repair of the posterior inguinal wall by the anterior approach in a succinct manner. At about the same time, Donald, in 1948,[5] described a similar use of this structure. Many of the current concepts of the anterior approach and the iliopubic tract should be credited to Griffith.[8] The works of Fruchaud depict the *bandelette iliopubienne* (iliopubic tract) in an exceptionally lucid manner.[6, 7]

The iliopubic tract is a strong fascial band which begins laterally along the crest of the ilium and at the anterior superior iliac spine. In this area it gives origin to the iliacus muscle and the lowermost fibers of the transversus abdominis muscle. The iliopubic tract arches over the psoas muscle and the femoral vessels, where it forms an integral part of the anterior femoral sheath. In its midportion it lies immediately subjacent to the inguinal ligament. It is, however, completely separated from the inguinal ligament and the relationship is one of proximity only. Continuing medially, the iliopubic tract inserts fanwise into the superior ramus of the pubis and into Cooper's ligament. The most inferior fibers of the iliopubic tract—those that insert most laterally into Cooper's ligament—are sharply recurved in the normal groin. It is this recurved portion of the iliopubic tract which defines the medial border of the femoral canal, not the lacunar (Gimbernat's) ligament of classic description.

The fundamental importance of the iliopubic tract in understanding the anatomy of groin hernias is appreciated when one realizes that the iliopubic tract forms one of the margins of the hernial defect in each of the common groin hernias. Direct and indirect inguinal hernial defects are limited on their posterior aspects by the fibers of the iliopubic tract; femoral hernial defects are similarly limited on their medial and anterior aspects.

Transversalis Crura and Sling of the Internal (Abdominal) Inguinal Ring

The internal ring is given an elliptic shape by the presence on its anterior and posterior aspects of a double fold of transversalis fascia, which cradles and supports the spermatic cord in this region. This sling appears to be open laterally; however, as is implied by the name (internal abdominal *ring*), transversalis fascia can be delineated on all sides of the defect. The posterior crus or arm of this sling consists of fibers that parallel the iliopubic tract and finally fuse with it. The anterior crus is a more dense band, which has an extensive origin in transversalis fascia above the internal ring. The two crura are, of course, continuous with each other on the medial aspect of the internal ring and the spermatic cord, and since they are more prominent at this level, a sling effect is given; thus the terminology, transversalis fascia sling of the internal abdominal ring.

Arch of the Transversus Abdominis Aponeurosis

The transversus abdominis muscle, at its lower border, forms a musculoaponeurotic arch clearly visible as a curved line when seen from the posterior aspect through the underlying transversalis fascia. This portion of the transversus abdominis is very important to the surgeon, since it is the superior border of most direct inguinal hernial defects.

Condon has re-emphasized the absence of a true *conjoined tendon* in most human dissections.[4] In over 135 dissections of fresh autopsy material, he found a fusion of transversus abdominis aponeurosis and internal oblique aponeurosis, which formed a true conjoined tendon in less than 3 per cent of the specimens. He concluded, "What the surgeon visualizes as 'conjoined tendon' is usually composed of fibers of only the transversus aponeurosis, and rarely is formed by a conjunction of fibers of both the transversus and internal oblique layers." The figure depicts these important anatomic structures in the posterior inguinal wall as viewed from the preperitoneal approach.

Observations on Operative Technique

Details of the technique for preperitoneal hernioplasty have been described recently.[11] The basic premise of treatment is to close the hole in the transversalis fascia lamina. Since the iliopubic tract is related to all hernial defects, and since it is regularly available for repair, this structure is sutured, in direct, indirect, and femoral hernias, to the arch of transversus abdominis, to anterior crus of the internal abdominal ring, and to Cooper's ligament, respectively.

Observations will be given concerning important facets of the technique instead of repeating the details of the procedure.

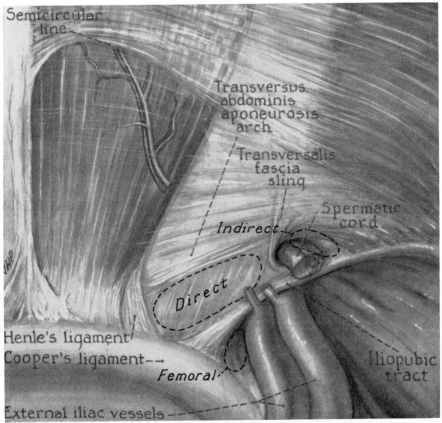

Fig. 1. The posterior inguinal wall viewed from the preperitoneal side. The peritoneum and all preperitoneal fat and lymphoid tissue have been excised, exposing the transversalis fascia. The areas through which the three common groin hernias occur are indicated, as are the transversalis fascia analogues, which are utilized in the iliopubic tract repair.

Incision

We have been very pleased with the transverse incision placed below the linea semicircularis and lateral to the rectus muscle. Although this has necessitated making two separate incisions (in contrast to the single vertical midline incision of the Cheatle-Henry approach) for bilateral hernioplasty, the advantage of proximity to the hernial defect outweighs this minor problem.

Care must be taken to avoid making the incision too far cephalad or caudad. A point approximately one and one half fingers' breadth above the symphysis pubis is usually satisfactory. The lateral border of the rectus muscle is an excellent landmark. Approximately three-fourths of the incision should be lateral to this structure.

Use of Relaxing Incision

A relaxing incision is *not* necessary.[10, 16] The incision preliminary to entering the preperitoneal space relaxes the tissues that are sutured together in the repair. Further, the distance (in a direct hernial repair) between the arch of transversus abdominis and the iliopubic tract is much less than between the arch and Cooper's ligament (structures sutured in a Cooper's ligament repair), thereby allowing the structures used in the iliopubic tract repair to be readily approximated.

Use of Prosthetics

It has been our goal to study this repair using the fascial tissues available, rather than prosthetics. It would be very simple to add the latter to our technique if indicated, but to date, prosthetic aids have not been deemed necessary.

Use of Inguinal Ligament in the Repair

The inguinal ligament is immediately adjacent to the iliopubic tract along much of its course. Undoubtedly, the iliopubic tract is mistaken for the shelving edge of Poupart's ligament on many occasions. The inguinal ligament is a much more impressive structure than the iliopubic tract, yet the inguinal ligament should not be used under these circumstances. The aponeurosis of the external oblique muscle is a structure of the anterior lamina of the inguinal wall; sutures placed into the inguinal ligament and transversalis fascia would prove to be ineffective, or would tear out or break due to natural pulls of force between these layers. It must be stated, however, that on a very few occasions this writer has been dissatisfied with the quality of the iliopubic tract, and has used the shelving edge of Poupart's ligament for a portion of the repair.

Wound Closure

At the time of wound closure, it is often difficult to find the transversalis fascia (endoabdominal fascia), which was originally cut to enter the preperitoneal space. The fascia is quite thin at this level. It is very important to suture this layer during final wound closure. It may be advantageous to mark this layer with sutures while performing the initial incision. Failure to close this layer may lead to a Spigelian hernia.

Current Impressions

We have now performed over 900 preperitoneal hernioplasties. The entire study has been one of evolution. Techniques used for repair in 1958 would not be accepted by us today. The concept of the iliopubic tract repair became a reality at the midportion of the study, 1959. We have recently reviewed our patients. When the primary hernial repairs are considered, the recurrence rate is 2.5 per cent. The recurrence rate following preperitoneal hernioplasty for recurrent hernia (not done originally by the preperitoneal technique) is 6.5 per cent.

These figures only give an impression of the current status of the study. The results are encouraging; however, with stabilization of the technique, we hope the results will improve.

The iliopubic tract repair *is* feasible from the anterior approach. This fact has been well documented. What advantage is there then to the preperitoneal approach?

The preperitoneal approach is an ideal method of circumventing the scar tissue in operations for recurrent hernia. This technique has been very advantageous in those patients with recurrence. In addition, we have been pleased to find the posterior inguinal wall usually untouched during the previous operation or operations, and therefore, the iliopubic tract repair has been feasible in every instance.

The sliding hernia, so frequently the cause for consternation, is readily recognized and handled. All incarcerated and/or strangulated hernias of the groin can be released with relative ease. The constricting ring can be cut with minimal danger to vital blood vessels and nerves. If the necessity for resection of necrotic bowel arises, the peritoneum may be opened and the appropriate resection and anastomosis undertaken. The problem of cryptorchidism is ideally suited for correction. Although hernioplasty and concomitant incidental appendectomy are currently the center of controversy, for those surgeons so inclined, the preperitoneal approach facilitates this maneuver.

As our techniques evolved, we became convinced that the approach was especially good for all complicated groin hernial problems. We have, moreover, expanded our indications to include all adult hernial problems, complicated and uncomplicated. We hope to continue this study until a definite answer can be given for this alternative viewpoint in the treatment of groin hernias.

References

1. Annandale, T.: Case in which a reducible oblique and direct inguinal and femoral hernia existed on the same side, and were successfully treated by operation. Edinburgh M. J., 21:1087, 1876.
2. Cheatle, G. L.: An operation for the radical cure of inguinal and femoral hernia. Brit. M. J., 2:68, 1920.
3. Clark, J. H., and Hashimoto, E. I.: Utilization of Henle's ligament, iliopubic tract, aponeurosis transversus abdominis and Cooper's ligament in inguinal herniorrhaphy. Surg., Gynec. and Obst., 82:480, 1946.
4. Condon, R. E.: Anatomy of the Inguinal Wall and Its Relationship to Groin Hernias. In Nyhus, L. M., and Harkins, H. N.: Hernia. Philadelphia, J. B. Lippincott Co., 1964.
5. Donald, D. C.: The value derived from utilizing the component parts of the transversalis fascia and Cooper's ligament in the repair of large indirect and direct inguinal hernias. Surgery, 24:662, 1948.
6. Fruchaud, H.: Anatomie Chirurgicale des Hernies de l'Aine. Paris, G. Doin & Cie, 1956.
7. Fruchaud, H.: Le Traitement Chirurgical des Hernies de l'Aine Chez l'Adulte. Paris, G. Doin & Cie, 1956.
8. Griffith, C. A.: Inguinal hernia: an anatomic-surgical correlation. S. Clin. North America, 39:531, 1959.
9. Henry, A. K.: Operation for femoral hernia by a midline extraperitoneal approach. Lancet, 230:531, 1936.
10. McVay, C. B.: The anatomy of the relaxing incision in inguinal hernioplasty. Quart. Bull. Northwestern Univ. M. School, 36:245, 1962.
11. Nyhus, L. M.: The Preperitoneal Approach and Iliopubic Tract Repair of All Groin Hernias. In Nyhus, L. M., and Harkins, H. N.: Hernia. Philadelphia, J. B. Lippincott Co., 1964.
12. Nyhus, L. M., Condon, R. E., and Harkins, H. N.: Clinical experiences with preperitoneal hernial repair for all types of hernia of the groin. Am. J. Surg., 100:234, 1960.
13. Nyhus, L. M., Condon, R. E., and Harkins, H. N.: Preperitoneal Hernioplasty: A Technic for the Repair of All Groin Hernias. A brochure presented at the Scientific Exhibit, 111th Annual Meeting of the American Medical Association, Chicago, Ill., June 1962.
14. Nyhus, L. M., Stevenson, J. K., Listerud, M. B., and Harkins, H. N.: Preperitoneal herniorrhaphy. A preliminary report in fifty patients. West. J. Surg., 67:48, 1959.
15. Tait, L.: Radical cure of exomphalos. Brit. M. J., 2:922, 1883.
16. Tanner, N. C.: A "slide" operation for inguinal and femoral hernia. Brit. J. Surg., 29:285, 1942.
17. Thomson, A.: Cause Anatomique de la Hernie Inguinale Externe. Jour. Conn. Méd. Prat., 4:137, 1836.
18. Ward, E. M.: Brit. M. J., 2: (July) 1886. (Quoted by Tait, 1891.)

Use of a Mesh Prosthesis

Francis C. Usher

Baylor University College of Medicine

Indirect and Direct Inguinal Hernias

The repair of the indirect inguinal hernia presents no difficult technical problem, and good results can be expected in 95 per cent of patients if the surgeon has a reasonable degree of skill in this field of surgery. The essential pathology here is the presence of the indirect sac and the defect in the transversalis fascia at the internal ring. A high ligation and removal of the sac and a secure closure of the transversalis fascia at the internal ring should result in a recurrence rate of less than 5 per cent. The conventional operations described by Bassini, Halsted, Ferguson, Andrews, McVay, and others should afford equally good results, provided care is taken to correct the two anatomical defects mentioned. The use of a mesh prosthesis is not necessary.

The direct inguinal hernia presents a different problem. Here the defect is the weakness and attenuation of the transversalis fascia in the floor of the inguinal canal, rather than the presence of the hernial sac. The sac of a direct hernia, unless it is large and pendulous, can be left undisturbed without ligation or removal. The correction of the defect in the inguinal floor is the all-important factor in the successful repair of this type of hernia. A careful dissection and search of the cord at the internal ring for the presence of an indirect sac should, of course, always be done, for many "recurrences" following the repair of direct inguinal hernias are overlooked indirect sacs.

The recurrence rate for direct inguinal hernias is considerably higher than for indirect hernias. Unfortunately in many reported series the authors fail to distinguish between the two types and give only the recurrence rate for the entire group of patients being reported. Zimmerman,[5] recognizing the importance of differentiating between these hernias, was able to present several large series satisfactorily classified, and found the recurrence rate for direct inguinal hernias to be 20 to 30 per cent.

Argument for Mesh Repair of Direct Hernias

Why should the recurrence rate be so high in direct hernias? The presence of an undiscovered indirect sac will account for some of these recurrences. But the majority are due to actual recurrence of a direct nature—a breakdown, partial or complete, of the repair of the floor of the inguinal canal. Regardless of the technique used to reconstruct the inguinal floor, and regardless of the sutures used, recurrence will take place if the tension on the approximated tissues exceeds the "holding power" of the tissues sutured. The recurrence may not be apparent for several months or years, but slowly, under the repeated stresses of increased abdominal tension, the individual sutures cut through the musculofascial tissues, and the fibrous tissue union of the approximated structures stretches and becomes attenuated until a true recurrent hernia has formed.

We feel that the best way to avoid tension in repairing these direct hernias is to use a mesh prosthesis to actually replace the defect rather than approximate tissues under tension. By this means the structures bordering the defect (conjoined tendon, internal oblique muscle, and Poupart's ligament) are not displaced from their normal relationship, and a new floor is created for the inguinal canal. This new structure replacing the defect is many times stronger than the original transversalis fascia, for it consists of a layer of white fibrous tissue 2 to 3 mm. thick reinforced by the mesh itself.

Polypropylene Mesh

We have used a knitted mesh of polypropylene to repair these defects,

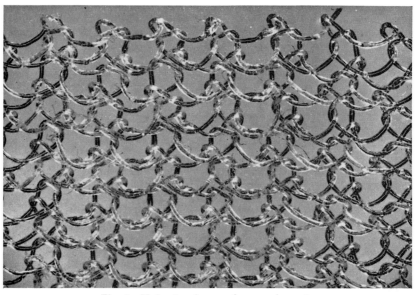

Fig. 1. Knitted polypropylene mesh. × 8.

using a monofilament suture of the same material to suture the mesh in place (Fig. 1). Polypropylene has the same degree of chemical and biological inertness as high-density polyethylene, but has a higher melting point (335° F.) permitting sterilization by autoclaving. This mesh has good tensile strength and flexibility, and exceptional resistance to work-fatigue. Experimental studies have shown that it causes very little foreign-body reaction and is inert in the presence of infection.[2, 3]

Technique of Mesh Repair

The conventional way of using a mesh prosthesis has been to first secure a primary repair of the tissues (usually conjoined tendon to Poupart's ligament), then implant the mesh over the repair as an onlay graft (Fig. 2). Fibrous tissue will grow through the mesh and reinforce the underlying tissues. The fault in this repair lies in the fact that the stress is borne by the approximated tissues rather than by the prosthesis. Tension is created by displacing these tissues to approximate them. The onlay graft is at a mechanical disadvantage in relieving this tension, as it is held in place with superficial interrupted sutures, which can easily pull away from the underlying structures.

We have found that greater mechanical advantage can be obtained by implanting the mesh beneath the transversalis fascia, allowing it to bridge the defect (Figs. 3 and 4). In order to do this, the transversalis fascia is incised from the internal ring to the pubic tubercle, the superior cut edge of the fascia is elevated, and the mesh secured to the under-surface of the transversalis fascia and conjoined tendon by through-and-through mattress sutures. The lower border of the mesh is sutured to Poupart's ligament, and a new internal ring is created by suturing the

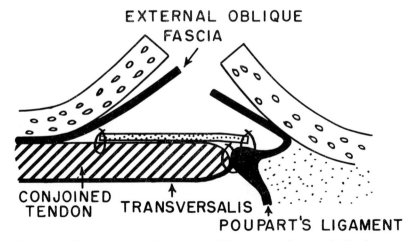

EXTERNAL OBLIQUE
FASCIA

CONJOINED
TENDON   TRANSVERSALIS
POUPART'S LIGAMENT

Fig. 2. Repair of direct inguinal hernia with polypropylene mesh. Used as an onlay graft to reinforce primary repair.

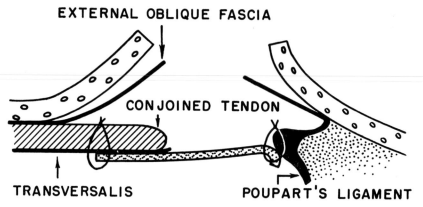

Fig. 3. Subfascial insertion of mesh, using the graft to bridge the defect.

lateral edge of the graft well under the arching fibers of the internal oblique muscle. The cord now has an oblique exit, lying between the internal oblique muscle and the graft, and the likelihood of recurrence at this point is greatly reduced. The cord is replaced over the newly created inguinal floor, and the external oblique fascia is closed over the cord.[1, 4]

Mesh Repair of Recurrent Hernias

Recurrent inguinal hernias may be repaired by the same subfascial technique described for direct hernias. The floor of the inguinal canal must be incised from the internal ring to the pubic tubercle to permit insertion of the graft beneath the transversalis fascia and conjoined tendon. The lower border of the mesh may be sutured to Cooper's ligament if the inguinal ligament has been destroyed.

Wound Complications

Many surgeons hesitate to use a mesh prosthesis in inguinal hernia repair because they fear wound complications. It is true that when large sheets of mesh are used in the repair of incisional hernias, serum accumulations may occur; in fact we routinely use suction drainage with catheters in these cases.

Such measures are not necessary in inguinal hernia repair if the mesh is implanted in a subfascial position as outlined. Because of the small size of the implant (1½ x 4 inches) and the deep position of the graft (lying beneath the transversalis fascia), no serum is formed, and it is not necessary to drain the wound. Because of the absence of serum accumu-

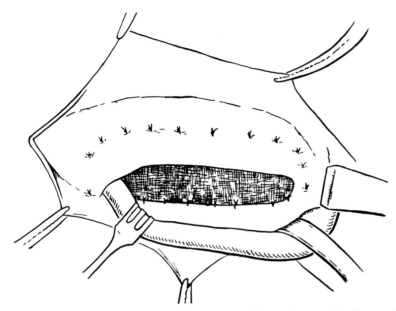

Fig. 4. Same as Figure 3. Graft replaces the direct defect and no tension is created.

lations, the incidence of wound infections is no greater than in the conventional repairs. If infection should occur, the wound may be opened and drained without fear that the mesh will cause a draining sinus, provided that monofilament sutures of polypropylene have been used to suture the mesh in place. Removal of the mesh is not necessary.

Summary

We feel that direct inguinal hernias can best be repaired by using a mesh prosthesis to bridge the defect, implanting it in a subfascial position. When used in this way no tension is created and recurrence is less likely. The mesh soon becomes infiltrated with a strong, pliable layer of white fibrous tissue, an excellent substitute for the attenuated transversalis fascia. Recurrent inguinal hernias may be repaired in a similar manner.

Wound complications are no more frequent with this type of repair than with the conventional operations.

References

1. Usher, F. C.: Further observations on the use of Marlex mesh: A new technic for the repair of inguinal hernias. Am. Surg., 25:792, 1959.
2. Usher, F. C.: Hernia repair with knitted polypropylene mesh. Surg., Gynec. and Obst., 117:239, 1963.

3. Usher, F. C., Allen, J. E., Jr., Crosthwait, R. W., and Cogan, J. E.: Polypropylene monofilament, a new biologically inert suture for closing contaminated wounds. J.A.M.A., *179*:780, 1962.
4. Usher, F. C., Cogan, J. E., and Lowry, T. K.: A new technic for the repair of inguinal and incisional hernias. A.M.A. Arch. Surg., *82*:847, 1960.
5. Zimmerman, L. M., and Anson, B. J.: Anatomy and Surgery of Hernia. Williams and Wilkins, Baltimore, 1953, pp. 204–213

Inguinal Hernioplasty in Infancy

Introduction

Opinions in the controversy whether the contralateral side should be explored in infants when a unilateral inguinal hernia is present have vacillated recently in surgical circles. At the present time, arguments for and against are continuing. Those differences of opinion may be based on conflicting reports of observations made of anatomical abnormalities during surgical exploration and specimen dissection. Differences of interpretation of developmental processes in the inguinal region, i.e., relationship of the unobliterated processus vaginalis to descent of the gonad, may also account for contradictory opinions of management. In the female infant a processus vaginalis forms, yet there is no gonadal descent; if there is obliteration of the processus vaginalis, no hernia develops and vice versa. In the male, arrest of testicular descent is associated with nonobliteration of the processus vaginalis, and a hernia sac is always found with undescended testis. The difference between a nonobliterated processus vaginalis and a hernia sac also is not always clear to observers. These relatively new concepts are discussed in the following two presentations to support contradictory opinions regarding the management of the infant with an inguinal hernia.

S. R. F.

Bilateral Exploration for
Unilateral Inguinal Hernia
in Male Infants and Children

C. Barber Mueller

State University of New York Upstate Medical Center

The presence of an inguinal hernia—demonstrable and definite—constitutes the indication for operation for its repair. In the adult this criterion applies without question. With adequate anesthesia, small instruments, fine technique and experience with the surgery of infants, the presence of an inguinal hernia in an infant or child is likewise an indication for immediate or early surgical repair. Gone are the days of the knitted yarn truss, hopeful expectation that the processus would close, and procrastination until the age of two or three years when the child became old enough to be operated on. However, with safe surgery now possible on newborn infants and young children, a secondary problem has arisen relative to care of the child with an inguinal hernia.

The Problem

Does the presence of one inguinal hernia constitute an indication for exploration of the opposite inguinal canal in the expectation that an additional unsuspected hernia will be found, thus sparing the patient a second hospital admission and a second operation with its attendant risks, discomfort, and costs?

The Background

In 1955, the first attempt was made to answer the question relating to contralateral exploration. Rothenberg and Barnett[10] reported a series of 50 patients in whom exploration of the contralateral side yielded a hernia or patent processus vaginalis in 74 per cent of the cases. Mueller and Rader reported a series of 75 cases with 60 per cent yield,[8] and McLaughlin and Kleager reported a yield of 52 per cent in 48 cases so explored.[7] These three reports touched off a series of observations relative to the subject of contralateral exploration.

A general review of the current literature suggests that of all infants and children presenting themselves with inguinal hernia, approximately 10 to 15 per cent will appear with bilateral hernias. It is the author's impression that the younger the patient, the more likely is there to be bilaterality. In the premature infant, it is far more common to find bilateral than unilateral hernia, and in infants, children, and adolescents, there are far more unilateral than bilateral hernias. However, in the reported series of bilateral exploration, the incidence of occurrence of an unsuspected hernia found by exploration of the contralateral or opposite side is not greatly decreased with increasing age.

Etiology

It is the generally held impression that defects in the transversalis fascia play no part in the pathogenesis of these juvenile hernias, but rather that incomplete or inadequate closure of the processus vaginalis is the most likely anatomic defect relating to the development of inguinal hernia in the child, and that with coughing, crying, straining, and walking, actual herniation of fluid or a viscus finally occurs. The bilateral development of such hernias is not necessarily simultaneous, and one side is likely to precede the other in those children who develop bilateral hernias. The current figures relating to laterality suggest that the right side is more likely to precede the left than vice versa; i.e., right inguinal hernias are more frequent than left by 5:3, yet in pooled data there is little to suggest that the probability of finding an unsuspected contralateral hernia is affected by the initial laterality of the evident hernia. This leaves the suggestion that there is no major intrinsic factor that produces right hernia rather than left. In some infants there is likely to be no closure of either side (bilateral hernias), and in those infants and children who are born without hernia, the left processus closes perhaps slightly better than the right so that if reopening occurs the right is apt to do so first, but regardless of which side reopens first, the incidence of bilateral anomaly is not greatly changed. There is thus an embryologic rationale for suspecting that the contralateral side may well contain a small congenital anomaly predisposing to a subsequent clinical herniation.

Observations

Several published observations and some unpublished series have confirmed the initial reports that careful exploration of the contralateral side yields an acceptable hernia or patent processus vaginalis in 50 to 60 per cent of cases.[1, 3, 5, 6, 11] All surgeons who operate on children have experienced the discomfiture that follows the appearance of a second hernia within days or weeks of repair of one side, yet 50 to 60 per cent of the patients do not return with a second hernia.

In Pickett's Syracuse studies of unilateral repair, 12 per cent returned with a second hernia within two years.[9] From a collection of several reports, it appears that about 15 per cent of children will subsequently develop a second hernia, i.e., one out of seven, though to be completely accurate, such a follow-up would require life-time observation. (In young and middle-aged adult life the inguinal hernias are almost always of the indirect type, anatomically identical to these hernias seen in children, and it is generally held that these, too, are a result of incomplete fusion of the processus.) Nevertheless, if we accept the thesis that contralateral exploration reveals an anomaly in approximately four of seven cases, it must be concluded that three of these four probably will *not* develop a second hernia. This logic accepts the unproved assumption that those who do develop subsequent hernias do so because they have a defect that might have been found and corrected if exploration had been carried out. By performing seven contralateral operations, therefore, we probably spare one of the children a second hospitalization and second procedure, at the expense of six unnecessary explorations, three of which will be unproductive and three of which will uncover some defect that may be called a hernia.

The morbidity of such an exploration is generally held to be negligible, and the development of inguinal hernia following a negative exploration is infrequent if related at all. In good hands, the extra time consumed is approximately 15 to 20 minutes. In infants there is not even a second incision, and the hospitalization is not extended by the procedure. There are European, but no American, reports that testicular atrophy or reduced testicular size occurred in 1 to 2 per cent of the cases.[2] All authors recommend that contralateral explorations be eliminated whenever there is apprehension regarding the condition of the child or the capacity of the surgeon to perform the meticulous surgery required.

Operation

The operation itself is designed for the sole purpose of extirpation of the sac and not for abdominal wall reconstruction. It consists of an incision in the suprapubic crease in infants, and bilateral incisions external to the abdominal inguinal ring in children over 12 to 15 months. The aponeurosis of the external oblique is identified and incised in the direction of its fibers and the lateral edge of the subcutaneous inguinal ring is left intact. The cremaster muscle is opened without removing the cord from its bed, and the structures within the cord are identified. A search is made for a hernia or patent processus vaginalis, and if none is present a tiny "tent" of peritoneum is pulled into the cord. This is always ligated with 4–0 silk, whether or not a hernia or patent processus is found. A fibrous remnant of the obliterated processus vaginalis is frequently present. The cremaster is closed with two or three sutures of 5–0 silk. The external oblique aponeurosis is approximated with interrupted 4–0 silk, as is Scarpa's fascia, and the skin closed with subcuticular 5–0 catgut on a cutting needle (eye suture). Flexible collodion is applied to the wounds of infants.

The Upper Limit

The age limits placed upon this contralateral procedure have not been well defined. Generally, most authors have not reported its use in patients over the age of eight or nine years. This is hardly surprising, since the incidence of hernia declines sharply following the age of 3 or 4 years, and I believe that contralateral exploration is to be discouraged whenever reconstruction of the canal is required, or when total hospitalization of more than 48 hours is anticipated. This latter condition merely suggests that if for some reason the care required for the repair of the presenting inguinal hernia is not a simple overnight hospital procedure, it is probably unwise to add the second side. In our hands, school children rarely are discharged on the first postoperative day, and with these two criteria in use, most of the children with bilateral exploration will be under the age of 5.

"In-Between" Approach

With the expectation that 15 per cent of the children with unilateral hernia will subsequently develop a contralateral hernia, there are currently only two ways of managing this group of patients. The first of these is to routinely repair the evident hernia and then detect the child with the contralateral hernia by waiting until a clinically evident hernia appears. The second of these is to explore the contralateral side on all patients, with the assumption that the risk is insignificant and the yield will be the elimination of the subsequent clinically evident hernia. The obvious ideal approach would be to determine, without exploring the canal, not only whether the contralateral hernia sac is present, but whether it is the one that will be a true clinical hernia in the future. Goodrich proposes that it is possible to determine the contralateral defect by using a Bakes dilator, which is passed through the evident hernia orifice; then from within the peritoneal cavity it is possible to identify the peritoneal out-pouching of the contralateral hernia by inserting the dilator tip into the defect.[4] This method is untested at this time. The alternative method is to increase the acumen of examination in learning to detect the "thickened cord" or "silk glove" sign. Pickett recorded his preoperative impressions regarding the presence or absence of a contralateral hernia in 500 consecutive cases of unilateral hernia.[9] Even with this large experience he was unable to predict the presence or absence of a hernia with enough certainty that it would be possible to construct a positive course of action regarding selective exploration.

Conclusion

It is the author's belief that in the case of an otherwise well male child under the age of five years with a single inguinal hernia, the contralateral inguinal canal should be explored. This exploration is for the sole purpose of extirpation of the hernial sac or patent processus vaginalis which may be found. The floor of the inguinal canal should not be disturbed; with expertise in the surgery of children, the hazards of such a procedure are negligible. This exploration is based upon the assumption that the presence of peritoneal anomalies in the cord predisposes to a clinically evident hernia in at least 25 per cent of those children that possess them.

References

1. Clausen, E. G., Jake, R. J., and Binkley, F. M.: Contralateral inguinal exploration of unilateral hernia in infants and children. Surgery, *44*:735, 1958.
2. Fischer, R., and Mumenthaler, A.: Ist bilaterale Herniotomie bei Sauglingen und Kleinkindern mit einseitiger Leisten-hernie angezeigt? Helvet. chir. acta, *24*:346, 1957.
3. Gilbert, M., and Clatworthy, H. W., Jr.: Bilateral operations for inguinal hernia and hydrocele in infancy and childhood. Am. J. Surg., *97*:255, 1959.
4. Goodrich, E. O., Jr.: Diagnosing the contralateral hernia without operative exposure. Surgery, *54*:432, 1963.
5. Kiesewetter, W. B., and Parenzan, L.: When should hernia in the infant be treated bilaterally? J.A.M.A., *171*:287, 1959.
6. McLaughlin, C. W., Jr., and Coe, J. D.: Inguinal hernia in pediatric patients. Am. J. Surg., *99*:45, 1960.
7. McLaughlin, C. W., Jr., and Kleager, C.: The management of inguinal hernia in infancy and early childhood. A.M.A. J. Dis. Child., *92*:266, 1956.
8. Mueller, C. B., and Rader, G.: Inguinal hernia in children. A.M.A. Arch. Surg., *73*:595, 1956.
9. Pickett, L. K.: Personal communication.
10. Rothenberg, R. E., and Barnett, T.: Bilateral herniotomy in infants and children. Surgery, *37*:947, 1955.
11. Santulli, T. V., and Shaw, A.: Inguinal hernia: infancy and childhood. J.A.M.A., *176*:110, 1961.
12. Sparkman, R. S.: Bilateral exploration in inguinal hernia in juvenile patients. Surgery, *51*:393, 1961.

Inguinal Hernioplasty
in Infancy: The Case against
Exploration of the Contralateral Side

Chester B. McVay

University of South Dakota School of Medicine

For many years surgeons have been aware of the fact that a hernia may appear on the opposite side following a unilateral hernioplasty. This has not caused any special comment for the adult patient, but for the infant a great deal has been written about this problem. Occasionally, the second hernia may appear before the child leaves the hospital, causing consternation for the parents and embarrassment for the surgeon. During the past 60 years this subject has been discussed from time to time, but in the past 10 years a large number of articles have appeared in support of the thesis that the side without the hernia should be explored.[1, 3, 5, 11, 12, 14, 15, 18] The reasons given are that a hernial sac is usually found and that it saves the child a second anesthetic and hospitalization. In recent years an equal number of articles have also appeared against exploring an inguinal region in which a hernia has never been demonstrated.[2, 6, 7, 9, 10, 13, 16, 19, 21] At one time this writer adhered to the teaching that the contralateral side should be explored, but since 1950 we have not operated on an inguinal region unless there is definite evidence of a hernia. Our reasons for change and the rationale of our current practice make up the text of this section.

Our first misgivings about exploration of the contralateral side were concerned with the question of unnecessary surgery. It is perfectly true that some remnant of the processus vaginalis is usually present among the cord structures of an infant and can be dissected free as a hernial sac. Occasionally, however, the diverticulum of peritoneum is so short that it is necessary to open the abdominal inguinal ring to find it, and it is likely that this represents nothing more than the dimple of peritoneum that is normally present at the lateral inguinal fovea. A short sac, just protruding through the abdominal inguinal ring, can be converted into a respectable appearing hernial sac by traction and dissection, but this additional hernial sac is only parietal peritoneum.

The fundamental etiology of the indirect inguinal hernia is the persistence of a diverticulum of peritoneum through the abdominal inguinal ring and into the inguinal canal. When the processus vaginalis is completely obliterated, it is impossible for the individual to develop an indirect inguinal hernia. In other words, an indirect inguinal hernial sac does not develop secondarily as do the sacs of the direct inguinal and the femoral hernia. An exception is the recurrent indirect inguinal hernia, in which the sac reappears at the abdominal inguinal ring and passes down the inguinal canal. However, this recurrent hernial sac does not bear the same relationship to the cord structures as the primary hernial sac does. If it does, then one can assume that the first hernial sac was not removed completely or was not removed at all. It is important to emphasize the congenital nature of the indirect inguinal hernial sac, whether the patient be an infant or an adult, because of the discrepancy between the overall incidence of bilaterality and the reported incidence of bilateral indirect hernial sacs in those infants who have been operated on for a unilateral hernia, and also have had the contralateral side explored.

The overall incidence of bilaterality in indirect inguinal hernias is variously stated, and the incidence of 18 per cent in our series is a fair average of published statistics. How then does one explain the difference between an average figure of 80 per cent bilateral presence of hernial sacs, which are called hernias if operated on, and the final incidence of bilateral indirect inguinal hernias in all large series? After all, infants become adults and are included in any series.

We may dispose of approximately 20 per cent of this group of 80 per cent on the basis of a finding, years ago, in the anatomy laboratory of Northwestern University. Of 100 cadavers examined, 20 were found to have a persistent processus vaginalis, but there was no evidence that a viscus had ever protruded into any of them. The mere presence of a sac does not constitute a hernia, since by definition, "a hernia is the protrusion of a viscus outside of its normal body cavity."

We must now account for roughly 40 per cent of the cases of alleged bilateral indirect inguinal hernial sacs. Some of this group must include those in which the small dimple of peritoneum at the abdominal inguinal ring is designated a hernial sac to justify the operation. The remainder, undoubtedly, represents newborn infants in whom the processus vaginalis is still in the process of obliteration. There is no direct laboratory proof of this latter opinion; however, we have all seen infants in whom a hernia has been demonstrated clinically, but the operation was deferred for one reason or another, and subsequently the hernia has never reappeared. A more common example is the communicating hydrocele, in which the sac fills with fluid during the day and empties back into the peritoneal cavity with recumbency at night. Many of these never develop a hernia, and some of them cease to have clinical evidence of a hydrocele. This is indirect evidence that the process of obliteration of the processus vaginalis is a gradual one, and that it may continue for several years after birth.

The report of Clausen, Jake and Binkley also supports this opinion.[2] They found a hernial sac on the contralateral side in 73.2 per cent of their cases six months of age or younger. In infants two years of age and older the incidence of a contralateral sac dropped to 37.5 per cent. The report of Rothenberg and Barnett also supports the theory of gradual postnatal obliteration.[18] They stated that, in their series, 100 per cent of infants under one year of age, with a unilateral hernia, had a contralateral sac, but that this figure dropped to 65.8 per cent when the children were older than one year.

The foregoing is this writer's attempt to explain the wide divergence of opinion among competent surgeons. Our incidence of 18 per cent bilaterality in the groin hernias includes direct inguinal and femoral hernias as well as the indirect variety, so that the true incidence of bilateral indirect inguinal hernias in our series is less than 18 per cent. However, for simplicity, if we assume that the incidence of bilateral indirect inguinal hernia is 20 per cent, then only one in five infants with a unilateral indirect inguinal hernia can be expected to develop a hernia on the contralateral side. If our reasoning is correct, then the advocates of exploration of the opposite side in all infants with a unilateral hernia are performing an unnecessary operation four out of five times. In other words, out of 100 infants with a unilateral indirect inguinal hernia, 20 can be expected to have, or to subsequently develop, a hernia on the opposite side. Eighty will not, and if all are explored on the contralateral side, this would constitute 80 unnecessary operations. This should not be taken lightly, especially when one contemplates the fact that there is considerable variation in the skill of the surgeons who perform hernioplasties the country over. Not only is there danger of damaging an intact inguinal wall with futile exploration, but even an occasional case of testicular atrophy. Very little has been written about the incidence of testicular atrophy following inguinal hernioplasty, and we do not have this information in our series. Iason quotes an incidence of 4 cases of testicular atrophy in 1600 operations for hernia performed at the Henry Ford Hospital, and records one case in his personal series of 1000 cases.[8] Swenson does not mention atrophy as a complication,[20] and Gross reports no cases of atrophy since 1940.[6] More recently, Fischer and Mumenthaler report 1 per cent atrophy and 2.9 per cent decrease in size of the testis.[4] They quote Perrot and Wachsmuth who report 2 per cent and 13 per cent, respectively, as the incidence of atrophy and diminution in size of the testis following inguinal hernioplasty in infants.

Most surgeons who perform infant hernia operations, and especially if the contralateral side is to be explored, do not mobilize the spermatic cord and cite this simplified technique and brief operating time as one justification for the bilateral operation. Early in our first 100 cases of infant hernioplasties, we missed bilateral femoral hernias in a case of bilateral indirect inguinal hernias. It is obvious that this case alone added 2 per cent to the recurrence rate. Since abandoning the bilateral operation, unless indicated, and since the isolated but distressing case cited above, we do the more time-consuming procedure of formally opening the inguinal canal. The spermatic cord is gently elevated from its bed so that the posterior inguinal wall may be properly evaluated for the concomitant presence of a direct inguinal or a femoral hernia. Since we adopted this procedure in 1950, we have found a coexistent direct inguinal hernia on two occasions, but no further instances of a femoral hernia. I may seem to be belaboring a very minor point, but in the consideration of recurrent hernia percentage, it assumes some importance. For example, in our first 100 infant hernioplasties we had one bonafide recurrence (12 years after operation), which is an acceptable recurrence rate. However, to this we must add the two missed femoral hernias, making a 3 per cent recurrence rate, which we consider too high. Had we missed the two direct inguinal hernias, our recurrence rate would have been 5 per cent, and this would certainly not be an acceptable recurrence rate for infant hernioplasty.

If the surgeon knows that one in five of his little hernia patients will develop a hernia on the contralateral side, how does he avoid the situation of an irate mother and father? Prior to the initial operation, we carefully explain the possibility, and the percentage chance, of a second hernia. Since the odds are 80 per cent against a second hernia and only 20 per cent in favor of a subsequent operation, parents invariably follow our advice to repair only the evident hernia.

In conclusion, we do not feel that the mere presence of a persistent processus vaginalis constitutes a hernia; that 20 per cent is a liberal estimate of the incidence of bilaterality; and, that the routine exploration of the contralateral side constitutes unnecessary surgery.

References

1. Clatworthy, H. W., Jr., Gilbert, M., and Clement, A.: The inguinal hernia, hydrocele, and undescended testicle problem in infants and children. Postgrad. Med., 22: 122, 1957.
2. Clausen, E. G., Jake, R. J., and Binkley, F. M.: Contralateral inguinal exploration of unilateral hernia in infants and children. Surgery, 44:735, 1958.
3. Duran, R., and Lizarralde, E.: Surgical exploration in the apparently normal side in inguinal hernia in children. Rev. Col. Med. Guatemala, 12:34, 1961.
4. Fischer, R., and Mumenthaler, A.: Is bilateral herniotomy indicated in unilateral inguinal hernia in infants and small children? Helvet. chir. acta, 24:346, 1957.
5. Gilbert, M., and Clatworthy, H. W., Jr.: Bilateral operations for inguinal hernia and hydrocele in infancy and childhood. Am. J. Surg., 97:255, 1959.
6. Gross, R. E.: The Surgery of Infancy and Childhood. Philadelphia, W. B. Saunders Co., 1953.
7. Hamrick, L. C., and Williams, J. O.: Is contralateral exploration indicated in children with unilateral inguinal hernia? Am. J. Surg., 104:52, 1962.
8. Iason, A. H.: Hernia. Philadelphia, Blakiston, 1941.
9. Lanzara, G.: The surgical therapy of congenital inguinal hernia (in consideration of

the opportunity for a systematic exploration of both inguinal canals). Minerva chir., *17*:278, 1962.

10. Larsen, R. M.: Inguinal hernia in childhood. J. Kentucky M. A., *53*:123, 1955.
11. Laufer, A., and Eyal, Z.: Contralateral inguinal exploration in child with unilateral hernia. Arch. Surg., *85*:183, 1962.
12. Lynn, H. B., and Johnson, W. W.: Inguinal herniorrhaphy in children (a critical analysis of 1000 cases). Arch. Surg., *83*:573, 1961.
13. Mascarella, A. A., and Stanley-Brown, E. G.: Inguinal hernia in infants and children. Am. J. Surg., *103*:453, 1962.
14. McLaughlin, C. W., Jr., and Kleager, C.: The management of inguinal hernia in infancy and childhood. Am. J. Dis. Child., *92*:266, 1956.
15. Mueller, C. B., and Radar, G.: Inguinal hernia in children. Arch. Surg., *73*:595, 1956.
16. Packard, G. B., and McLauthlin, C. H.: Treatment of inguinal hernia in infancy and childhood. Surg., Gynec. and Obst., *97*:603, 1953.
17. Pinto, V. A., Adde, F., Moraes, R. V., Modesto, G., Curti, P., and Arra, M.: Clinical evaluation of the bilaterality of inguinal hernia in the child. Rev. Assoc. Med. Brasil, 7:283, 1961.
18. Rothenberg, R. E., and Barnett, T.: Bilateral herniotomy in infants and children. Surgery, *37*:947, 1955.
19. Shidler, F. P.: The surgical treatment of inguinal hernia in infants and small children. Stanford M. Bull., *15*:83, 1957.
20. Swenson, O.: Pediatric Surgery. New York, Appleton-Century-Crofts, Inc., 1958.
21. Williams, C., Jr.: Inguinal hernia in infants and children. Virginia M. Month., *86*:314, 1959.

Acute
Thrombophlebitis

Introduction

There has been a shifting pattern in controversies in the management of thrombophlebitis. At one time the diverse approaches to the problem included sympathetic blocks, peripheral venous ligations, rigid immobilization, antibiotics, and anticoagulant therapy. The lack of accord stemmed (and still does) in part from the fact that the pathogenesis of thrombophlebitis has not been thoroughly understood, and the abnormal coagulation mechanisms in this condition have been even less precisely delineated. Apparently the degree of inflammation at the site of thrombophlebitis is inversely proportional to the danger of embolic phenomena, so that in the bland type of the disease, sometimes called phlebothrombosis, when emboli may go to the lung, other forms of management are considered. In the second volume of Current Surgical Management (1960), the controversy regarding the management of thromboembolism pertained to whether inferior vena caval ligation or anticoagulants should be used. In the absence of embolic phenomena in patients with acute thrombophlebitis, the problem at the present time revolves around methods of rendering the blood incoagulable or reversing the tendency toward intravascular venous thrombosis. The following three presentations describe different methods of doing this: the use of anticoagulants, the use of heparin principally, and the relatively new concept of the use of dextran in acute thrombophlebitis.

S. R. F.

Heparin in the
Treatment of Thrombophlebitis

Harold Laufman

Northwestern University Medical School

Among the unresolved questions in the therapy of thrombophlebitis, two remain uppermost. One is the question whether anticoagulant therapy holds any advantage over ancillary care alone; the other is concerned with a comparison of the therapeutic effects of heparin and prothrombin inhibitors.

Despite repeated attempts by many investigators to provide answers to these questions, the available data are still inconclusive and even conflicting. Any one of several therapeutic points of view can be supported by statistically valid evidence, depending upon how a study is carried out. As a result, one can find studies to support the view that "anticoagulants" are valuable in the treatment of thrombophlebitis, and studies to demonstrate that they are not. Most often, no distinction is made between heparin and prothrombin inhibitors in such studies. Yet, other investigations, in which a comparison of these two classes of anticoagulants is made, usually demonstrate decided differences in therapeutic action.

At least two sets of variables must be distinguished if one is to come to a conclusion in this dilemma. One is the great variability in the natural history of venous thrombosis and its sequelae. The second is related to documentation of the type of anticoagulant therapy employed, adequacy of treatment, and complications of therapy.

The great variability in the course of thrombophlebitis and its sequelae creates difficulties in the comparison of cases, let alone in comparison of patient-response to therapy. Peripheral venous thrombosis presents several paradoxes, depending on its location, extent, degree of inflammatory involvement, and rate of progression. At times, it may be virtually impossible to diagnose; other times, it is all too obvious. Most of the time, its course is benign, responding gratifyingly to almost any type of supportive care; yet, on occasion, it may cause severe complications, lifelong invalidism, or sudden death. Because we have no simple test which can inform us of impending danger or of the body's response to an established thrombus, we are compelled to employ therapy without really knowing how much of it is necessary, or whether it is proper for a given patient. Even with a successful result, we cannot be sure that our treatment was responsible or that it was necessary.

Much of our therapeutic approach to thrombophlebitis might be classified as cultism.[17] A routine of treatment is set up which experience has shown to be satisfactory, or at least acceptable. For example, it has become both popular and convenient, but not necessarily correct, for the physician to initiate anticoagulant therapy with injections of heparin for a day or two while prothrombin-inhibitor therapy is coadministered. With this method, heparin is discontinued after 48 hours, or when the Quick time for prothrombin reaches "therapeutic levels," after which the oral prothrombin-inhibitor drug is administered alone. This method continues to be popular, despite the fact that proof from a number of investigators demonstrates that quantitative prothrombin values cannot be equated with Quick times until at least five days of anticoagulant administration. After five to seven days, the Quick time is more dependable, provided certain other features of the test are controlled. Nonetheless, if heparin is discontinued before quantitative prothrombin values are adequately depressed, one could expect a recrudescence of the thrombotic process during this interval. This and other problems in anticoagulant therapy will be elucidated in this section.

Case material for this discussion was obtained from our recently published series of 404 patients.[18] The pertinent literature is reviewed in the subsequent discussion.

Analysis of 404 Cases

In a retrospective study extending over some 15 years, 404 cases of patients with a variety of venous thromboembolic phenomena were analyzed. After collation of the data, many of the same elusive variables that prevented other investigators from reaching valid conclusions became obvious. Individual case histories often contained information not reflected in the accumulated data. For example, in addition to its anticoagulant action, heparin was observed to exert significant secondary effects other than those on coagulation. In instances of acute exacerbation of postphlebitic syndrome with tumescence, eczematoid dermatitis, and inflammation, heparin administration was generally followed by rapid resolution of symptoms and findings. When lipemic serum was present, heparin rapidly cleared the serum, usually with subsidence of thrombophlebitic symptoms. In contrast, prothrombin depressants exerted none of these actions in our patients. Many other individual observations, to be discussed later, appeared in favor of heparin. But these observations, placed in tabular form, were open to many of the same criticisms mentioned previously.

The case material was divided into four broad categories: (1) acute thrombophlebitis of superficial veins; (2) acute noninflammatory thrombosis of deep veins (so-called phlebothrombosis) with or without embolization; (3) combined deep and superficial thrombophlebitis with or without embolization; and (4) postphlebitic syndrome with recurrent symptomatic thrombophlebitis or other acute inflammatory phenomena. The location of the disease was the lower extremity in every instance.

Treatment could be divided into five groups: (1) heparin for a day or two followed by prothrombin-depressant therapy alone; (2) prothrombin-depressant therapy alone; (3) prothrombin-depressant therapy replaced by heparin; (4) heparin alone, and (5) no anticoagulants. It must be emphasized that patients in all treatment categories were placed at bed rest with elevation of the affected part. Except very early in the series, no heat of any kind was used. The only additional treatment for these patients was occasional salicylates for pain, and sleeping medication, which also appeared on the order sheets of most other patients.

Every patient in the series was seen by the author, either throughout the entire course of the disease, or in consultation after treatment had been initiated by another physician. Most patients treated with the prothrombin inhibitors fell into the latter group. All patients were adults, ranging in age from 23 to 78. There were 218 males and 186 females, comprising the total of 404 patients.

GROUP 1. Heparin was administered initially, ranging in dosage from one injection of 50 mg. to eight injections given over a 24-hour period. Route of administration included the intravenous, intramuscular, and subcutaneous routes, depending upon the preference of the attending physician who initiated therapy. Prothrombin-inhibitor therapy was usually begun concurrently with the initial heparin therapy and continued for periods up to 58 days.

GROUP 2. Prothrombin-depressant drugs were administered from the start without initial heparin treatment. Type of drug included bishydroxycoumarin, warfarin sodium, and phenindione.

GROUP 3. Treatment was started with or without heparin, but prothrombin depressant therapy was in effect when therapy was considered unsatisfactory, either because of progression of the disease process, or bleeding (hematuria, hemoptysis) in the presence of unsatisfactory clinical response. The switch to heparin and discontinuance of prothrombin depressant therapy was invariably made in the presence of accepted therapeutic levels of prothrombin time.

GROUP 4. In the early years of this series, beginning in 1946, heparin was administered intravenously to patients whose entire treatment was my responsibility. A few patients in this group received heparin in a long-acting menstruum intramuscularly under the direction of other physicians.

TABLE 1.   RESULTS OF TREATMENT

Group No.	Treatment	Deep		Superf.		Deep and Superf.		Postphlebitic Syndrome		Total
		+	−	+	−	+	−	+	−	
1.	Heparin and pro-thrombin depressants	27	7 (3E)	16	4	7	2	21	5 (1E)	89 (4E)
2.	Prothrombin depressant alone	2	3 (2E)	1	2	2	4 (2E)	7	5 (1E)	26 (5E)
3.	Prothrombin de-pressant followed by heparin	2	0	3	0	4	0	5	0	14
4.	Heparin alone	76	1 (1E*)	43	0	21	0	54	0	195 (1E)
5.	No anticoagulant	8	5 (1E)	21	7	2	3	26	8	80 (1E)
	Totals	115	16 (6E)	84	13	36	9 (2E)	113	18 (2E)	404 (10E)
		131		97		45		131		404

+ = satisfactory subsidence and no recrudescence
− = poor response, recrudescence or
E = thromboembolism
* = death from pulmonary embolism from iliac vein following lapse in heparin control

In the past five years, heparin has been administered as the pure aqueous solution by deep subcutaneous, intermittent injections, as described below.

GROUP 5.   Patients in all groups were placed at bed rest with varying degrees of elevation of the affected extremities. Patients in Group 5 differed from those in other groups only in that they received no anticoagulants at any time. Elastic compression was applied only after it could be tolerated. Ambulation was usually permitted as tolerated after subsidence of acute symptoms.

Table 1 includes all the case material. Results of treatment were considered positive (+) if they included satisfactory subsidence of symptoms and no recrudescence. A negative (−) result consisted of failure to arrest propagation of thrombosis, failure to cause subsidence in inflammation, recrudescence of symptoms during therapy, and occurrence of embolization during therapy.

Analysis of the information set forth in Table 1 revealed that although the total number of patients was appreciable, the fractionation into uneven categories of disease and treatment made comparison of groups invalid. Therefore, it was decided that one question would be posed, "How does heparin therapy compare with prothrombin-depressant therapy in the treatment of venous thromboembolic disease?"

A direct answer to this question could be obtained by analysis of the smallest group in the series, Group 3, in which patients on therapeutic dosage of prothrombin-depressants were switched to heparin because of complications or poor results, in the hope that the course of the disease could be altered.

Each patient in this group suffered extension of the disease process while receiving "adequate" coumarin-type therapy. The diseases for which patients were treated are shown in Table 2. These include: acute inflammatory thrombophlebitis of superficial veins (four patients); post-operative deep vein thrombosis (three patients); combined deep and superficial thrombophlebitis with repeated emboli and pulmonary infarction (2 patients), and acute exacerbation of postphlebitic syndrome (five patients).

Table 3 lists the type of prothrombin-inhibitor therapy these patients received. Patients who had received obviously inadequate anticoagulant therapy before introduction of heparin therapy were excluded, because the improvement produced by heparin in such cases could be construed as substitution of adequate for inadequate therapy rather than administration of a more effective drug. The criterion for adequacy of treatment with prothrombin inhibitors was the one customarily employed—a Quick time of 20 to 30 seconds, using a commercial thromboplastin with a control time of 12 seconds.

Nine of the 14 patients had been initially treated with intravenous heparin for one or two days while a prothrombin drug was coadministered, then heparin was continued alone. Five patients received no heparin initially, but received a coumarin-type drug from the beginning. Bishydroxycoumarin (Dicumarol) was used in seven instances, warfarin sodium

TABLE 2. DISEASES TREATED BY PROTHROMBIN DEPRESSANT
FOLLOWED BY HEPARIN

Acute inflammatory thrombophlebitis, superficial	4
Postoperative deep thrombosis	3
Repeated emboli and infarction, combined deep and superficial thrombophlebitis	2
Acute exacerbation postphlebitic syndrome	5

TABLE 3. TYPES OF PROTHROMBIN DEPRESSANT USED IN PATIENTS LATER
TREATED WITH HEPARIN

Bishydroxycoumarin (Dicumarol)	7
Warfarin sodium (Coumadin)	2
Phenindione (Hedulin)	5

Quick time—14–48 sec., usually over 20 sec.
Duration Rx—3–22 days, average 7½ days
Hematuria—2; hemoptysis—1

(Coumadin) in two, and phenindione (Hedulin) in five (Table 3). Duration of treatment was three to 22 days, averaging 7½ days before the change to heparin. In all 14 of these patients treatment had been initiated by a physician other than the author, and the switch to heparin was made after the author saw the patients in consultation.

Two preparations of heparin were used,* both described by the manufacturers as exceeding U.S.P. standards for purity. This type of highly refined concentrated aqueous heparin is as slowly absorbed from the deep subcutaneous tissues as repository material injected intramuscularly, but tends to produce more dependable responses, is less painful, easier to administer, and less expensive. A large variety of dosage forms is available, ranging from 1000 to 40,000 U.S.P. units per cc., making it convenient to give virtually any desired dose in 1 cc. volumes. The usual initial dosage given was 10,000 units (100 mg.) intravenously, followed by the same dose in six or eight hours by deep subcutaneous injection, depending on the response, then usually maintained at a dose of 10,000 units administered by deep subcutaneous injection every 8 to 12 hours after the first two or three days. The injections were usually made in the subcutaneous tissues of the abdomen at about waist level.

Lee-White coagulation times, done two hours after intravenous administration, and six, eight, or 10 hours after deep subcutaneous injection, were maintained at more than 20 minutes in virtually all instances; the lowest temporary level was 11 minutes, observed in one patient with extremely acute inflammation, and corrected by increasing the dosage. Despite occasional peak prolongations of coagulation time to over 50 minutes (in one instance 110 minutes), bleeding was not noted in any patient in this group. In fact, all three patients who experienced hematuria or hemoptysis during prior prothrombin-inhibitor therapy stopped bleeding when therapy was switched to heparin.

Although symptoms began to subside within 12 to 24 hours after heparin administration (Table 4), the duration of heparin therapy averaged

TABLE 4. RESULTS OF TREATMENT WITH HEPARIN

Lesion	Response to Heparin	Number of Patients
Acute inflammation, superficial	Subsidence of pain, tenderness and inflammation in 24 hours. Gone in 72 hours (3 treated surgically).	4
Deep thrombosis (Bleeding in 1 pt.)	Subsidence of edema and tenderness in 24 hours. Gone in 72 hours. Bleeding stopped.	3
Repeated emboli; infarction and effusion (Bleeding in 2 pts.)	Cessation of emboli; rapid resolution and absorption effusion. Bleeding stopped.	2
Exacerbation postphlebitic syndrome	Anti-inflammatory effect noted in 24–72 hours (4 treated surgically)	5

* Lipo-Hepin (Riker) was used in 11 patients.
  Panheprin (Abbott) was used in 3 patients.

8 days, ranging from 5 to 16 days. The time for discontinuance was determined by observing complete subsidence of major symptoms and findings. Six of the patients were subjected to extirpative vein surgery 3 to 10 days after the acute process had completely subsided with heparin therapy. Elastic support was applied to the lower extremity only after tenderness had subsided enough to permit it. Ambulation with elastic support was permitted 48 hours after application of the elastic. Surgical procedures consisted of removal of thrombosed superficial leg veins in 3 patients, and extensive vein strippings in 4 of the patients with postphlebitic disease.

Heparin administration was never stopped abruptly. After subsidence of clinical findings, the dose was halved for one day, then quartered for another, before discontinuance. If diminution in dosage resulted in symptomatic recurrence, as it did in 2 patients, full dosage was resumed for another 5 days. Occasionally, long-term anticoagulation with heparin was continued on a self-administration basis. This regimen became necessary in patients with recurrent thromboembolic disease who were either sensitive to coumarins, or could not be maintained on them without recurrences of disease.

Neither vena cava nor femoral vein ligations were done on any patients in this group. Vena cava ligation was seriously considered in the case of one patient, but consideration was dropped when the embolizations ceased and the patient improved on heparin therapy.

Review of Pertinent Literature

Because of wide variations in the natural history of thrombophlebitis and its sequelae, retrospective analysis of a series of patients treated in various ways is open to legitimate criticism. However, in the reported group of patients unsuccessfully treated with adequate doses of prothrombin-depressant drugs, the switch to heparin made each patient his own control regardless of the type of venous disease he had. The contention is made that the rapid and marked improvement which ensued after heparin therapy was instituted demonstrates the superiority of heparin over prothrombin-inhibitor drugs in the treatment of venous thromboembolic disease. This contention is borne out by experimental work and by certain other clinical studies.

The experimental studies of Wessler and associates showed that when serum fractions prepared from dog's blood were infused into another dog, massive thrombosis occurred in areas of retarded blood flow despite pretreatment of either or both donor and recipient animal with large doses of bishydroxycoumarin.[25, 26] In contrast, the deposition of thrombi was completely blocked by heparin injected into either dog in amounts merely sufficient to double the clotting time. Williams and Elliott were able to prevent thrombus propagation with heparin when the Lee and White clotting time was elevated to at least one and one-half times the preheparin level.[27]

Failure to maintain this elevated clotting time allowed thrombus propagation. Dicumarol, Tromexan, and Coumadin were ineffective unless prothrombin times were held at dangerously low levels.

Among the several reports of series of patients treated with anticoagulants, the one by Fuller, Robertson, and Smithwick appeared to offer clearcut evidence of the superiority of heparin.[9] The two main forms of anticoagulant therapy were compared in a survey of 744 cases of venous thromboembolism. These investigators observed that ". . . bishydroxycoumarin appeared to have little to offer in the therapy of pulmonary embolization, prevention of recurrence of the thrombotic process or speed of subsidence of the inflammatory process." A number of investigators, including Griffith and co-workers,[13] and Engelberg,[8] have found that heparin permits more adequate anticoagulation and results in lower mortality than bishydroxycoumarin in the treatment of patients with coronary disease.

Eliot and co-workers compared the efficacy of daily heparin injections as anticoagulant therapy with the possibility of self-treatment on an outpatient basis.[7] These investigators used an instrument called the thromboelastograph. Patients on subcutaneous heparin injections were compared with a group on Dicumarol or Coumadin. Heparin was found to delay both the onset and progress of fibrin formation, and the duration of anticoagulant action depended upon the dosage used. Twenty hours of anticoagulant action could be obtained with a single subcutaneous injection of 4 mg./kg. of heparin. On the other hand, although all patients on prothrombin inhibitors had a prothrombin activity of 15 to 20 per cent of normal, their coagulograms showed only a small deviation from normal. The prothrombin time, upon which the physician bases the dosage of prothrombin-depressing agents, did not reflect the true degree of anticoagulation. About 50 per cent of the patients on a therapeutic level of prothrombin activity did not show a significant decrease in coagulability. Patients maintained within therapeutic range of activity in this series had bleeding problems.

In contrast to these reports are those of Butcher, whose data are interpreted by him to indicate that neither heparin nor coumarin-type drugs hold any advantage over the avoidance of anticoagulants in the treatment of venous thromboembolic disease.[3] In a third camp are those, including Milch and associates[20] and Thomes and co-workers,[24] who are convinced from their data that the use of prothrombin-inhibitor drugs has materially reduced the incidence of thromboembolic phenomena.

Various investigators have pointed out a number of faults with the administration of prothrombin inhibitors. Sise has performed experiments to show that the Quick value is a poor reflection of quantitative prothrombin;[22] that whereas the Quick time may fall to therapeutic range within 48 hours after the drug is administered, the prothrombin content of the blood may not reach therapeutic range for 5 or 6 days (Fig. 1). This finding has important clinical implications. It may mean that unless heparin and a prothrombin-inhibitor drug are co-administered for at least 5 days before discontinuance of the heparin, the thrombotic process may progress un-

impeded for several days before prothrombin values are sufficiently low to
be effective, yet during which time the Quick values are well within "therapeutic" range.

Another fault with prothrombin-inhibitor therapy lies in the test used
to determine the narrow margin between ineffectiveness and bleeding levels,
a range measured by a test so crude that Armand Quick himself has said:

It has been observed that the free prothrombin remains normal until the prothrombin
time is increased to 20 seconds.[21] It is the reduction of the prothrombin which is probably
the actual determinant of both the therapeutic effect and the bleeding tendency. . . . The
therapeutic range which has been clinically found optimal is 20–25 seconds. In this range
the true prothrombin is reduced to about 40 per cent of normal. Only when the one-stage
test is carried out with precision and with a thromboplastin that yields a value of 12 seconds
on fresh human plasma do these values hold. It is my belief that any patient whose prothrombin time is shorter than 19 seconds is receiving little or no benefit, except that the
periodic encounter with the needle reminds him that he has a cardiac condition, and that
he must observe the rules.

According to Hartert,[15] a considerable amount of laboratory work is
required if optimal efficiency of anticoagulant therapy with prothrombin-
depressants is to be combined with optimal security against hemorrhage. He
acknowledges that the rapidly-reacting clotting factors can be verified by
the Quick test, which chiefly concerns prothrombin and factor VII. The
Quick test, however, is blind to the slowly responding thromboplastic
factors, which are best verified with the aid of a thromboelastogram; this
in turn is less sensitive to the rapidly responding factors. Thus, the margin
between dangerous bleeding and dangerous clotting is often obscured by
falsely secure tests. For these reasons, in Hartert's clinic in Heidelberg two
tests are systematically used in all patients on anticoagulant therapy: the
thromboelastogram and the Quick test.

In contrast to the dangers and pitfalls inherent in prothrombin depres-

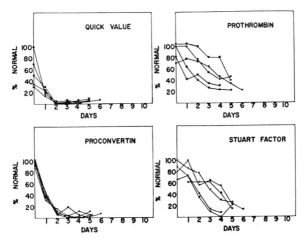

Fig. 1. Activity measured by the Quick test as compared to proconvertin, prothrombin, and Stuart factor after 300 mg. of Warfarin intravenously. (From Sise et al.: New
England J. Med., *259:266*, 1958.)

sant therapy, one has but to ponder the statement of de Takats,[4] "The clotting time, no matter how crude and simple or how complicated the methods used, strictly parallels the heparin levels in the blood."

When oral anticoagulants originally became available, they were hailed because they would "simplify" anticoagulant therapy, and would be "less expensive" than the injections of heparin. Today, it appears that these advantages are somewhat less overwhelming than they had seemed in the beginning.

Benditt reviewed the actions of heparin other than those on coagulation and cited a large body of evidence documenting the actions of heparin as an anti-allergic, anti-inflammatory, lipemia-clearing, and complement-inhibiting agent.[1] Some of these actions appear to have been important in the clinical management of our patients.

It is well known that a hypercoagulable state may accompany inflammatory lesions, and that thrombosis almost invariably gives rise to phlebitis. De Takats, in 1943, observed that the patient's heparin tolerance fluctuates with the acuteness of the disease.[5] The more acute the thrombophlebitis, the larger the dose generally required. This same relationship usually does not hold for the prothrombin depressant drugs. The reciprocal relationship between heparin dosage and acuteness of inflammation is reflected in the demonstrable subsidence of the inflammation once adequate dosage of heparin is reached. The type of periphlebitic inflammation occurring in thrombophlebitis is probably more closely allied to a histamine-release reaction than it is to bacterial varieties of inflammation. Experimentally, heparin exerts little or no effect on the latter.[22] This anti-inflammatory action of heparin, not shared by prothrombin-inhibitors, appears to be important in the management of established thrombophlebitis.

The antiallergic effects of heparin are considered to be the result of inhibition of histamine release at the cellular level.[6] These effects have been amply documented experimentally,[11] and were apparent in our patients with postphlebitic dermatitis. Because the anti-allergic action of heparin is not as potent as that of corticosteroids, the steroids have been coadministered with heparin in severe hypersensitivity reactions in postphlebitic disease. None of these cases fell into the group of patients reported in this paper.

The lipemia-dispersing effect of heparin[14] is apparently due to activation of lipoprotein lipase by the drug.[12] Although we have never observed clearance of serum lipids by prothrombin-depressants, George and associates recently reported that several oral anticoagulants stimulate in vivo fat clearance, as measured by levels of I^{131}-labeled triglycerides.[10] These drugs appeared to exert approximately two-thirds of the lipemia-clearing action of intravenous heparin administered every 4 hours. We did not perform actual lipid determinations on the patients described in this report, but data from a general group of 35 of our patients with acute thrombophlebitis showed them to have somewhat elevated serum cholesterol levels ranging from 285 to 420 mg. per cent.[19] Brown and co-workers recently showed that heparin given systemically produced a much improved or normal response in patients with slow lipid-clearing after meals. Whether or not hyperlipemia is conducive to acute thrombophlebitis is uncertain at present.[2]

Despite these many apparent advantages of heparin over prothrombin inhibitors, an unknown number of patients with thrombophlebitis do improve with only prothrombin-inhibitor therapy. Such improvement may be due to (1) ancillary care such as elevation and bed rest,[16] (2) spontaneous subsidence, or (3) specific effects of bishydroxycoumarin, thus far not reproducible experimentally.

Regimen of Treatment

From our experiences, we have arrived at the following regimen for the treatment of thromboembolic disease: bed rest and moderate elevation of the legs; determination of control Lee-White coagulation time (if performed at 37.5°C, control values are normally 10 to 12 minutes; if performed at room temperature, 5 to 7 minutes); administration of 15,000 units of heparin deep subcutaneously or 10,000 units intravenously for the first dose; thereafter, 10,000 units are administered deep subcutaneously at 8-hour intervals for the first 24 hours, then 10,000 units at 12-hour intervals; Lee-White times need only be done every 24 hours, 2 hours before the next dose (if 10 A.M. and 10 P.M. dosages are given, Lee-White time is checked at 8 A.M. daily while the patient is in the hospital); adjustments in dosage are usually made in 5000-unit amounts (Lee-White coagulation times should be over 20 minutes); treatment is continued for a minimum of 5 days but usually 10 days; if patient is to be placed on long-term coumarin therapy, heparin should be coadministered with the coumarin drug for 5 to 7 days before discontinuing heparin. For patients on long-term heparin therapy, 10,000 to 20,000 units per day is self-administered in the deep subcutaneous abdominal fat just above the belt line. Lee-White determinations may be done as seldom as once weekly, as a rule 10 to 12 hours after the injection.

Surgical intervention depends on individual case selection. In general, superficial thrombophlebitis is treated by early excision; deep thromboses are removed early in the disease by thrombectomy. Later, after clots have become fixed, ligation procedures may become indicated if embolization occurs despite adequate heparin therapy.

Conclusions

A group of 14 patients were chosen from a series of 404 with various manifestations of acute thrombophlebitis and its sequelae, because the disease process in this group either progressed or did not respond favorably in the face of what is commonly considered to be adequate prothrombin-inhibitor therapy. This select group afforded an excellent opportunity to compare effects of prothrombin-depressant therapy with those of heparin therapy. Three patients on prothrombin-inhibitor therapy experienced hematuria or hemoptysis at the same time that their thrombotic disease was propagating. After therapy was changed to heparin, a favorable response was noted in a relatively short time, usually within 24 hours; patients who had bled during prothrombin-inhibitor therapy did not bleed after receiving heparin, although the thrombotic process was arrested.

Analysis of these data and application of pertinent material from the literature appears to support a clear superiority for heparin over prothrombin depressants in the treatment of thrombophlebitis and its sequelae.

References

1. Benditt, E. P.: Actions of heparin other than those on coagulation. Ann. Rev. Med., 8:407, 1957.
2. Brown, D. F., Heslin, A. S., and Doyle, J. T.: Postprandial lipemia in health and in ischemic heart disease: a comparison of three indexes of fat absorption and removal and their modification by systemic heparin administration. New England J. Med., 264:733, 1961.
3. Butcher, H. R.: Anticoagulant and drug therapy for thrombophlebitis in lower extremities: valuation. A.M.A. Arch. Surg., 80:864, 1960.
4. deTakats, G.: Letters to the Editor. New England J. Med., 264:728, 1931.
5. deTakats, G.: Heparin tolerance: a test of clotting mechanism. Surg., Gynec. and Obst., 77:31, 1943.
6. Dragstedt, C. A., Wells, J. A., and deSilva, R.: Inhibitory effect of heparin upon histamine release by trypsin, antigen, and protease. Proc. Soc. Exper. Biol. and Med., 51:191, 1942.
7. Eliot, R. S., von Kaulla, K. N., and Blount, S. G., Jr.: Thromboelastographic studies with a 24-hour schedule for subcutaneous heparin: a comparison of its efficiency with prothrombin-depressing agents. Circulation, 24:1204, 1961.
8. Engelberg, H.: Heparin in acute myocardial infarction. California Med., 91:327, 1959.
9. Fuller, C. H., Robertson, C. W., and Smithwick, R. H.: Management of thromboembolic disease. New England J. Med., 263:983, 1960.
10. George, E. P., Hall, G. V., and Farkas, G. S.: Lipemia clearing action of artificial anticoagulants. Nature, 187:782, 1960.
11. Good, R. A., and Thomas, L.: Studies on generalized Shwartzman reaction. IV. Prevention of local and generalized Shwartzman reactions with heparin. J. Exper. Med., 97:871, 1953.
12. Graham, D. M., Lyon, T. P., Gofman, J. W., Jones, H. B., Yankley, A., Simonton, J., and White, S.: Blood lipids and human atherosclerosis. II. The influence of heparin on lipoprotein metabolism. Circulation, 4:666, 1951.
13. Griffith, G. C., Zinn, W. J., Engelberg, H., Dooley, J. V., and Anderson, R.: Heparin versus heparin-bishydroxycoumarin anticoagulant therapy. J.A.M.A., 174:1157, 1960.
14. Hahn, P. F.: Abolishment of alimentary lipemia following injection of heparin. Science, 98:19, 1943.
15. Hartert, H.: International symposium: myocardial infarction. Abbottempo, 1:14, 1963.
16. Laufman, H.: Ancillary care in postphlebitic syndrome. S. Clin. North America, 39:183, 1959.
17. Laufman, H.: Cultism in thromboembolic therapy. Editorial. Surg., Gynec. and Obst., 114:747, 1962.

18. Laufman, H.: Superiority of heparin over prothrombin depressants in the treatment of thrombophlebitis and its sequelae. S. Clin. North America, 44:195, 1964.

19. Laufman, H.: Unpublished data.

20. Milch, E., Berman, L., and Egan, R. W.: Bishydroxycoumarin (Dicumarol) prophylaxis. A.M.A. Arch. Surg., 83:132, 1961.

21. Quick, A. J.: Letters to the Journal. J.A.M.A., 178:1119, 1961.

22. Rigdon, R. H., and Wilson, H.: Capillary permeability and inflammation in rabbits given heparin. A.M.A. Arch. Surg., 43:64, 1941.

23. Sise, H. S., Lavelle, S. N., Adamis, D., and Becker, R.: Relation of hemorrhage and thrombosis to prothrombin during treatment with coumarin-type anticoagulants. New England J. Med., 259:266, 1958.

24. Thomes, A. B., Scallen, R. W., and Savage, I. R.: Value of long-term anticoagulant therapy in coronary disease. J.A.M.A., 176:181, 1961.

25. Wessler, S., and Reimer, S. M.: The role of human coagulation factors in serum-induced thrombosis. J. Clin. Invest., 39:262, 1960.

26. Wessler, S., Ballon, J. D., and Katz, J. H.: Studies on intravascular coagulation: V. A distinction between the anticoagulant and antithrombotic effects of Dicumarol. New England J. Med., 256:1223, 1957.

27. Williams, R. D., and Elliott, D. W.: Effect of heparin and coumarin derivatives on a standardized intravenous thrombosis. Surgical Forum, 9:138, 1959.

Anticoagulant Therapy in the
Management of Acute Thrombophlebitis

John A. Spittell, Jr.

Mayo Clinic and Mayo Foundation

Introduction

Venous thrombosis continues to be a frequent problem in clinical practice. Despite extensive studies by many investigators, understanding of pathogenetic mechanisms remains incomplete, objective measures of diagnosis are lacking, and differences of opinion regarding therapy persist.

Virchow, more than a century ago, postulated three factors—stasis of blood flow, damage to the vascular endothelium, and alteration in blood coagulability—as important in the development of intravascular thrombi. Although the relative importance and interdependence of these factors are not understood, they can be used as the basis for a therapeutic approach to venous thromboembolism. Equally important in formulating a program of treatment is a consideration of the goals of therapy; these include prevention of further thrombosis and pulmonary embolism, relief of venous congestion, and restoration of venous flow to as near normal as possible.

At present no unanimity of opinion exists concerning definitive treatment of acute venous thrombosis. There are advocates of anticoagulant therapy, fibrinolytic therapy, and vein ligation with or without thrombectomy.

Anticoagulant therapy has certain advantages over the other types of treatment. Assuming that hypercoagulability of the blood is a factor in intravascular thrombosis, effective anticoagulant therapy should prevent further thrombosis. In addition, experimental evidence indicates that anticoagulant therapy hastens recanalization of thrombi. Although bleeding is a calculated risk during anticoagulant therapy, sufficient experience with the anticoagulant drugs has been accumulated to minimize this risk, provided the dosage of the anticoagulant drugs is regulated by adequate laboratory tests.

The dissolution of thrombi by fibrinolytic enzymes is a promising approach to the management of venous thrombosis, but at present limited experience with this type of therapy indicates that it is best suited for investigative rather than general use.

Ligation of an involved femoral or iliac vein has the advantage of trapping the thrombus and thus preventing pulmonary embolism, provided additional thrombi do not develop proximally or in the other leg. The latter is a distinct possibility if alteration of blood coagulability plays some role in the development of intravascular thrombi. Ligation of the inferior vena cava is a more formidable procedure and, in addition to the limitations mentioned for femoral vein ligation, has the added disadvantage of producing chronic venous insufficiency of the lower extremities in many cases. Ligation of veins in the treatment of venous thrombosis thus seems best reserved for those cases in which anticoagulant therapy is contraindicated or has proved ineffective.

More recently thrombectomy has been advocated in the treatment of deep venous thrombosis. Advocates of this procedure think that it has the advantage of minimizing the incidence of postphlebitic venous insufficiency. A review of cases of iliofemoral thrombophlebitis treated with anticoagulant therapy has shown that the incidence of chronic deep venous insufficiency is no greater after anticoagulant therapy than that reported after thrombectomy.

Anticoagulant Drugs

Anticoagulant drugs produce changes in the clotting mechanism of the blood; the physician employing them, therefore, must balance the risk of thrombosis or its complications without anticoagulant therapy in each case against the risk of bleeding from the use of anticoagulants.

Heparin, a mucopolysaccharide, is a potent anticoagulant that has multiple effects on the coagulation mechanism, the chief of which appears to be as an antithrombin (Table 1). The anticoagulant effect of heparin immediately follows intravenous injection; its greatest application, therefore, is in emergency situations. Since it must be administered parenterally and is expensive, its use for the most part is limited to emergency situations to

TABLE 1. SCHEME OF BLOOD COAGULATION

Step I. Factor XII, Factor XI, Factor VIII, Factor IX + Platelets $\xrightarrow{Calcium}$ Plasma thromboplastin

Step II. Plasma thromboplastin $\xrightarrow{\text{Factor V, Factor VII, Factor X}}$ Activated plasma thromboplastin

Step III. Prothrombin $\xrightarrow{\text{Activated plasma thromboplastin}}$ Thrombin

Step IV. Fibrinogen $\xrightarrow{Thrombin}$ Fibrin

produce and maintain an anticoagulant effect until the slower acting coumarin drugs have induced an adequate anticoagulant effect. The proper laboratory test for the control of heparin therapy is the whole blood clotting time. Heparin may be administered by continuous intravenous infusion of a dilute solution, or by intermittent intravenous injection or intermittent deep subcutaneous injection of a concentrated aqueous solution. My colleagues and I prefer intermittent intravenous injection of heparin in doses of 5000 units every 4 hours.

A number of coumarin and indandione anticoagulant drugs are available (Table 2). It is probably best for each physician to select and become thoroughly familiar with one or two of these drugs, since all have essentially the same mode of action. Some of the drugs produce an anticoagulant effect more rapidly and of shorter duration than others. Only one of the coumarin anticoagulants, warfarin sodium, is available for parenteral use. Anticoagulant drugs presently available for oral use depress four coagulation factors: prothrombin, factor VII, factor X, and factor IX (Table 1). Changes in the first three of these factors are measured by the prothrombin time of Quick, but changes in factor IX are not. Nonetheless, the one-stage prothrombin time of Quick remains the most practical and reliable test for the regulation of oral anticoagulant therapy in our opinion.

Since a variety of thromboplastins are available for use in determining the prothrombin time, the normal prothrombin time varies in different laboratories from 11 to 20 seconds. This variation of normal leads to some confusion. To avoid this confusion, some physicians have advocated converting the prothrombin time to a percentage and have recommended a "therapeutic" anticoagulant range of 10 to 30 per cent of normal. As a generalization the therapeutic range of the prothrombin time can be con-

TABLE 2. ORAL ANTICOAGULANT DRUGS*

Drug	Trade Name	Usual Dose (mg.)	
		Initial	Daily Maintenance
Coumarin derivatives			
Bishydroxycoumarin	Dicumarol	300	25 to 200
Ethyl biscoumacetate	Tromexan	1200	600 to 900
Warfarin sodium†	Coumadin, Panwarfin, Prothromadin	40 to 45	2.5 to 10
Warfarin potassium	Athrombin-K	40 to 45	2.5 to 10
Phenprocoumon	Liquamar	21	1.5 to 4.5
Acenocoumarin	Sintrom	24	4 to 5
Indandione derivatives			
Phenindione	Hedulin, Danilone, Eridone	300	50 to 150
Diphenadione	Dipaxin	20 to 30	3 to 6
Anisindione	Miradon	400	75 to 100

* Modified from Owen, Spittell, and Thompson: Am. J. Cardiol., *12:*309, 1963.
† Parenteral preparations also available.

TABLE 3. CONTRAINDICATIONS TO ANTICOAGULANT THERAPY*

Heparin and coumarin and indandione derivatives
    a. Hemorrhagic diatheses
    b. Operations on the brain, spinal cord, or eye
    c. Active hemorrhage
Coumarin and indandione derivatives
    a. Hepatic insufficiency
    b. Inability to obtain accurate prothrombin times

* Modified from Owen, Spittell, and Thompson: Am. J. Cardiol., *12*:309, 1963.

TABLE 4. CONDITIONS REQUIRING ADDED CAUTION IN THE USE OF ANTICOAGULANTS*

Heparin and coumarin and indandione derivatives
    a. Ulcerating lesions or open wounds
    b. Recent hemorrhage
    c. Tube drainage of body cavities
Coumarin and indandione derivatives
    a. Renal insufficiency
    b. Prolonged dietary deficiency
    c. External biliary drainage
    d. Treatment with broad spectrum antibiotics

* Modified from Owen, Spittell, and Thompson: Am. J. Cardiol., *12*:309, 1963.

sidered to be one and one-half to two and one-half times the normal prothrombin time in a given laboratory.

As mentioned earlier, since use of anticoagulant drugs necessarily involves a risk of bleeding, certain conditions are considered contraindications
to the use of anticoagulant therapy because of the increased risk or the
serious consequence of bleeding (Table 3). In some cases, anticoagulant
therapy, when indicated, can be utilized, but with extra caution (Table 4).

Treatment of Superficial Thrombophlebitis

Superficial thrombophlebitis is rarely complicated by pulmonary embolism, although the thrombotic process may extend from the superficial
to the deep veins. Ordinarily, rest in bed and the application of warm, moist
packs to the involved extremity is all that is necessary for superficial
thrombophlebitis. Phenylbutazone (Butazolidin) in a dose of 100 mg. four
times a day for 3 to 4 days may help reduce the inflammation. Oral anticoagulant therapy is utilized only when superficial thrombophlebitis is extensive or when superficial thrombophlebitis extends despite use of the
measures mentioned previously. For varicose vein and chemical thrombophlebitis, warm moist packs and rest are usually all that is necessary.

Treatment of Deep Venous Thrombosis

For deep venous thrombosis heparin is administered initially for immediate anticoagulant effect, and its use is continued until adequate anticoagulant effect has been established by the orally given anticoagulant drugs (usually 24 to 48 hours). Thereafter, oral anticoagulant therapy is used for maintenance. Other measures employed in the management of deep venous thrombosis include rest in bed with elevation of the involved extremities and application of warm moist packs to the involved extremity. Rest in bed is continued until all signs and symptoms of the deep venous thrombosis have cleared, and anticoagulant therapy is continued until the patient is fully ambulatory. The duration of therapy for acute deep venous thrombosis depends on the vein involved and the clinical response of the patient, but in general varies from 1 to 2 weeks. When edema and tenderness have disappeared, the patient is allowed out of bed. An adequate elastic support (from ankle to knee) must be worn whenever he is up, for at least a month. Its use can be discontinued then, unless chronic venous insufficiency is present.

Prophylactic Anticoagulant Therapy

One should not leave the subject of anticoagulant therapy for venous thrombosis without consideration of prophylactic anticoagulant therapy, particularly in the postoperative patient. Clinical experience has shown that the risk of venous thrombosis is increased by certain conditions (Table 5). In such patients, prophylactic therapy with orally administered anticoagulant drugs is effective in preventing venous thromboembolism. The oral administration of an anticoagulant is started usually on the second postoperative day, and an effort is made to attain the desired anticoagulant effect by the fifth day, since venous thrombosis occurs most commonly between the fifth and fourteenth postoperative days. Oral anticoagulant therapy is usually continued until the patient is fully ambulatory or until he leaves the hospital. Heparin is not used for prophylactic anticoagulant therapy because it must be administered parenterally and it is expensive.

TABLE 5.   CONDITIONS ASSOCIATED WITH INCREASED RISK OF
VENOUS THROMBOEMBOLISM*

During the postoperative period
   a. History of venous thrombosis
   b. Cardiac disease
   c. Trauma to legs
   d. Polycythemia vera
   e. Obesity
Specific surgical procedures
   a. Pelvic operations
   b. Splenectomy
   c. Abdominal operations for malignant lesions

* Modified from Owen, Spittell, and Thompson: Am. J. Cardiol., 12:309, 1963.

Vitamin K and Its Use

The most effective antidote for reversal of the effect of orally administered anticoagulant drugs is phytonadione (vitamin K_1) which is available for both oral and parenteral use. Should the prothrombin time become unduly prolonged, the simple measure of reducing or omitting a dose or doses of the anticoagulant may be adequate, or a small dose (1.25 to 5 mg.) of vitamin K_1 may be administered orally to return the prothrombin time to the therapeutic range. Should minor bleeding such as epistaxis or hematuria occur, a similar program of management will usually suffice. Should more serious bleeding develop, administration of the anticoagulant should be discontinued and vitamin K_1 in a larger dose (25 to 50 mg.) is administered orally or parenterally to return the prothrombin time to normal as soon as possible.

Summary

Anticoagulant therapy is an effective and rational means of treatment of acute deep venous thrombosis. Assuming that hypercoagulability of the blood plays at least some role in the development of thrombosis, anticoagulant therapy with heparin or with the anticoagulant drugs for oral use, although it does not attack directly any specific alteration of clotting, suppresses coagulation to such a degree that its effect tends to counteract hypercoagulability and thus prevent thrombosis. The prophylactic and therapeutic use of anticoagulant drugs will continue to be important in the treatment of venous thrombosis until the specific causes of thrombosis have been more clearly defined and more specific therapy becomes available.

References

1. Alexander, B., and Wessler, S.: A guide to anticoagulant therapy. Circulation, *24:* 123, 1961.
2. Allen, E. V., Barker, N. W., and Hines, E. A., Jr.: Peripheral Vascular Diseases. Third Edition. Philadelphia, W. B. Saunders Company, 1962.
3. Coon, W. W., and Willis, P. W., III: Deep venous thrombosis and pulmonary embolism. Am. J. Cardiol., *4:*611, 1959.
4. McCallister, B. D., Shick, R. M., and Kvale, W. F.: Iliofemoral thrombophlebitis: a ten-year study of conservative treatment. (Abstr.) Circulation, *28:*766, 1963.
5. Owen, C. A., Jr., Spittell, J. A., Jr., and Thompson, J. H., Jr.: The surgical patient on anticoagulant therapy. Am. J. Cardiol., *12:*309, 1963.
6. Sawyer, W. D., Alkjaersig, N., Fletcher, A. P., and Sherry, S.: Thrombolytic therapy: basic and therapeutic considerations. Arch. Int. Med., *107:*274, 1961.
7. Shirger, A., Spittell, J. A., Jr., and Ragen, P. A.: Small doses of vitamin K_1 for correction of reduced prothrombin activity. Proc. Staff Meet. Mayo Clin., *34:*453, 1959.
8. Spittell, J. A., Jr.: Thrombophlebitis and pulmonary embolism. Circulation, 27:976, 1963.

The Use of Dextran in the
Therapy of Acute Thrombophlebitis

John A. Moncrief, Colonel, MC, and Joseph C. Darin

Brooke Army Medical Center; Marquette University School of Medicine

Introduction

Thrombophlebitis has been recognized for a long time as a difficult clinical problem. Results of therapeutic regimens have been disputable, and relief of thrombotic episodes often incomplete. The morbidity associated with chronic involvement and the mortality of thromboembolic phenomena have been sufficient reason for fearing this complication of surgical illnesses.

In view of the widely accepted though erratically successful role of anticoagulants in the therapy of thrombophlebitis, one must have more than simply a desire to improve therapy before discarding a method with so many adherents. It is necessary to have not only a different approach to the problem, but one that offers a greater chance of success with no more, and preferably fewer, disadvantages. The use of "clinical dextran," average molecular weight 75,000, in the treatment of thrombophlebitis meets such criteria by virtue of its success and simplicity.

Etiology of Thrombophlebitis

The onset of thrombophlebitis may be insidious or dramatic, and the clinical course is completely unpredictable. Symptomatology may be clearly typical or deceptively obscure. The pathophysiology is not completely known, and concepts of etiology are controversial.

Intimal damage, stasis, and alterations in coagulability of the blood are generally conceded to play a part in the etiology of the disease process. While there is no doubt that damage to the intima is a prime factor in obviously traumatic phlebitis, the cases ordinarily seen are spontaneous and unassociated with known trauma. In addition, identification of intimal damage by light microscopy is rarely accomplished in such cases. However, it is possible that electron microscopy may reveal a different picture.

Page 508

Stasis alone cannot cause thrombosis. This is classically demonstrated by ligation of a vein in two places in so gentle a fashion as to prevent intimal damage. Nor can changes in coagulability alone cause thrombus formation. However, stasis and hypercoagulability combined can routinely cause rapid clot formation. It is likely that stasis and minimal intimal damage combined will result in thrombosis also. Thus, stasis and hypercoagulability combined offer the greatest possibility for clinical development of thrombophlebitis. Minor intimal trauma is a likely contributing factor in many cases, particularly if flow is not maintained.

It is of significance to note also that resolution of new clots can and does occur spontaneously with extreme rapidity in the laboratory animal. There is clinical evidence that this occurs in man as well. Mature thrombi, however, require prolonged periods for revascularization and resolution.

Inadequacy of Anticoagulant Therapy

While anticoagulant therapy has been widely used by many and enthusiastically supported by some, the distressing facts are that there is little conclusive evidence that use of heparin and/or dicumarol alone have significantly contributed to the therapy of the disease. Reports vary widely in the results obtained, indicating not only inconsistency in interpretation, but wide variations in the course of the disease.

Anticoagulant therapy of thrombophlebitis is aimed at altering favorably only one of the triad of factors responsible for the onset of the disease, namely, hypercoagulability. Stasis (or increased viscosity) and intimal damage, even minimal lesions, are overlooked or ineffectively combated in such treatment. Possibly this can explain the variation in results reported. The favorable reports with anticoagulant therapy may include a great percentage in which hypercoagulability is a dominant factor.

Properties of Dextran Suggesting Its Value in Thrombophlebitis

In contrast to the anticoagulants, which possess a limited potential for effective counteraction, dextran has unique properties that are of potential value in the therapy of thrombophlebitis.

Dextran is known to effect blood viscosity by two means: (1) The aggulutination of red blood cells is either prevented or reversed, particularly by the lower molecular weight fractions, and (2) these fractions, while increasing viscosity of normal plasma slightly, decrease whole blood viscosity by simple dilution. In addition, abnormally viscous plasma is made more fluid (though not normally so) by the presence of the lower molecular fractions of dextran. It would thus appear logical to utilize dextran to inhibit the stasis factor in thrombophlebitis.

Molecular coating of intimal surfaces by dextran has been well demonstrated. This film of molecular dextran impedes the flow of current across a vessel when applied by electrodes in an animal. This property could be expected to impair the thrombotic effect of any local injury currently existing secondary to intimal damage. Thus, dextran may obviate some of the effects of local intimal injury.

The bleeding tendency long reported, particularly with the administration of more than 1000 cc. of dextran, has been well documented as to occurrence, but not as to etiology. When clinically apparent, the condition may exist with or without demonstrable defects in bleeding and clotting times. It would appear that such a property could be used to advantage in combating a state of hypercoagulability.

Laboratory studies utilizing dextran as the only mode of therapy have confirmed the premise that the known properties of dextran are successful in preventing experimental venous thrombosis. That dextran can also effectively inhibit propagation of preformed clots is readily demonstrable. Resolution of thrombi subsequent to dextran administration has been neither confirmed nor disproved in the laboratory.

Choice of Type of Dextran

Dextran is available in solutions of three different molecular weight aggregations, either in saline or dextrose-water. The average molecular weight of these solutions is either 42,000 (low molecular dextran), 75,000 (clinical dextran), or 185,000 (high molecular dextran). Efficiency and duration of volume expansion vary directly with molecular size, while flow-promoting qualities vary indirectly. Bleeding tendencies, red blood cell agglutination, and antigenicity also are directly related to molecular size.

The high molecular weight solution is obviously a bad choice for such therapy. The lowest weight is theoretically the best, but is yet to be approved by the Food and Drug Administration for human use. The clinical dextran (average weight 75,000), which is approved by FDA, is thus a more logical selection. Laboratory experiments indicate that the clinical dextran is more effective in obviating experimental thrombosis than is the low molecular dextran. While clinical dextran is preferred at this time, subsequent events may prove the lower molecular weights to have advantages.

Method of Therapy

The diagnosis of thrombophlebitis is made on the clinical basis of edema, pain, tenderness, and often accompanying erythema and increase in local temperature. Calf pain on dorsiflexion of the foot is common in deep vein involvement. Palpable thrombosed vessels are readily appreciated when the superficial component is significant. Our experience to date has been with unilateral disease.

Once the diagnosis is established, several factors are recorded:

1. Circumference of both extremities is measured in several areas above and below the knee, care being taken to secure bilaterally symmetrical measurements with the level readily reproducible.

2. The distribution and degree of edema, erythema, and increased temperature are determined as related to the opposite extremity.

3. The Lowenberg test is done. This is accomplished by placing a blood pressure cuff about the involved calf and inflating it until definite pain is perceived by the patient. With acute thrombophlebitis the pressure is below 100 mm. Hg and usually near 50 to 60 mm. Hg. Pain is perceived in the normal leg usually at 150 mm. Hg or more.

This is the most objective and reproducible means of determining the effectiveness of therapy and has proved quite reliable.

Therapy is instituted as follows:

1. Six per cent dextran (average weight 75,000) is administered as 1 per cent of the body weight (TBWt) by volume the first day (e.g., a 70-kg. man receives 700 ml. dextran). This is 600 mg./kg. On each succeeding day, 0.5 per cent TBWt is given (300 mg./kg.). The rate of infusion is 1000 ml. per hour. Dextran in saline is preferred since red blood cell agglutination may sometimes occur with exposure of red blood cells to high concentrations of dextran in sugar solutions.

2. Antibiotic therapy is not instituted unless there are specific indications other than thrombophlebitis.

3. The patient may ambulate *ad libitum*, but is not permitted to sit or stand still for more than very brief periods.

4. No specific laboratory tests are done. Coagulation tests are not necessary.

Dextran continues to be given at 300 mg./kg. daily until all signs and symptoms of the disease have cleared, particularly in the Lowenberg test, which is considered normal when the involved leg pressures are the same as those of the opposite extremity.

Results

Clinical studies have demonstrated dextran to be of great value in the therapy of acute thrombophlebitis. The response to therapy is rapid and often dramatic. The subjective symptoms resolve in most instances within 24 hours, with the patient frequently remarking that the rest pain disappeared in a few hours. Erythema and edema clear with similar speed, though the latter may persist beyond 48 hours in some cases. With extensive edema, resolution is associated with diuresis, although dextran is not an osmotic diuretic.

Local tenderness, and particularly the Lowenberg, are slower to return to normal, but in no case to date has the test been abnormal more than 96 hours after beginning therapy. Dextran has been discontinued when the Lowenberg returned to normal, even though some edema may have persisted beyond this time.

This mode of therapy has not been utilized for a long enough period to allow any observations of long-term results or the impact on the post-phlebitic syndrome. Limited experience with chronic thrombophlebitis treated with dextran indicates that such therapy influences only the acute exacerbations. In these cases recurrent episodes have been noted several weeks after successful treatment of the acute disease process. However, on each occasion response to therapy was prompt and complete.

Others have successfully utilized a long term program of weekly administration of dextran in such chronic cases.

Cases resistant to heparin or dicumarol have responded promptly to dextran therapy. No bleeding problems have been encountered.

Advantages of Dextran Therapy

With dextran therapy there is: (1) prompt and consistent resolution of signs and symptoms of disease; (2) ease of administration (daily single dose without need of bleeding, clotting, or prothrombin times); (3) effectiveness in cases resistant to anticoagulant therapy; (4) in the dose range utilized, absence of hemorrhagic complications.

Caution

1. Allergic reactions, though uncommon and mild, may occur. These disappear with cessation of administration.

2. Dextran is a volume expander. This should be noted when it is used in patients with cardiopulmonary disease, but is not a contraindication. In fact, it is being used in the treatment of acute myocardial infarction.

References

1. Moncrief, J. A., Darin, J. C., Canizaro, P. C., and Sawyer, R. B.: Use of dextran to prevent arterial and venous thrombosis. Ann. Surg., 158:553, 1963.
2. Wessler, S., and Deykin, D.: Theory and practice in acute venous thrombosis. Circulation, 18:1190, 1958.

Index of Contributors

Page numbers in *italics* indicate introductory material.

Index of Subjects